Beta-Blockers and Cardiac Arrhythmias

FUNDAMENTAL AND CLINICAL CARDIOLOGY

Series Editor

Samuel Z. Goldhaber, M.D.

Cardiovascular Division
Department of Medicine
Harvard Medical School
and Brigham and Women's Hospital
Boston, Massachusetts

1. *Drug Treatment of Hyperlipidemia,* edited by Basil M. Rifkind
2. *Cardiotonic Drugs: A Clinical Review: Second Edition, Revised and Expanded,* edited by Carl V. Leier
3. *Complications of Coronary Angioplasty,* edited by Alexander J. R. Black, H. Vernon Anderson, and Stephen G. Ellis
4. *Unstable Angina,* edited by John D. Rutherford
5. *Beta-Blockers and Cardiac Arrhythmias,* edited by Prakash C. Deedwania

Additional Volumes in Preparation

Exercise and the Heart in Health and Cardiac Disease, edited by Roy Shephard and Henry S. Miller, Jr.

Cardiopulmonary Physiology in Critical Care, edited by Steven M. Scharf

Adjunctive Therapy for Acute Myocardial Infarction, edited by Eric Bates

Beta-Blockers and Cardiac Arrhythmias

edited by

Prakash C. Deedwania

University of California at San Francisco
School of Medicine
San Francisco, California
and
Veterans Affairs Medical Center
Fresno, California

Marcel Dekker, Inc. New York • Basel • Hong Kong

Library of Congress Cataloging-in-Publication Data

Beta blockers and cardiac arrhythmias / edited by Prakash C.
Deedwania.
p. cm. -- (Fundamental and clinical cardiology; 5)
Includes bibliographical references and index.
ISBN 0-8247-8450-2 (alk. paper)
1. Adrenergic beta blockers. 2. Myocardial depressants.
3. Arrhythmia--Chemotherapy. I. Deedwania, Prakash C.
II. Series: Fundamental and clinical cardiology; v. 5.
[DNLM: 1. Adrenergic Beta Receptor Blockaders--pharmacology.
2. Adrenergic Beta Receptor Blockaders--therapeutic use.
3. Arrhythmia--drug therapy. W1 FU538TD v. 5 / WG 330 B562]
RM347.B46 1992
616.1'28061--dc20
DNLM/DLC
for Library of Congress 91-46942
CIP

This book is printed on acid-free paper.

MARCEL DEKKER, INC.
270 Madison Avenue, New York, New York, 10016

Current printing (last digit):
10 9 8 7 6 5 4 3 2 1

PRINTED IN THE UNITED STATES OF AMERICA

To my wife, Cathy
and my children, Anne and Ravi
who are my inspiration

Series Introduction

Marcel Dekker, Inc., has focused on the development of various series of beautifully produced books in different branches of medicine. These series have facilitated the integration of rapidly advancing information for both the clinical specialist and the researcher.

In this series, Fundamental and Clinical Cardiology, my goal as Series Editor is to assemble the talents of world-renowned authorities to discuss virtually every area of cardiovascular medicine. In the current monograph, Dr. Deedwania has edited an extraordinary book, *Beta-Blockers and Cardiac Arrhythmias*. Because we have recently learned that beta-blockers are much safer than most type IA antiarrhythmia agents, his book is especially timely and relevant to contemporary clinical practice.

Samuel Z. Goldhaber

Foreword

One of the major challenges facing physicians today is the management of serious cardiac arrhythmias. Over the years it has been very difficult to demonstrate that any antiarrhythmic agent can prolong life in patients. Even though many agents are effective in suppressing ventricular arrhythmias, their proarrhythmic effects can be deleterious. The Cardiac Arrhythmia Suppression Trial (CAST) study demonstrated this dramatically when it showed that encaine and flecainide, which are effective in suppressing VPCs, actually increased mortality in patients after a myocardial infarction. This has emphasized the importance of beta-blockers in this setting, since they reduced mortality, reinfarction, and sudden death. This latter result suggests that the sympathetic nervous system and elevated catecholamines are adverse in a number of cardiac conditions, especially ischemic heart disease.

Thus, this volume is very timely as a summary of the effects of beta-blockers in the management of cardiac arrhythmias. Readers will find that it is an excellent comprehensive overview of this topic—covering basic mechanisms, comparative pharmacology, and clinical studies. The clinical studies review the effects of beta-blockers in a wide variety of settings including post-myocardial infarction. The effects of beta-blockers on the circadian pattern of ischemia and sudden death are of special interest. Traditional beta-blockers are discussed as well as the new unique beta-blocker, sotalol. The concept of combined beta-blocking and class III antiarrhythmic effects make sotalol of considerable interest. Similarly, the combination of beta-blockers with class I antiarrhythmic agents offers a promising approach to antiarrhythmic therapy.

As we rely more on beta-blockers as a proven class of antiarrhythmic agents, clinicians will appreciate the content of this book which nicely summarizes an important body of data in one place.

William W. Parmley, M.D.
Chairman, Cardiology Division
University of California at San Francisco Hospitals
and Professor of Medicine
University of California School of Medicine
San Francisco, California

Preface

Sudden cardiac death remains a leading cause of cardiac mortality. Although considerable progress has been made in understanding the electrophysiologic mechanisms or arrhythmias, the treatment of patients with cardiac arrhythmias is one of the most difficult issues facing the clinician today. During the last decade, several new antiarrhythmic agents with varying electrophysiologic properties have been approved for clinical use in the treatment of patients with ventricular tachyarrhythmias. Although many of these new antiarrhythmic drugs are highly effective in suppressing the ventricular ectopic activity, their efficacy in reducing the risk of sudden cardiac death has been disappointing. As a matter of fact, results of the recently published Cardiac Arrhythmia Suppression Trial (CAST) clearly indicate that treatment with class IC agents, flecainide and encainide, is associated with an increase in the risk of cardiac mortality, particularly arrhythmic death in the survivors of acute myocardiac infarction who have frequent ventricular premature contractions. These findings and the results of several other clinical studies demonstrating the proarrhythmic effects of class I antiarrhythmic agents are in clear contrast with the well-documented cardioprotective effects of therapy with beta-blocking agents. Several large clinical studies have established the benefits of beta-blocker therapy in patients with acute myocardial infarction by reducing the risk of sudden cardiac death as well as cardiac mortality due to recurrent infarction. Although it is not clear whether these beneficial effects of beta-blockers are secondary to their antiarrhythmic effect or the anti-ischemic actions, there is little doubt that beta-blockers possess unique and significant antiarrhythmic properties.

The primary purpose of this book is to provide an in-depth and comprehensive review of available data regarding the antiarrhythmic actions of beta-blocking agents and their clinical applications in patients with cardiac tachyarrhythmias. Combining the expertise of 16 distinguished authorities in this field, the book provides the latest information regarding the basic mechanisms of action of these drugs as well as their role in various clinical subsets of patients with cardiac arrhythmias. The book is unique because it is the first collection of articles with clinically meaningful information regarding the use of beta-adrenergic blocking drugs as antiarrhythmic agents. The authors of various chapters in this book were selected based on their long-standing interest and established investigative experience in their respective fields. Each author has provided an up-to-date review of the subject area with special emphasis on the clinical application of the findings.

In the first chapter, Kupersmith describes the electrophysiologic basis of cardiac action potentials and the effects of beta-agonists, thereby establishing a strong base for defining the cellular mechanisms of the antiarrhythmic action of beta-blockers. The second chapter, by Anderson, deals with an equally important area and examines a possible mechanism of cardioprotective effects of beta-blockers by illustrating their often ignored but significant effect on ventricular fibrillation threshold. In the third chapter, Coumel describes the rational basis for the antiarrhythmic actions of beta-blocking drugs and provides a succinct review of their application in various clinical settings. Although beta-blockers as a class share the beta-adrenergic blocking property, they differ considerably in many aspects. Frishman (Ch. 4) provides a comprehensive review of comparative pharmacologic properties of various beta-blocking agents with special reference to cardioselectivity, intrinsic sympathomimetic activity, and membrane stabilizing activities as they relate to the antiarrhythmic actions of these drugs.

Chapters 5, 6, and 7 deal with the well-demonstrated cardioprotective effects of beta-blockers in the survivors of acute myocardial infarction. In Chapter 5, Singh discusses the mechanisms and rationale of beta-blocker therapy in patients with acute emyocardial infarction and compares the efficacy of beta-blockers with that of calcium channel blockers. He emphasizes the importance of the differing effects of these agents on the 24 hour heart rate and relates the cardioprotective effects of such action. Although the precise mechanism of the cardioprotection by beta-blockers is not established, it is thought to be partly related to their antiarrhythmic action. This is examined in detail in Chapter 6 by Lichstein, primarily based on the BHAT experience. It is now well established that both acute myocardial infarction and sudden cardiac death have a demonstrable circadian rhythm with a clustering of these events in the morning (6 A.M. to noon) hours. Peters (Ch. 7) discusses the available data in this regard and provides some intriguing analysis of the BHAT data demonstrating the benefit of beta-blocker therapy in reducing the risk of cardiac death in the morning hours.

The role of beta-blockers as primary antiarrhythmic agents is discussed in the remaining six chapters. It is well known that ventricular arrhythmias can be triggered by physical exercise or emotional stress. In Chapter 8, Sung and co-workers describe the mechanisms of exercise-induced tachyarrhythmia and compare the effects of verapamil with that of beta-adrenergic blockade in this setting. In Chapter 9, Moore and Cruickshank provide a detailed account of clinical experience with the cardioselective beta-blocker, atenolol, in patients with ventricular and supraventricular tachyarrhythmias as well as for arrhythmias in special settings such as perioperative period, mitral valve prolapse, and long QT syndromes. Beta-blockers have also played a significant role as a combination therapy with other antiarrhythmic drugs. The rational basis and clinical efficacy of such combination therapy are discussed at length in Chapter 11. Chandraratna and co-workers (Ch. 12) provide data regarding comparative antiarrhythmic actions of class IA antiarrhythmic agents and beta-blockers in the treatment of ventricular arrhythmias.

Finally, Chapter 13 provides a comprehensive review of sotalol, a unique beta-blocker that, in addition to its class II antiarrhythmic properties, also produces selective lengthening of the action potential duration in all cardiac tissues (class III antiarrhythmic action). These electrophysiologic properties make it a novel antiarrhythmic agent. Chapter 13 examines the pharmacologic properties of sotalol, and the clinical experience with sotalol in patients with supraventricular and ventricular tachyarrhythmias. It will be evident from the discussions in Chapters 10 and 13 that sotalol appears to be more effective than other beta-blockers, particularly in patients with life-threatening ventricular arrhythmias refractory to conventional antiarrhythmic agents.

It is hoped that this comprehensive state-of-the-art review of the role of beta-blockers in treatment of cardiac arrhythmias will not only be of use to clinicians in their current practice, but also stimulate investigators interested in pursuing research in this area.

I am grateful to the contributors for their efforts in providing excellent reviews of their subject area. I would also like to express my sincere appreciation to all my staff and the staff at Marcel Dekker, Inc., for assisting me in the preparation of this volume. Finally, I wish to acknowledge the support, encouragement, and endurance of my family during the time I spent editing this book.

Prakash C. Deedwania

Contents

Contributors

JEFFREY L. ANDERSON, M.D. Professor, Department of Medicine, University of Utah, and Chief, Division of Cardiology, LDS Hospital, Salt Lake City, Utah

VIJAY BHASIN, M.D. University of Southern California Medical Center, Los Angeles, California

P. ANTHONY CHANDRARATNA, M.D., M.R.C.P. Bauer and Bauer Rawlins Professor of Medicine, University of Southern California School of Medicine, and Associate Chief, Division of Cardiology, and Director, Echocardiography/Graphics, Los Angeles County & University of Southern California Medical Center, Los Angeles, California

SATISH K. CHOUDHARY, M.D. University of Southern California Medical Center, Los Angeles, California

PHILIPPE COUMEL, M.D. Professor, Department of Cardiology, Hôpital Lariboisière, Paris, France

JOHN MALCOLM CRUICKSHANK, D.M., F.R.C.P.* Consultant in Cardiovascular Medicine, ICI Pharmaceuticals, Macclesfield, Cheshire, England

PRAKASH C. DEEDWANIA, M.D., F.A.C.C. Clinical Professor of Medicine, University of California at San Francisco School of Medicine, San Francisco, and Chief, Division of Cardiology, Department of Medicine, Veterans Affairs Medical Center, Fresno, California

WEI FAN, M.D. Wadsworth Veterans Affairs Medical Center, and University of California at Los Angeles School of Medicine, Los Angeles, California

WILLIAM H. FRISHMAN, M.D. Professor and Associate Chairman, Department of Medicine, The Albert Einstein College of Medicine, and the Hospital of the Albert Einstein College of Medicine/Montefiore Medical Center, Bronx, New York

MOTONOBU HAYANO, M.D. Wadsworth Veterans Affairs Medical Center and University of California at Los Angeles School of Medicine, Los Angeles, California

JOEL KUPERSMITH, M.D. Chairman, Department of Medicine, College of Human Medicine, Michigan State University, East Lansing, Michigan

EDGAR LICHSTEIN, M.D. Director, Department of Medicine, Maimonides Medical Center, and Professor of Medicine, Department of Medicine, State University of New York—Health Science Center at Brooklyn, Brooklyn, New York

VALERIE E. MOORE, B.Sc., Ph.D. Department of Medical Affairs, ICI Pharmaceuticals, Macclesfield, Cheshire, England

ROBERT W. PETERS, M.D. Chief, Division of Cardiology, Veterans Affairs Medical Center, and Associate Professor of Medicine, University of Maryland School of Medicine, Baltimore, Maryland

*Present affiliation: Wythenshawe Hospital, Winslow, Cheshire, and Royal Brompton and National Heart and Chest Hospital, London, England.

BRAMAH N. SINGH, M.D. Chief, Cardiology Section, Veterans Affairs Medical Center of West Los Angeles, and Professor of Medicine, University of California at Los Angeles School of Medicine, Los Angeles, California

RUEY J. SUNG, M.D.* Professor in Residence, Departments of Medicine and Cardiology, San Francisco General Hospital, and The Cardiovascular Research Institute, University of California at San Francisco, San Francisco, California

---

*Present affiliation: Director of Electrophysiology and Cardiac Arrhythmia Service, Stanford University Medical Center, and Professor, Division of Cardiovascular Medicine, Department of Medicine, Stanford University School of Medicine, Palo Alto, California

Beta-Blockers and Cardiac Arrhythmias

I

Basic and Clinical Pharmacology of Beta-Blockers as Antiarrhythmic Agents

1

Cellular Mechanisms of the Antiarrhythmic Action of Beta-Blockers

Joel Kupersmith
College of Human Medicine, Michigan State University, East Lansing, Michigan

This chapter will deal with the cellular electrophysiologic effects of beta-adrenergic blockers that are pertinent to their effects on arrhythmias. To understand effects of agents, we have to first review relevant aspects of basic electrophysiology. Our understanding of basic electrophyusiology derives mainly from studies using intracellular microelectrodes which record electrical activity in individual myocytes. A technique derived from this called "voltage clamp" has provided the bulk of information on the types of ionic currents that implement electrical activity. More recently, molecular techniques have begun to shed light on the biochemistry underlying these ionic currents. Studies have begun to elucidate the form and structure of the channels, mediators involved in generating the currents, and mediators involved in transferring information from beta and other receptors. Overall our knowledge of the cellular mechanisms of beta-blockers is based on data and concepts derived from the above three levels of understanding: direct electrophysiological, ionic, and molecular.

CARDIAC ACTION POTENTIAL

Normal Action Potential

The basic unit of cardiac electrical activity is the action potential. Each type of cardiac tissue has its own characteristic action potential, and they are of two types. One type, a "fast response," is found in the atrium, His-Purkinje system, and ventricle (Fig. 1A). It is characterized by a rapid upstroke during which the cell depolarizes, a plateau phase of varying duration (longest in Purkinje fiber, shortest in atrium), and repolarization at which time membrane potential returns to baseline. By convention, the action potential is divided into five phases. Phase 0 (so called because it is so rapid as to have been unrecordable by the earliest electrophysiological techniques) represents depolarization. In this phase membrane potential moves from a baseline (or "resting potential") of about −90 to about +30 mV. Phase 1 is a slight movement of membrane potential in a negative direction toward baseline. Phase 2 is the plateau, phase 3 repolarization, and phase 4 electrical diastole.

Another type of action potential exists in sinoatrial and AV nodes. As seen in Figure 1B, it is slower in upstroke and smaller and has been labeled "slow response" in contrast to the above "fast response." Phase 0

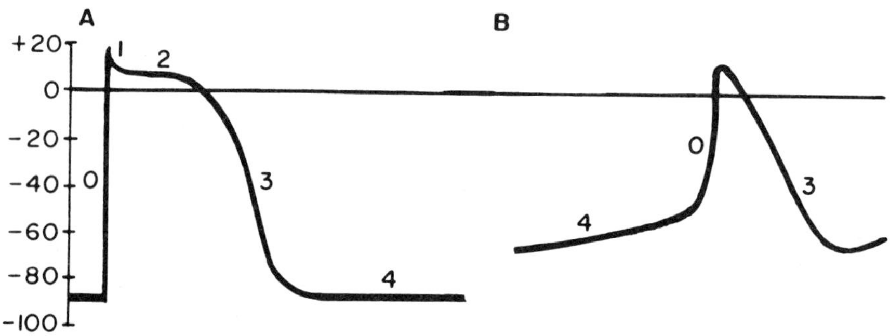

Figure 1 Types of action potentials in the heart: (A) the "fast response" that exists in normal atrium, ventricle and His-Purkinje tissue; (B) the "slow response" that occurs in the sinus and AV nodes. Here the upstroke is slower and smaller than in the "fast response" in A. Fast response action potentials (A) are mediated by a rapid inward movement of Na^+ ions, whereas slow responses (B) are mediated by a slow inward movement of mainly Ca^{2+} ions. See text for further discussion.

is slow and small, phase 2 is highly abbreviated, and phase 3 is rather gradual. While the fast upstroke of the myocardial and His-Purkinje action potentials are mediated by a rapid inward movement of Na^{+} ions, the slow response upstrokes are mediated by a slow inward movement of mainly Ca^{2+} ions.

The sinoatrial and AV nodes are also the major sites with the ability to act as the initiators of cardiac electrical activity. This property of self-excitation, called "automaticity," is mediated by a gradual depolarization of phase 4, which brings the cell to the threshold of generation of the upstroke (Fig. 1B). Cells of the sinus node, which possess the most rapid phase 4 depolarization, are the primary rhythm generators of the heart. Next is the AV node (or AV junction). His-Purkinje cells also have this capacity and are the last resort for rhythm generation when the other two fail or when there is complete heart block.

Temporally the sinus node upstroke occurs just before the P wave. The P wave then coincides with atrial depolarization, the P-R segment with AV nodal and His-Purkinje depolarization, the QRS with depolarization of the ventricle. The ST-segment represents the plateau phase of the ventricular action potential and the T-wave repolarization. His-Purkinje action potentials are longer than ventricular muscle, and their repolarization appears to occur either during the T wave or to be independently represented by the U wave of the ECG.

Interventions that slow the upstroke of the ventricular action potential also prolong the QRS of the ECG and those that slow the atrial upstroke prolong the P wave. Interventions that prolong the ventricular action potential duration (APD) also prolong the Q-T interval, while those that prolong the His-Purkinje action potential probably induce or intensify the U wave.

One peculiarity regarding the Q-T interval reflects the fact that it does not represent "repolarization" per se, but potential differences created by the fact that repolarization occurs at different times within the ventricle, i.e., repolarization moves in an epicardial to endocardial direction. If repolarization occurred simultaneously throughout the ventricle, there would be no T wave. Thus, interventions that shorten action potentials nonuniformly and serve to make repolarization even more discordant than normal in fact prolong and intensify the Q-T interval. For example, sympathetic stimulation does this (see below) (1).

Action Potential Abnormalities

Apart from normal action potentials, there are certain well-described and well-studied action potential abnormalities. Afterdepolarizations, leading to triggered activity, comprise one group of abnormalities. Afterdepolarizations are classified into two types: early and delayed (2). Early afterdepolarizations (EADs) occur during very prolonged and rather bizarre appearing action potentials, i.e., they occur prior to repolarization (Fig. 2) (3-5). They are defined as depolizations that occur during or delay repolarization (3-5). EADs can give rise to triggered activations (Fig. 3). These may be responsible for rapid tachycardias and are almost surely responsible for Torsade de Pointes ventricular arrhythmias (3,6). EADs are induced by class I and III antiarrhythmic drugs (see below) among other interventions.

Delayed afterdepolarizations (DADs) are low-level depolarizations that follow the action potential (7) (Fig. 3) and also can give rise to triggered activations. They characteristically occur in digitalis toxicity.

Slow responses (i.e., action potentials similar to those in the AV node), when they are elicited in His-Purkinje or myocardial tissue, represent another type of abnormal action potential. The common method of eliciting slow response action potentials in these tissues is to first depolarize tissue (e.g., in high K^+ to completely inactivate inward Na^+ current) and then add catecholamines to induce slow responses (8-11). Here slow I_{Ca} is in the main responsible for the upstrokes. Slow response action poten-

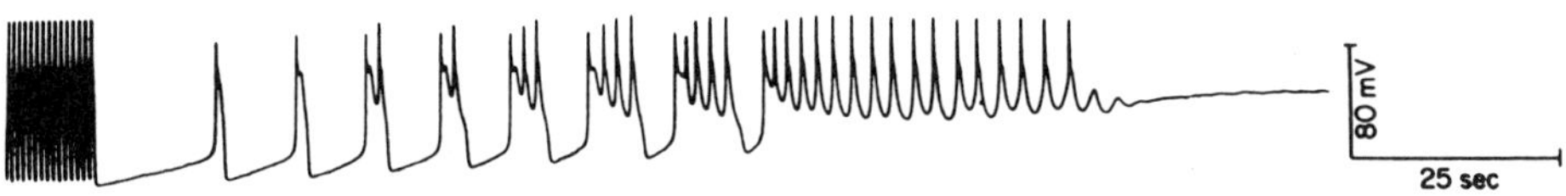

Figure 2 Repolarization failure, abnormal action potential prolongation, and the occurrence of early afterdepolarizations (EADs) in canine Purkinje fiber exposed to hypoxia, acidic Tyrode's solution. Following a train of rapid pacing (close action potentials on the left) there is further and further prolongation of action potential duration (APD) with occurrence of EAD-induced triggered activations, i.e., activations occurring before repolarization. These increase in number up to 4. Finally, in the last action potential there is complete failure to repolarize with a sequence of 16 activations and then arrest and a depolarized membrane potential. (From Ref. 5.)

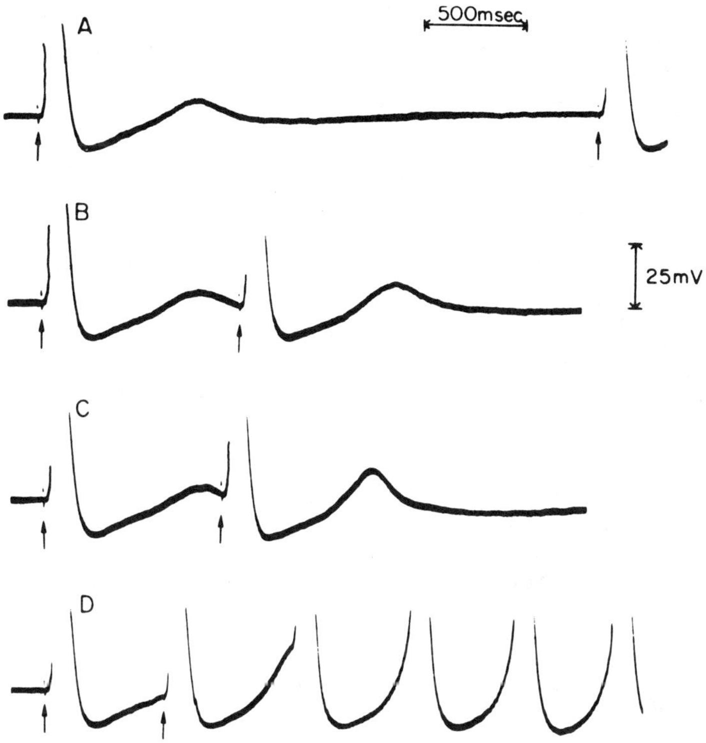

Figure 3 Triggered activity due to delayed afterdepolarizations, in this case in the fiber of the monkey mitral valve in Tyrode's solution. Note that in D an early premature stimulus triggers a train of sustained activity. This behavior is typical for DADs. (From Ref. 7.)

tials, which of course resemble those in the sinus and AV nodes, are believed to play a role in arrhythmias in ischemia (12).

Ionic Currents

A number of ionic currents that explain the various components of the action potential have been described and studied. Rapid inward sodium current (I_{Na}) leads to the upstroke of the action potential in atrium, His-

Purkinje tissue, and ventricle. When the threshold for activation of this inward current is reached through transmission of current from a neighboring cell in the process of conduction of an impulse, via phase 4 depolarization or via external stimulation, there is a rapid inward movement of ions to create the upstroke. The upstroke in "fast" myocardial, and His-Purkinje tissue (Fig. 1) is predominantly I_{Na}. However, the very last part (0 to +30 mV) also includes I_{Ca}. In "slow response" sinus and AV node tissue, the upstroke is all slow inward current.

A brief outward current called I_{to} follows the upstroke and explains phase 1. This is caused by either outward K^+ or Cl^- current.

During phase 2, I_{ca} maintains depolarization of cells in the plateau and is the first step in excitation contraction coupling. Recently I_{Ca} has been divided into two types: a "T" type I_{Ca}, which activates at a rather negative membrane potential and appears to play a role in automatic activity, and a "L" type I_{Ca}, which is larger and is responsible for the major inward Ca^{2+} movement during the plateau (13). Besides I_{Ca}, a portion of the I_{Na} (called "window I_{Na}") also plays a role in maintaining phase 2.

K^+ currents (inwardly rectifying I_{K1} and the delayed rectifier I_K) (14) are the main outward currents in the heart. Among the factors that mediate repolarization are a decline in I_{Ca} and window I_{Na} and the occurrence of outward I_K. We have also shown that extracellular K^+ accumulation, which in turn increases the conductance to I_K to favor outward current is important in mediating repolarization (15).

Certain currents play a role in automaticity (phase 4 depolarization) in part depending upon the tissue involved. In early phase 4 there is a decline in outward I_K, favoring depolarization, and in later phase 4 there is activation of both the depolarizing Na^+ pacemaker current (I_f) (16) and I_{Ca} (17).

Ion exchanges provide additional current. The Na-K pump, which exchanges 3 Na^+ (outward) for 2 K^+ (inward), results in net outward current, favoring both repolarization and a more negative resting potential (15,18). The Na-Ca exchange mechanism (which exchanges 1 Ca^{2+} for 3 or 4 Na^+) adds inward current when removing Ca^{2+} from the cell (19).

DRUG EFFECTS ON THE ACTION POTENTIAL

In evaluating the effects of beta-blockers and other drugs, one examines certain parameters in particular. The maximum rate of rise of the upstroke is one such parameter as it correlates with the speed of conduction and therefore QRS duration.

Resting potential or the membrane potential at which the action potential initiates is relevant here. The more depolarized (i.e., less negative, more positive) the resting potential, the slower the rate of rise of the action potential (20). If the resting potential is depolarized beyond (positive to) the threshold for inward sodium current (about −60 mV), the cell is completely inactivated and action potentials dependent on rapid inward sodium current cannot occur.

When resting potential is depolarized to levels less positive than this (i.e., up to −60 mV), the cell is said to be "partially" rather than completely inactivated. That is, upstrokes related to I_{Na} still occur but are slower because I_{Na} has been partially inactivated (i.e., fewer Na^+ ions are available). Here not only is movement of Na^+ into the cell diminished and slower but, in addition, the I_{Ca} component of the upstroke is proportionately greater. Thus, drug effects on resting potential are as important for the upstroke as are the direct actions on I_{Na}. Such effects are particularly important in ischemia, which is characterized by membrane depolarization and partial or complete inactivation of myocardial and His-Purkinje cells.

APD and effective refractory period (ERP) (i.e., the time from onset of the action potential to the earliest new action potential that can be elicited) are other important parameters, as is the slope of phase 4 depolarization. Depression of this slope means slower automatic activity (and vice versa).

Threshold and excitability are also important here. Lowering of the thresholds for I_{Na} (in His-Purkinje or myocardial cells) or for slow inward Ca^{2+} current (in sinoatrial, AV nodal, and slow response tissue) or enhancement of excitability serves to improve conduction (adjacent cells are excited earlier) and enhance automaticity (self-excitation occurs earlier).

In terms of ionic currents, their modification will have the following effects: diminution of I_{Na} for fast response and I_{Ca} for slow response slows the upstroke of the action potential, therefore, slows conduction of the impulse in the heart (and when ventricular muscle is involved prolongs QRS duration). Diminution of I_{Ca} or I_f depresses automaticity. Enhancement of the Na-K exchange pump, as occurs with rapid rates, increases outward current, therefore favors repolarization, shortens APD (18,21), and via ventricular muscle effects, shortens Q-T interval. Beta-blockers influence a number of these currents to exert their electrophysiological and antiarrhythmic effects.

MECHANISMS OF ARRHYTHMIA

Arrhythmias are believed to occur via the mechanisms of reentry and automaticity, and perhaps repolarization failure. Reentry is illustrated in Figure 4. Here slowing of conduction and one-way block has occurred in a segment of abnormal tissue. Impulses from the contiguous normal segment proceed into the abnormal segment in a retrograde direction to complete a reentrant cycle and thus initiate a reentrant tachycardia. Reentry may occur anywhere in the heart. For example, in the AV node it causes paroxysmal atrial tachycardia; in the His-Purkinje system or ventricle it causes ventricular tachycardia. Figure 5 shows an example of one-way block due to slow response (9).

In the main, drugs eliminate reentry by depressing conduction or prolonging refractoriness in the abnormal segment thereby converting one-way (Fig. 4 and 5) to two-way block and aborting the reentrant cycle. For this reason drug cellular effects on upstroke (conduction), APD, and ERP (refractoriness) are important in considering their antiarrhythmic effects. It is also easy to see that drug-induced slowing or block of conduction can cause or worsen arrhythmias as well as suppress them. In fact, this drawback is the major dilemma for antiarrhythmic drug therapy.

A second mechanism of arrhythmia is automaticity. This may take the form of either enhanced normal automaticity, i.e., a major increase in

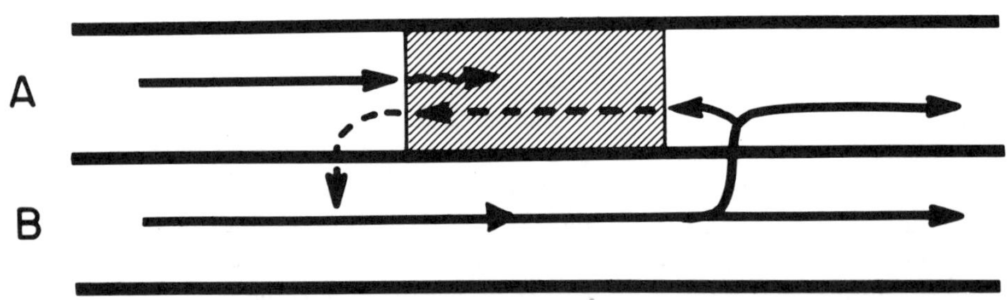

Figure 4 Model of reentry. The cross-hatched zone is a zone of slow conduction and one-way block. Impulses proceed in an antegrade direction into this segment and are blocked. Impulses proceed in the contiguous normal segment to reenter in a retrograde direction through the depressed segment completing a reentrant cycle. (See also Fig. 5 for an example of one-way block due to slow response activity.)

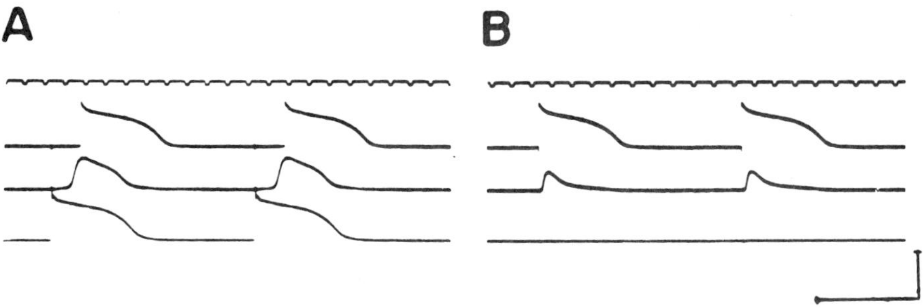

Figure 5 One-way block through a segment displaying slow response action potentials. The upper and lower tracings show normal action potential. The middle tracing shows a zone of slow response activity induced by a high K^+-catecholamine medium. Note that in A with stimulation from the lower trace, conduction proceeds to the upper, while in B with stimulation from the upper trace, conduction is blocked and does not proceed to the lower. One-way block is the essential element in reentry (see also Fig. 4). (From Ref. 9.)

the slope of phase 4 depolarization in AV nodal or His-Purkinje times, or abnormal automaticity, described above, e.g., DADs (see Fig. 3).

A third possible mechanism is repolarization failure in which there is abnormal action potential prolongation or complete failure to repolarize (4,5). This leads to the occurrence of EADs and triggering (see Fig. 2). Although they can be considered a form of abnormal automaticity, it is of value to indicate that repolarization failure can be the initiating factor in their occurrence since APD shortening in addition to suppression of automaticity or upstroke is a method of reversal (5).

EVALUATING ELECTROPHYSIOLOGICAL EFFECTS OF BETA-BLOCKERS

There are certain pitfalls in evaluating the antiarrhythmic effects of beta-blockers by strictly in vitro electrophysiological criteria. For one, in vitro tissue is obviously devoid of both sympathetic innervation and circulating catecholamines as exist in situ. Here one depends upon the level of intrinsic sympathetic activity, which may not be high (22). On the other hand, one cannot achieve the same precision of analysis in situ as one does in in vitro studies (though certain kinds of data regarding action potentials can be acquired in ischemia and other states) (23,24).

Another interpretive problem is the fact that alpha-adrenergic activity exerts electrophysiologic effects (25-28). In many instances these effects are opposite those of beta-agonists (e.g., on APD, see below) (28,29). In situ certain electrophysiological effects of beta-blockers may be via a loss of beta-inhibition and consequent unmasking of the now unopposed alpha-effects. This phenomenon is analogous to adrenergic effects on vasomotor tone whereby withdrawal of beta-vasodilator properties leaves alpha-vasoconstrictive properties unopposed. Also, the fact that intrinsic alpha- as well as beta-activity is low in vitro makes for another difficulty in extrapolating in vitro data to the in situ state.

Beta-blockers have antiischemic as well as electrophysiological effects. Amelioration of ischemia is obviously of great potential importance in the antiarrhythmic properties. For example, although it is clear that following myocardial infarction beta-blockers prevent sudden death (30,32), it has never been clarified whether this benefit results from antiischemic or direct antiarrhythmic electrophysiological properties (or a combination of the two that may display considerable interpatient variability).

Antiarrhythmic effects of beta blockers may also occur via peripheral $beta_2$ rather than direct cardiac mechanisms. $Beta_2$-agonist activity tends to lower serum K^+ (primarily via effects on the large mass of skeletal muscle), a factor disposing to ventricular arrhythmias (32,33). Catecholamine-induced hypokalemia may be especially important to Torsade de Pointes, occurring in the long Q-T syndrome (see below). Nonselective beta blockade tends to reverse hypokalemia induced in this manner (32,33) and thus exert antiarrhythmic effects in a way that cannot be directly evaluated in vitro.

Other issues regarding extrapolation of in vitro data apply more generally to the evaluation of any agent. There are questions regarding proper in vitro concentrations versus in situ dose and serum level (e.g., protein binding is not replicated in presently used in vitro solutions; there may be altered drug delivery to ischemic zones; also there appears to be local neuron accumulation of at least some beta blockers in excess of serum levels) (34). In addition, in vitro concentrations that block effects of added catecholamines may be different (less) than concentrations that antagonize effects of intrinsic sympathetic activity.

Active metabolites may be important relative to the parent compound in situ, though this is less of an issue in evaluating generic beta-blocking properties. Since most studies evaluate normal tissue in vitro, effects on abnormal tissue may be less examined. However, this issue has become well understood, and drugs have been studied in a wide variety of pertinent abnormal models.

NON-BETA-BLOCKING ELECTROPHYSIOLOGIC EFFECTS

A further complexity is that several beta-blockers have additional membrane-active electrophysiological properties. Table 1 shows the Vaughan Williams classification of antiarrhythmic drug (with the Harrison modification) (35,36). In this, Class I includes the local anesthetics. These agents block I_{Na} and therefore slow conduction and prolong refractoriness. Class I agents are subclassified into IA, IB, and IC depending primarily on the degree of blockade of inward current (IC agent the most, and IB the least). In addition, IA agents prolong, IB shorten, and IC have no effect on APD. Class II agents are the beta-blockers. Class III agents greatly prolong APD, and Class IV agents are calcium channel blockers.

Several beta-blockers exhibit Class I or Class III properties in addition to beta blockade. Propranolol, acebutolol, and pindolol (of those used in the United States) exhibit Class I actions (called "membrane-stabilizing activity") (MSA) (37). Often MSA resides primarily or strictly in the D-isomer. In the case of propranolol, the D-isomer exhibits MSA (38-41) and no important beta-blocking properties, while the L-isomer exhibits both properties (42).

Officially MSA is evaluated using in vitro nerve models (e.g. frog sciatic nerve) (43), though effects demonstrated in that model are not always great enough to translate into relevant MSA in use. To which subclassification (IA, B, or C) the local anesthetic properties of any of the beta-blockers belong remains for the most part unstudied.

Sotalol has Class III properties (44-48)—D-sotalol is exclusively a Class III agent completely devoid of beta-blocking (or Class I) (49) actions.

MSA and Class III actions add another dimension to the electrophysiological and clinical evaluation of beta-blockers. These agents may have

Table 1 Classification of Antiarrhythmic Drugs

Class I	—	Local anesthetic agents
IA	—	Agents that depress I_{Na} and prolong APD
IB	—	Agents that moderately depress I_{Na} and shorten APD
IC	—	Agents that greatly depress I_{Na} and have little effect on APD
Class II	—	Beta-blockers
Class III	—	Agents that greatly prolong APD
Class IV	—	Calcium channel blockers

Source: Refs. 35, 36.

antiarrhythmic actions beyond that associated with beta blockade. In some cases D-isomers have been thought to completely explain antiarrhythmic actions, and both D-propranolol and D-sotalol have been used as antiarrhythmic drugs on their own. Our work suggests an antiarrhythmic and electrophysiological role for the local anesthetic properties of propranolol in ischemia (23,24). However, it is also true that, for example, in post-MI sudden death trials, it is not possible to distinguish differences in result among agents with and without this property (30,31).

Drug levels are important to consider in evaluating MSA. For some agents with this property (e.g., practolol and pindolol) (49a) concentrations required for MSA are so much above that required for beta blockade that MSA has no practical importance. For others, such as propranolol, where MSA concentrations are within the clinical range, as the concentration increases, the local anesthetic effects become more and more prominent in relation to beta blockade. One eventually reaches a dose or concentration of complete or nearly complete beta blockade beyond which local anesthetic properties begin to play the major electrophysiological role (38). For example, propranolol has been found to be effective against ventricular premature beats at very high doses beyond which beta blockade has already been achieved and at which local anesthetic properties seem to play the major role (50).

Several beta-blockers have "intrinsic sympathomimetic activity" (ISA). That is, in the presence of complete beta blockade they act as sympathomimetic agents. Of drugs available in the United States, pindolol has the most prominent ISA (37) as does acebutolol. Agents with ISA may exhibit blunting of their beta-blocking actions at higher concentrations (24). Agents with prominent ISA are probably not as useful for arrhythmias.

BETA-EFFECTS ON IONIC CURRENTS

Beta-effects on ionic currents will be considered from the point of view of both agonist and blocking activity. Beginning with I_{Na}, there are multiple influences as indicated earlier. I_{Na} mediates the upstroke in His-Purkinje and myocardial tissue. Its rapidity depends on both direct effects on the current itself and indirect effects on its initial state of activation, which in turn depends on resting potential. A lowering of (positive shift in) resting potential will cause partial inactivation of I_{Na} and a slower upstroke (20).

In the past, determining the direct influence of the beta-receptor in I_{Na} has been somewhat confounded by coexisting MSA, which serves to inhibit I_{Na}, e.g., for propranolol (51). When studied, the currently available agents either inhibit I_{Na} and slow upstroke velocity, usually due to coexisting MSA, or have no detectable effects on these parameters (52).

More recent studies on the interaction of beta-receptors with Na^+ channel have yielded somewehat unexpected results. Beta-agonists may in fact *depress* I_{Na} (53). This inhibitory effect was more pronounced in partially inactivated (depolarized) cells. The extent and significance of the effect for arrthythmias is as yet unclear. In addition, to what extent or even whether beta-blockers may directly enhance I_{Na} is at present unknown. At present such an effect would appear to be beyond the sensitivity of studies performed.

Regarding indirect effects on I_{Na}, beta-agonists increase (make more negative) resting potential (54) via the enhancement of Na-K pump and outward I_K (55). Beta-agonists also lower threshold and make myocytes more excitable (i.e., easier to excite or, in other words, easier to induce an action potential via I_{Na}) (54). This will serve to improve conduction (adjacent cells excited earlier) and enhance automaticity (self-excitation occurs earlier).

In the case of I_{Ca}, beta-agonists clearly enhance (56-58) and blockers suppress the current. Effects of the beta-receptor appears to be primarily on the L-type I_{Ca} (57). This action will cause beta-agonists to enhance (and blockers to depress) the upstroke in sinoatrial node, AV node, and slow response tissues. Beta-agonists enhance I_f the inward pacemaker Na^+ current (to enhance automaticity) (59). Beta-agonists also enhance outward I_K to favor repolarization as well as increasing resting potential (57).

An important effect of beta-agonists is to enhance the Na-K pump (60-62). Since this ion exchange mechanism also provides outward current (see above), it is an important electrophysiological property for both beta-agonists and blockers with relevance to resting potential and APD 15,18,60).

POSSIBLE ARRHYTHMOGENIC EFFECTS OF BETA-AGONISTS

Apart from promoting ischemia (via increased heart rate and inotropy), beta-agonists may favor arrhythmogenicity by a variety of actions in automaticity and reentry models. Beta-agonists enhance both normal and abnormal automaticity. They increase the normal slope of phase 4 depolarization in all automatic tissues (via increased I_f and/or I_{Ca}) (Fig. 6) (61,62) to favor or induce arrhythmias based on this mechanism.

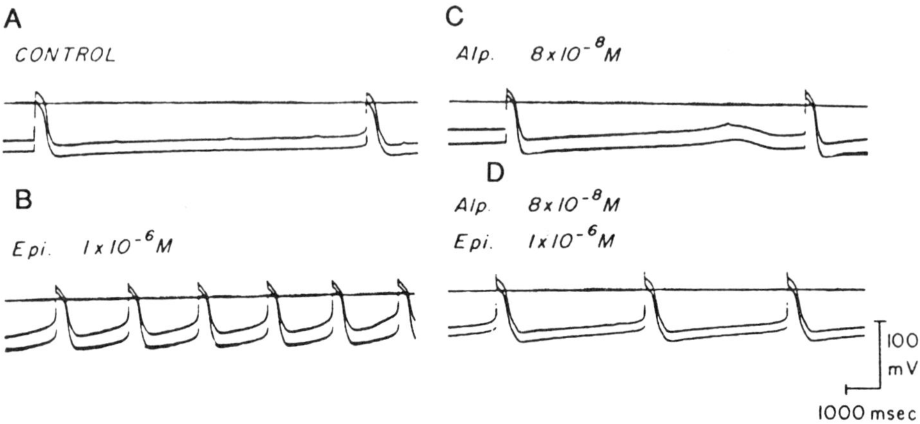

Figure 6 Effect of catecholamines and the beta-blocker on automaticity in canine Purkinje fiber. (A) Spontaneous automatic activity with phase 4 depolarization. (B) Addition of epinephrine (1×10^{-6} M) causes enhanced automaticity with more rapid beating. (C) Fiber after washout of epinephrine and addition of alprenolol, a beta-blocker (8×10^{-8} M). Note that there is little difference in automatic activity at this concentration of alprenolol from that of control, i.e., this low concentration of beta-blocker has little effect presumably because of the low intrinsic sympathetic activity in the in vitro Purkinje fiber. (D) Readdition of epinephrine. Note that automatic activity is considerably slower than that of the bottom left. Thus a low concentration of alprenolol effectively opposes enhanced automaticity induced by catecholamine. (From Ref. 62.)

Beta-agonists enhance DADs and thereby play a role in digitalis-induced arrhythmias. They also favor EAD-induced triggered activity, but this effect is a bit more complex. In mammalian tissue, depending on heart rate and concentration, beta-agonists tend to shorten APD, which might prevent triggered activity from occurring. However, if APD is prolonged by other factors (e.g., low pH as in ischemia), triggering is enhanced by beta-agonists (4,5). Enhancement of EADs and DADs is related to enhanced I_{Ca}.

Beta-agonists have little effect on upstroke and conduction in normal His-Purkinje tissue and myocardium. However, in abnormal tissue, effects on conduction depend on the initial situation of the membrane. In ischemic zones, for example, myocardial and His-Purkinje tissue may be either completely or partially inactivated. Completely inactivated tissue is inert and therefore does not participate in arrhythmias. Beta-agonists may adversely change this by (1) inducing the occurrence of slow responses (abnormal action potentials which resemble those in the AV node) (see Fig. 4) via enhancement of I_{Ca}, or (2) increasing resting potentials and thereby converting a completely inactivated to a partially inactivated site. In either instance, previously inert tissue is recruited into possible arrhythmogenic activity with the slow sites of conduction thereby created acting as substrate for reentry.

In the partially inactivated tissue, the upstroke is mediated by a less vigorous movement of I_{Na} than usual and a proportionately more prominent I_{Ca}. Beta-agonists may promote the I_{Ca} component of the action potential or may slow the I_{Na} component. However, they may also restore resting potential to a more activated state. Thus, depending on the specifics of the situation, reentry may be favored. Or, in a seeming paradox, reentry may also be abolished. For example, beta-agonists may restore the cell to complete activation and a normal fast response (54). This is probably a mechanism for *anti*arrhythmic effects that may occur with intravenous catecholamines in cardiac arrest and in certain other situations.

Effects of beta-agonists on resting potential may have consequences for automaticity. Automatic cells, as they move to more depolarized resting potentials, first display enhanced automaticity; then with more positive potentials, no automaticity; and then with even more positive potentials display automaticity again. This increase in automaticity at positive potentials is called "depolarization-induced automaticity," and its rate becomes faster with even further depolarization (63,64).

Although beta-agonists tend to favor automaticity at all levels of membrane potential (via increased I_f and/or I_{Ca}), they could also influence it via a change in resting membrane potential. That is, by promoting a more negative potential, beta-agonists may enhance or even suppress automaticity.

Sympathomimetic effects on APD have also been considered a possibility for arrhythmia induction. Beta-agonists tend to shorten APD (though not always). Circulating beta-agonists do so uniformly. However, sympathetic innervation of the heart is not uniform, and it is thought that during sympathetic stimulation myocytes adjacent to the neurons have much more marked APD shortening than those that are distant. Thus, APD disparities would be created. Such disparities favor reentry because they make it possible for a premature impulse to find refractory cells creating one way block (1). In addition, boundary currents flowing into cells with shortened APD might also induce arrhythmias. Finally, systemic $beta_2$ agonist activity may promote arrhythmias via induction of hypokalemia as indicated earlier (32,33).

ELECTROPHYSIOLOGICAL EFFECTS OF BETA BLOCKADE

Sinoatrial and AV Nodal Effects

The sinoatrial and AV nodes have the richest sympathetic innervation in the heart. Beta-blockers slow the slope of phase 4 depolarization and somewhat raise the threshold for activation in sinus and AV nodal cells (see Fig. 6). Both of these actions serve to suppress automaticity. Suppression of I_f and I_{Ca} and perhaps direct or indirect effects on the timing of I_K underlie this effect.

Beta-blockers also depress or abolish the upstrokes in both sinoatrial and AV nodes via suppression of I_{Ca}. Thus conduction in both of these structures is slowed.

The above effects cause slowing of sinus as well as of subsidiary AV nodal pacemaker (61,62,65), prolongation of sinoatrial conduction time (an effect that may only be apparent in patients with sick sinus syndrome) (66), and slowing of conduction through the AV node with prolongation of A-H intervals and increased likelihood of Wenckebach block (39,65, 67,68). In addition, beta-blockers cause prolongation of AV nodal effective and functional refractory periods (65).

His-Purkinje and Myocardial Effects

In spite of some differences, beta-blocker actions in atrium, ventricular, and His-Purkinje systems are similar enough to be considered together (though Purkinje fiber tends to be more reactive).

UPSTROKE AND CONDUCTION

Beta-effects on upstrokes (and therefore on conduction of impulses) have been discussed above. Among factors to consider are differences in normal, partially, inactivated, and slow response tissues, direct beta-effects on I_{Na} and I_{Ca} versus indirect effects on resting potential, co-existing MSA, and in situ alpha effects.

These factors sort out as follows:

1. Beta blockade alone has little or no direct effect I_{Na}, i.e., beta-blockers do not alter membrane responsiveness curves (which compare upstroke velocity to resting potential) (52,69). However, agents with MSA (by definition) reduce I_{Na} (51,70). This effect is generally of little significance in normal tissue where agents do not substantially

alter conduction, but it may play a role in depressing conduction in abnormal (partially inactivated) tissue (23,71). (Note that sotalol with co-existing Class III actions has no effect on upstroke).

2. Beta-blockers depress I_{Ca}. Thus they will depress or abolish conduction of slow responses and, to some degree, responses in partially inactivated tissue.
3. Beta-blockers tend to reduce resting potential (via I_K and the Na-K pump) thereby indirectly depressing or abolishing the upstroke (though again probably little detectable effect in normal tissue) (72).
4. Unopposed alpha-stimulation reduces membrane potential and also tends to block conduction in partially inactivated tissue (25).

Overall, beta-blockers have little effect on normal but slow conduction in abnormal tissue in situ especially in situations in which sympathetic activity in high, e.g., ischemia (23,24). The propranolol-induced prolongation of H-V intervals in abnormal but not in normal hearts also exemplifies this phenomenon (73).

ACTION POTENTIAL DURATION

Studies of beta-blocker effects on APD are somewhat variable. Considerations here are:

1. Relative effects on the various ionic currents. Direct suppression of I_K and the Na-K pump will tend to lengthen APD, while direct suppression of I_{Ca} will shorten it. In abnormal states, effects on one or another current may be more important.
2. Unopposed alpha-stimulation lengthens APD (11,28,29,74).
3. Class III actions in the case of satolol lengthen APD (44-47).
4. Reduction of the resting potential might shorten APD.
5. In some instances variable effects of beta-blockers in a given situation depend on concentration and heart rate.

In vitro studies of beta-blockers have been contradictory. Propranolol, for example, has been found to shorten APD in Purkinje fibers (70,75), shorten or lengthen APD in atrium (75), and either have no effect on or lengthen APD in ventricular muscle (70). (Shortened APD in vitro may be secondary to its non-beta-blocking, possibly IB, effects (76).) Other agents have either prolonged or had little influence on APD. Tissues exposed to beta-blockers chronically have displayed APD prolongation (35).

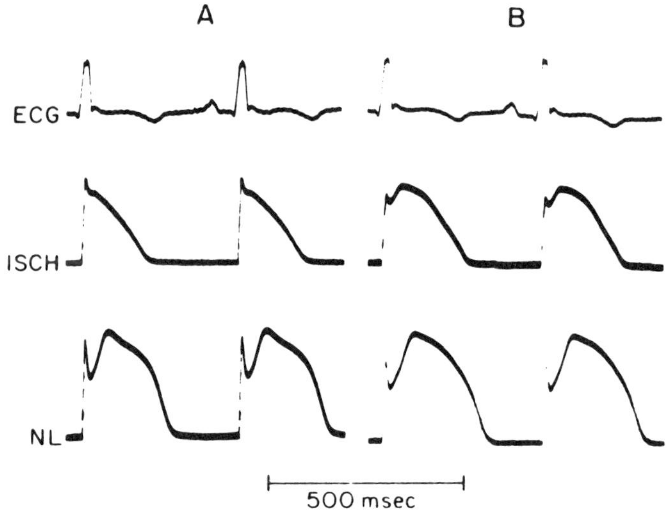

Figure 7 Effects of the beta-blocker practolol on monophasic action potential duration in situ. The top trace shows ECG lead II, the middle and bottom traces show monophasic action potentials recorded from an ischemic zone (ISCH) induced by ligation of the left anterior descending coronary artery and a normal (NL) zone in the right ventricle. (A) Control ligation. (B) Ligation after which 0.4 mg/kg of practolol was administered. Note that practolol prolongs APD (equally) in both ischemic and normal zones (213-267 msec in NL vs. 175-233 msec in ISCH). Thus the beta-blocker practolol prolonged APD to approximately the same degree in ischemic and normal zones. See text for further discussion. (From Ref. 24.)

In situ studies more consistently show that beta-blockers prolong APD, and functionally this should be considered the beta-blocker effect (23, 24,29). One study showed that practolol (a beta-blocker with MSA) prolongs monophasic APD equally in ischemic and normal zones in situ (Fig. 7), while propranolol (which has MSA) more greatly prolonged APD in ischemic zones (23,24). It is likely that unopposed alpha-stimulation plays an important role in APD prolongation in situ (23).

EFFECTIVE REFRACTORY PERIOD

Studies of beta blockade on ERP in vitro have tended to show little effect or prolongation. ERP is defined as the time from the onset of the action potential to the earliest time that a new propagated action potential can be elicited. This new action potential is elicited during the latter part of phase 3. ERP is thus a function of both APD and of the status of inward currents which would create the early propagated impulse. If APD is prolonged, then the time to the earliest possible new activation would also be prolonged. If inward currents are reduced or threshold elevated, a very early stimulus or impulse (which would occur at reduced membrane potential during phase 3) would be less likely to initiate a propagated response. These earliest responses are mediated by partially inactivated I_{Na} with substantial I_{Ca}. Thus prolongation of APD and reduction of I_{Ca} via beta blockade (or I_{Na} via MSA) would tend to prolong ERP.

In addition, primary reduction in I_{Ca} would prolong ERP to a greater extent than APD (i.e., increase the ERP/APD ratio). The functional importance of this last effect is that earliest slow impulses are abolished making reentry less likely. Studies of beta-blockers in general have shown an increase in ERP, but effects on ERP/APD are less certain. For example, our studies show that propranolol, which has MSA, altered this ratio while practolol, with absent MSA, did not (23,24).

AUTOMATICITY

It is very clear that beta-blockers reduce phase 4 depolarization in all automatic tissue at any level of potential (e.g., Fig. 6). This action occurs at rather low concentration in preparations in which automaticity had previously been increased by catecholamines (Fig. 6). Alpha-stimulation also tends to reduce automaticity. Thus, in situ both direct effects and unopposed alpha-stimulation (27) suppress automaticity.

As indicated previously, beta-blockers also tend to diminish automatic triggering due to DADs or EADs.

ELECTROPHYSIOLOGICAL EFFECTS OF BETA-BLOCKERS IN SPECIFIC ARRHYTHMIAS

Overall Considerations

In this section we will consider how the above electrophysiological effects of beta-blockers serve to prevent, reduce, or abolish arrhythmias in specific situations. First, however, some overall considerations: The mechanism of arrhythmia is important. Reentry may be abolished by one of a variety of actions that serve to alter the pattern of conduction either via direct effects on conduction or effects on refractoriness. Automaticity is generally suppressed by direct effects on phase 4 depolarization, DADs, or EADs with the last (i.e., repolarization failure) also suppressible by APD shortening.

Indirect effects on arrhythmia substrate via antiischemic properties also are important. These occur via negative inotropy, negative chronotropy, and perhaps effects on arteriosclerotic plaques. As discussed earlier, the relative roles of antiarrhythmic and antiischemic properties in arrhythmia situations, e.g., post-MI prevention of sudden death, is still a subject of debate. In addition, recently described improvement in mortality in congestive cardiomyopathy via beta blockade may also result from indirect effects in addition to or apart from antiarrhythmic effects. One hypothesis is that benefit here results from upregulation of beta receptors. $Beta_2$-blocking properties also play a role in suppressing arrhythmia that result from or are furthered by catecholamine-induced hypokalemia.

To what degree sympathetic activity plays a role in a given arrhythmia is another factor. This is especially pertinent for arrhythmias related to heightened emotional activity or exercise no matter what the underlying cause or "catecholamine storm" as in phenochromocytoma or severe emotional reaction (e.g., a person in an airplane about to crash). In vitro, even low concentrations of beta-blockers antagonize effects of added catecholamines (especially on automaticity) (49,77).

Specific Arrhythmia Settings

Reentry

Beta-blockers are effective in general via converting one-way (Figs. 4,5) to two-way block. Suppression of I_{Ca}, I_K, or the Na-K pump (causing alterations in resting potential, prolongation of APD and therefore refractory period) would be possible mechanisms.

Automaticity

Beta-blockers suppress normal automaticity (at rather lower concentrations if induced by catecholamines) and also automatic triggering due to EADs (Figure 7) or DADs. Indirect effects on automaticity via changes in resting potential may also occur.

Paroxysmal Atrial Tachycardia

This arrhythmia is caused by reentry within the AV node (most commonly), sinoatrial node, or in the case of Wolff-Parkinson-White syndrome a pancardiac pathway involving the AV node. The "slow" arm of the reentrant pathway in these arrhythmias depends on slow response action potentials. Beta-blockers suppress this arrhythmia by suppressing AV nodal or sinus nodal I_{Ca} thus blocking reentry. Atrial arrhythmias due to automaticity are generally not effectively suppressed by beta-blockers.

Arrhythmias Due to DADs

Digitalis-induced tachycardias result mainly from DADs, which can be suppressed by beta-blockers (16) (though MSA may also play a role here) (43). At present the evidence for DAD involvement in other arrhythmias is scattered.

Long Q-T Syndrome

This syndrome is characterized by bursts of Torsade de Pointe type ventricular arrhythmias, occurrence of sudden death, induction of arrhythmias with emotion or other sympathetic activity, and diminution of arrhythmia by this beta-blockade. Two mechanisms have been postulated for this suppression. For many years it has been thought that arrhythmias in the long Q-T syndrome are due to enhanced sympathetic nervous stimulation causing nonuniform shortening of, and therefore disparity in, APD (see above as to why this sequence of events may prolong Q-T interval) (1). Beta-blocker effectiveness would be via antagonism of APD shortening making APDs more nearly equal.

Another, and more perhaps likely, scenario is that arrhythmias result from APD prolongation and EADs. Myocardial cells in patients with long Q-T syndrome may have K^+ channel abnormalities that under certain circumstances lead to abnormal action potential prolongation (and thus long Q-T intervals). Arrhythmias would then occur via repolarization failure with EADs (1,6,78). In this scenario increased sympathetic activity causes arrhythmias directly by inducing EADs or indirectly by causing hypokalemia (see above), which favors APD prolongation and EADs. Beta-blockers would suppress arrhythmias directly via suppression of the EADs (79) or indirectly via $beta_2$-blockade of hypokalemic effect (32,33). It is possible that Torsade de Pointe from other causes (e.g., antiarrhythmic drugs) may also be influenced by these elements.

Ischemia

This is one of the more intricate situations. In ischemia, among elements to consider (besides effects on ischemia per se) are reduction of resting membrane potential leading to partial inactivation of I_{Na}, quiescence, or slow responses. These last may be induced in otherwise quiescent tissue by catecholamines. There is also intracellular Ca^{2+} loading, which is believed to favor several arrhythmogenic mechanisms as well as transiently elevated local K^+, which favors outward currents. In addition, in later ischemia, there may be EADs, DADs, or possibly enhanced normal automaticity.

Therefore, to suppress arrhythmias beta-blockers in ischemia may:

1. Reduce resting potential to cause partially inactivated tissue to revert to quiescence (diminution of I_K and Na-K pump) and become inert with regard to arrhythmogenesis.
2. Reduce upstroke in partially inactivated tissue (diminution of the I_{Ca} component).
3. Inhibit slow response (diminished I_{Ca}).
4. Reduce intracellular Ca^{2+} loading (diminished I_{Ca}).
5. Prolong refractoriness (diminished I_K, Na-K pump, I_{Ca}, and with MSA, I_{Na}).
6. Diminish excitability.

All of these actions will tend to abolish reentry via conversion of one-way to two-way block. In addition, beta-blockers may suppress both normal and abnormal automaticity (Figure 7) directly or perhaps indirectly via change of resting potential.

MSA may also participate in depressing conduction. Our study suggests a role for propranolol's local anesthetic properties in ischemia (23, 24) as have certain clinical studies (50). In addition, the Class III properties of sotalol certainly seem pertinent to its antiarrhythmic effects. However, as indicated above there is no apparent distinction among beta-blockers with and without intrinsic sympathomimetic activity in prevention of postmyocardial infarction sudden death (30,31).

PROARRHYTHMIA

Proarrhythmia is a pertinent issue for antiarrhythmic drugs as documented in the recent Cardiac Arrhythmia Suppression Trial (CAST) (80). Beta-blockers have been reported to display proarrhythmia in chronic ventricular arrhythmias (81). Certain of the above properties that lead to zones of slow conduction could promote reentry or disorganization of electrical activity. On the other hand, antiischemic as well as antiautomatic properties would not appear to have this liability. While post-MI studies show increased mortality and therefore important proarrhythmia for several Class I antiarrhythmic drugs (81,82), they show only benefit for beta-blockade at least in the overall populations (30,31). Although the data is as yet incomplete and one presumes some similar electrophysiologic mechanisms for Class I as for beta-blocking drugs in certain situations, it is the overall impression that proarrhythmia in the case of beta-blockers is less prominent.

MOLECULAR BASIS OF BETA-EFFECTS

Recent work has considerably increased our understanding of the biochemical basis of beta-blocker actions. Beta-effects occur in the following sequence: Attachment of beta-agonists to the beta-receptor activites membrane-bound adenyl cyclase, which in turn increases cAMP, the intracellular messenger for beta-stimulation. cAMP then enhances I_{Ca}, I_K, and probably I_f via a cAMP-dependent protein kinase.

Recent work on the Ca^{2-} channels has shown that the beta-induced increase in I_{Ca} is via cAMP (83,84) and a signal transducing protein (G_s). G_s stimulates I_{Ca} via two separate pathways—fast and slow. In the fast pathway, Gs couples beta-receptors to Ca^{2+} channels directly in the membrane, while the slow (cytoplasmic) pathway is indirect and utilizes adenyl cyclase. Propranolol inhibits both pathways. Interestingly, the presence of a fast pathway (which has a time constant of 150 msec) explains how sympathetic activation can change heart rate with a single beat (85).

As indicated earlier, G_s can also directly couple the beta-receptor to the Na^+ channel. In this case G_s may serve to inhibit I_{Na} especially in partially inactivated cells (53). Thus beta-agonist activity via G_s may have different effects on I_{Na} (inhibitory) from that of I_{Ca} (enhancing).

Over the next few years we can expect a substantial increase in our understanding of the biochemical mediators of beta-actions.

REFERENCES

1. Surawicz B, Knoebel SB. Long QT: good, bad or indifferent? J Am Coll Cardiol 1984; 4:398-408.
2. Cranefield PF. Action potentials, afterpotentials, and arrhythmias. Circ Res 1977; 41:415-25.
3. Brachmann J, Scherlag BJ, Rosenshtraukh LV, Lazzara R. Bradycardia-dependent triggered activity: relevance to drug-induced multiform ventricular tachycardia. Circ 1983; 68:846-56.
4. Kupersmith J, Hoff P. Occurrence and transmission of repolarization abnormalities in vitro. J Am Coll Cardiol 1985; 6:152-60.
5. Kupersmith J, Hoff P, Guo S. In vitro characteristics of repolarization abnormality—a possible cause of arrhythmias. J Electrocardiol 1986; 19:361-70.

6. Schechter E, Freeman CC, Lazzara R. Afterdepolarizations as a mechanism for the long QT syndrome: electrophysiologic studies of a case. J Am Coll Cardiol 1984; 3:1556-67.
7. Cranefield PF. The conduction of the cardiac impulse. The slow response and cardiac arrhythmias. Mount Kisco, NY: Futura Publishing Co., 1975.
8. Cranefield PF, Klein HO, Hoffman BF. Conduction of the cardiac impulse. Circ Res 1971; 28:199-219.
9. Cranefield PF, Wit AL, Hoffman BF. Genesis of cardiac arrhythmias. Circulation 1973; 47:190-204.
10. Davis LD, Helmer PR. Electrophysiological effects of norepinephrine on slow responses induced in isolated canine cardiac Purkinje fibers by reduced extracellular pH. J Pharmacol Exp Ther 1980; 214:94-100.
11. Pappano AJ. Propranolol-insensitive effects of epinephrine on action potential repolarization in electrically driven atria of the guinea pig. J Pharmacol Exp Ther 1971; 177:85-95.
12. Kupersmith J, Cohen R. Differing electrophysiologic effects of slow response inhibiting agents manganese and verapamil in ischemic, infarcted and normal tissue in situ. J Pharmacol Exp Ther 1980; 215:394-400.
13. Hirano Y, Fozzard HA, January CT. Characteristics of L- and T-type Ca^{++} currents in canine cardiac Purkinje cells. Am J Physiol 1989; H1478-H1492.
14. McDonald TF, Trautwein W. The potassium current underlying delayed rectification in cat ventricular muscle. J Physiol (London) 1978; 274:217-46.
15. Kline RP, Kupersmith J. Effects of extracellular potassium accumulation and sodium pump activation on automatic canine Purkinje fibers. J Physiol (London) 1982; 324:507-33.
16. Dohadwalla AN, Freedberg AS, Vaughan Williams EM. The relevance of β-receptor blockade to ouabain-induced cardiac arrhythmias. Br J Pharmac 1969; 36:257-67.
17. Noma A, Kotake H, Irisawa H. Slow inward current and its role mediating the chronotropic effect of epinephrine in the rabbit sinoatrial node. Pflugers Arch 1980; 388:1-9.
18. Gadsby DC, Cranefield PF. Direct measurement of changes in sodium pump current in canine cardiac Purkinje fibers. Proc Nat Acad Sci USA 1979; 76:1783-7.
19. Mullins LJ. Ion transport in heart. New York: Raven Press, 1981.
20. Weidmann S. The effect of the cardiac membrane potential on the rapid availability of the sodium-carrying system. J Physiol 1955; 127:213-24.
21. Kline RP, Cohen I, Falk R, Kupersmith J. Activity dependent extracellular K^+ fluctuation in canine Purkinje fiber. Nature 1980; 286:68-71.
22. Parmley WW, Braunwald E. Comparative myocardial depressant and antiarrhythmic properties of d-propranolol, dl-propranolol and quinidine. J Pharmacol Exp Ther 1967; 158:11-21.
23. Kupersmith J, Shiang H, Litwak RS, Herman MV. Electrophysiological and antiarrhythmic effects of propranolol in canine acute myocardial ischemia. Circ Res 1976; 38:302-7.

24. Kupersmith J, Shiang HS. Electrophysiologic effects of beta adrenergic blockade with practolol in canine acute myocardial ischemia. J Pharmacol Exp Ther 1979; 207:976-82.
25. Cranefield PF, Hoffman BF, Wit AL. Block of conduction in partially depolarized cardiac Purkinje fibers induced by an A-adrenergic agent. Nature New Biology 1971; 234:159-60.
26. Dukes JD, Vaughan Williams EM. Electrophysiological effects of α-adrenoceptor antagonists in rabbit sino-atrial node, cardiac Purkinje cells and papillary muscles. Br J Pharmacol 1984; 83:419-26.
27. Rosen MR, Hordof AJ, Ilvento JP, Danilo P Jr. Effects of adrenergic amines on electrophysiological properties and automaticity of neonatal and adult canine Purkinje fibers. Circ Res 1977; 40:390-400.
28. Giotti A, Ledda F, Mannaioni PF. Effects of noradrenaline and isoprenaline, in combination with α- and β-receptor blocking substances, on the action potential of cardiac Purkinje fibres. J Physiol 1973; 229:99-113.
29. Amlie JP, Refsum H, Landmark K. Acebutolol-induced changes in refractoriness and monophasic action potential of the right ventricle of the dog heart in situ. Cardiovasc Res 1978; 12:493-6.
30. Norwegian Multicenter Study Group. Timolol induced reduction in mortality and reinfarction in patients surviving acute myocardial infarction. N Engl J Med 1981; 304:801-12.
31. The Beta-Blocker Heart Attack Trial Research Group. A randomized trial of propranolol in patients with acute myocardial infarction. JAMA 1982; 247:1707 17.
32. Lockwood RH, Lum RBB. Effects of adrenergic agonists and antagonists on potassium metabolism. J Pharmacol Exp Ther 1974; 189:119-29.
33. Vincent HH, Boomsma F, Man in't Veld AJ, Derkx FHM, Wenting GJ, Schalekamp MADH. Effects of selective and nonselective β-agonists on plasma potassium and norepinephrine. J Cardiovasc Pharmacol 1984; 6:107-14.
34. Pruett JK, Walle T, Walle UK. Propranolol effects on membrane repolarization time in isolated canine Purkinje fibers: threshold tissue content and the influence of exposure time. J Pharmacol Exp Ther 1980; 215:539-43.
35. Vaughan Williams EM. A classification of antiarrhythmic actions reassessed after a decade of new drugs. J Clin Pharmacol 1984; 24:129-47.
36. Harrison CD. Antiarrhythmic drug classification: new science and practice applications. Am J Cardiol 1985; 56:185.
37. Squire A, Kupersmith J. Beta adrenergic blocking agents, review and update. Mt Sinai Med J 1985; 52:553-8.
38. Dawson AK, Reele SB, Wood AJJ, Duff HF, Woosley RL, Smith RF. Electrophysiological effects of high-dose propranolol in dogs: evidence in vivo for effects not mediated by the beta adrenoceptor. J Pharmacol Exp Ther 1984; 229:91-7.

39. Smithen CS, Balcon R, Sowton E. Use of bundle of His potentials to assess changes in atrioventricular conduction produced by a series of beta-adrenergic blocking agents. Br Heart J 1971; 33:955-61.
40. Howe R, Shanks RG. Optical isomers of propranolol. Nature (Lond) 1966; 210:1336-8.
41. Jaillon P, Heckle J, Weissenburger J, Cheymol G. Cardiac electrophysiologic properties of dl-propranolol, d-propranolol, l-propranolol and dl-pindolol in anesthetized dogs. J Pharmacol Exp Ther 1980; 212:347-53.
42. Barret AM, Cullum VA. The biological properties of the optical isomers of propranolol and their effects on cardiac arrhythmias. Br J Pharmacol 1968; 34:43-55.
43. Lucchesi BR, Whitsitt LS, Stickney JL. Antiarrhythmic effects of beta adrenergic blocking agents. Ann NY Acad Sci 1967; 134:940-51.
44. Strauss HC, Bigger JT Jr, Hoffman BF. Electrophysiological and beta-receptor blocking effects of MJ 1999 on dog and rabbit cardiac tissue. Circ Res 1970; 26:661-78.
45. Singh BN, Vaughan Williams EM. A third class of anti-arrhythmic action. Effects on atrial and ventricular intracellular potentials, and other pharmacological actions on cardiac muscle, of MJ 1999 and AH 3474. Br J Pharmacol 1970; 39:675-87.
46. Kato R, Ikeda N, Yabek SM, Kannan R, Singh RN. Electrophysiologic effects of the levo- and dextrorotatory isomers of sotalol in isolated cardiac muscle and their in vivo pharmacokinetics. J Am Coll Cardiol 1986; 7:116-25.
47. Manley BS, Alexopoulos D, Robinson GJ, Cobbe SM. Subsidiary class III effects of beta blockers? A comparison of atenolol, metoprolol, nadolol, oxprenolol and sotalol. Cardiovasc Res 1986; 20:705-9.
48. Carmeliet E. Electrophysiologic and voltage clamp analysis of the effects of sotalol on isolated cardiac muscle and Purkinje fibers. J Pharmacol Exp Ther 1985; 232:817-25.
49. Hiromasa S, Coto H, Li ZY, Maldonado C, Kupersmith J. Dextrorotatory isomer of sotalol: electrophysiologic effects and interaction with verapamil. Am Heart J 1988; 116:1552-7.
49a. Shimizu T, Iwamura N, Kodama I, Toyama J, Yamada K. Effects of beta-adrenergic blocking drug pindolol (LB46) on cardiac fibers in relation to its membrane effects. Jpn Heart J 1978; 19:865-75.
50. Woosley RL, Kornhauser D, Smith R, Reele S, Higgins SB, Nies AS, Shand DG, Oates JA. Suppression of chronic ventricular arrhythmias with propranolol. Circulation 1979; 60:819-27.
51. Coltart DJ, Meldrum SJ. The effect of racemic propranolol, dextro-propranolol and racemic practolol on the human and canine cardiac transmembrane action potential ([1]) (beta blockade and the cardiac action potential). Arch Int Pharmacodyn 1971; 192:188-97.

52. Bagwell EE, Custy J, Steen RG, Newman WH. Beta receptor blocking and antiarrhythmic properties of totamolol. J Pharmacol Exp Ther 1974; 191: 496-505.
53. Schubert B, Van Dongen AMJ, Kirsch GE, Brown AM. β-Adrenergic inhibition of cardiac sodium channels by dual G-protein pathways. Science 1989; 245:516-19.
54. Hoffman BF, Singer DH. Physiological and clinical aspects of beta adrenergic blockade. Appraisal of the effects of catecholamines on cardiac electrical activity. Ann NY Acad Sci 1967; 139:914-39.
55. Boyden PA, Cranefield PF, Gadsby DC. Noradrenaline hyperpolarizes cells of the canine coronary sinus by increasing their permeability to potassium ions. J Physiol (London) 1983; 339:185-206.
56. Reuter H. Localization of beta adrenergic receptors and effects of noradrenaline and cyclic nucleotides on action potentials, ionic currents and tension in mammalian cardiac muscle. J Physiol (London) 1974; 242:429-51.
57. Walsh KB, Begenisich TB, Kass RS. β-Adrenergic modulation of cardiac ion channels. J Gen Physiol 1989; 93:841-54.
58. Carmeliet E, Vereecke J. Adrenaline and the plateau phase of the cardiac action potential. Importance of Ca^{++}, Na^{+} and K^{+} conductance. Pflugers Arch 1969; 313:300-15.
59. Earm YE, Shimoni Y, Spindler AJ. A pace-maker-like current in the sheep atrium and its modulation by catecholamines. J Physiol 1983; 342:569-90.
60. Vassalle M, Barnabei O. Norepiniphrine and potassium fluxes in cardiac Purkinje fibers. Pflugers Arch 1971; 322:287-303.
61. Wit AL, Hoffman BF, Rosen MR. Electrophysiologic and pharmacology of cardiac arrhythmias IX. Cardiac electrophysiologic effects of beta adrenergic receptor stimulation and blockade. Part A. Am Heart J 1975; 90: 521-33.
62. Wit AL, Hoffman BF, Rosen MR. Electrophysiologic and pharmacology of cardiac arrhythmias IX. Cardiac electrophysiologic effects of beta adrenergic receptor stimulation and blockade. Part C. Am Heart J 1975; 90: 795-803.
63. Katzung BG, Hondeghem LM, Grant AO. Cardiac ventricular automaticity induced by current of injury. Pflugers Arch 1975; 360:193-203.
64. Aronson RS, Cranefield PF. The effect of resting potential on the electrical activity of canine cardiac Purkinje fibers exposed to Na-free solution or to ouabain. Pflugers Arch 1974; 347:101-16.
65. Seides SF, Josephson ME, Batsford WP, Weisfogel GM, Lau SH, Damato AN. The electrophysiology of propranolol in man. Am Heart J 1974; 88: 733-41.
66. Tsuchioka Y, Matsumoto K, Fujii H, Masaoka S, Yuasa A, Tateishi H, Matsuura H, Sato H, Kajiyama G. Electrophysiological effects of propranolol in patients with sinus node dysfunction. Jpn Heart J 1980; 29:319-24.

67. Whitsitt LS, Lucchesi BR. Effects of beta-receptor blockade and glucagon on the atrioventricular transmission system in the dog. Circ Res 1968; 23: 585-95.
68. Fitzgerald JD, Wale JL, Austin M. The hemodynamic effects of (±)-propranolol, dexpropranolol, oxprenolol, practolol and sotalol in anesthetized dogs. J Pharmacol 1972; 17:123-34.
69. Gibson JK, Gelband H, Bassett AL. Direct and beta adrenergic blocking actions of nadolol (SQ 11725) on electrophysiologic properties of isolated canine myocardium. J Pharmacol Exp Ther 1977; 202:702-10.
70. Davis LD, Temte JV. Effects of propranolol on the transmembrane potentials of ventricular muscle and Purkinje fibers of the dog. Circ Res 1968; 22:661-77.
71. Weiner I, Mindich B, Distefano D, Kupersmith J. Regional differences in the effects of propranolol on intramyocardial conduction in patients with coronary artery disease. Clin Pharm Ther 1979; 26:696-700.
72. Vaughan Williams EM. Mode of action of beta receptor antagonists on cardiac muscle. Am J Cardiol 1966; 38:399-405.
73. Kirkorian G, Touboul P, Atallah G. Electrophysiologic effects of propranolol in intraventricular conduction disturbance. Am J Cardiol 1988; 61:341-51.
74. Boachie-Ansah G, Kane KA, Parratt JK. Cardiac electrophysiological effects of isoprenaline, phenylephrine, and noraderenaline on normal and mildly "ischaemic" sheep Purkinje fibers. J Cardiovasc Pharm 1989; 13: 291-8.
75. Raine AEG, Vaughn Williams EM. Adaptation to prolonged β-blockade of rabbit atrial, Purkinje, and ventricular potentials, and of papillary muscle contraction. Circ Res 1981; 48:804-12.
76. Wu CH, Narahashi T. Mechanism of action of propranolol on squid axon membranes. J Pharmacol Exp Ther 1973; 184:155-62.
77. Kumakura S, Somani P. The effect of LB-46, a β-adrenoreceptor blocking drug, on isolated normal and ouabain-intoxicated Purkinje fibers of the dog. Eur J Pharmacol 1974; 25:335-50.
78. Bonatti V, Rolli A, Botti G. Monophasic action potential studies in human subjects with prolonged ventricular repolarization and long QT syndromes. Eur Heart J 1985; 6(Suppl D):131-7.
79. Arnsdorf MF. The effect of antiarrhythmic drugs on triggered sustained rhythmic activity in cardiac Purkinje fibers. J Pharmacol Exp Ther 1977; 201:689-700.
80. Cardiac Arrhythmia Suppression Trial. Preliminary report: effect of encainide and flecainide on mortality in a randomized trial of arrhythmia suppression after myocardial infarction. N Engl J Med 1989; 321:406-12.
81. Velebit V, Podrid P, Lown B, Cohen BH, Graboys TB. Aggravation and provocation of ventricular arrhythmias by antiarrhythmic drugs. Circulation 1982; 65:886-94.

82. Hine LK, Laird NM, Hewitt P, Chalmers TC. Meta-analysis of empirical long-term antiarrhythmic therapy after myocardial infarction. JAMA 1989; 262:3037-40.
83. Bean BP, Nowycky MC, Tsien RW. β-Adrenergic modulation of calcium channels in frog ventricular heart cells. Nature 1984; 307:371-5.
84. Tsien RW. Calcium channels in excitable cell membranes. Ann Rev Physiol 1983; 45:341-58.
85. Yatani A, Brown AM. Rapid β-adrenergic modulation of cardiac calcium channel currents by a fast G protein pathway. Science 1989; 245:71-4.

2

Effects of Beta-Blockers on Ventricular Fibrillation Threshold

Jeffrey L. Anderson
University of Utah and LDS Hospital, Salt Lake City, Utah

Various experimental models have been developed to assess the potential of pharmacologic and other interventions to reduce the propensity for ventricular fibrillation (VF), particularly in the setting of myocardial ischemia. The most basic model employs the introduction during cardiac pacing in open chest, anesthetized animals, of premature electrical stimuli in single beats or trains and of increasing current strength. The current strength at which VF is induced is defined as the VF threshold (VFT). Beta-blockade substantially increases VFT both under nonischemic and ischemic conditions. In contrast, nitroglycerin showed negligible effects on VFT in a comparative trial, and diltiazem (calcium channel blocker) had more modest effects. Section of the stellate ganglion, which supplies sympathetic neuronal traffic to the heart, also increased VFT. In another series of experiments, a correlation was found between the effects of beta-blockade on experimental VFT and inducibility of sustained ventricular tachyarrhythmias after subacute myocardial infarction. In a more sophisticated model of VF and other life-threatening arrhythmias induced by acute myocardial ischemia in concert with sympathetic hyperactivity, beta-blockade was effective and Class I antiarrhythmic therapy ineffective. Other agents with antisympathetic activity, including amiodarone, verapamil, and prazosin, also showed beneficial activity. Finally, in a conscious canine model of sudden coronary death caused by VF associated with acute coronary thrombosis, beta-blockade, but not Class I antiarrhythmic therapy, was shown to be effective. Similarly, other agents with effects on sympathetic tone, including bretylium and amiodarone, were effective. Although extrapolation of experimental results to the clinical setting should be done cautiously, the correlation between these experimental findings and the outcome of clinical trials is of note, and suggests that VFT effects may be a better predictor of outcome than traditional measures of antiectopic activity. The antifibrillatory effects of beta-blockers may be an important mechanism of their clinical action in ischemic heart disease.

ANTIFIBRILLATORY VERSUS ANTIECTOPIC ACTIVITY

Relationships Among Sudden Death, Ventricular Ectopy, and Antiarrhythmic Therapy

It has been well established that cardiac arrest and sudden cardiac death are caused by ventricular tachycardia/ventricular fibrillation in the vast majority of patients (1-4). Studies over the past decade have also identified spontaneous ventricular ectopy as a risk factor for cardiac arrest/sudden cardiac death, especially in patients with associated structural heart disease such as myocardial infarction or congestive heart failure (5-10). This had led to the hypothesis that suppression of the risk marker, ventricular ectopy, may lead to a reduction in the adverse outcome, ventricular fibrillation (11-13). However, this hypothesis has been dealt a serious blow by the results of the ongoing Cardiac Arrhythmia Suppression Trial (CAST) (14). In CAST, the Class IC antiarrhythmic agents encainide and flecainide suppressed ventricular ectopy in postinfarction patients to a high degree (greater than 80%) and yet *increased* both total cardiac mortality (risk ratio 2.5) and sudden death/cardiac arrest risk (risk ratio 3.6). Previous studies with Class IA and Class IB antiarrhythmic agents, although not as compelling, have also suggested an adverse rather than beneficial outcome (15). In contrast, the beta-blockers (Class II antiarrhythmic agents) have consistently demonstrated the potential to reduce total mortality (16) and specifically sudden death rates (17). Postinfarction patients in these studies were not selected for the presence of ventricular arrhythmias, and therapy was not guided by effects on ventricular ectopy. These clinical considerations suggest the importance of differentiating antifibrillatory from antiectopic effects (18,19).

Distinction Between Antifibrillatory and Antiarrhythmic Actions

The distinction between antifibrillatory and antiarrhythmic (antiectopic) actions has become increasingly recognized in recent years (18). An antiarrhythmic (antiectopic) drug action leads to a decrease in the frequency of ventricular ectopic beats. In contrast, an antifibrillatory action increases myocardial electrical instability, decreasing the propensity for ventricular fibrillation. Of course, some antiarrhythmic agents, such as the beta-blockers, may display both antifibrillatory and antiectopic activity. However, the relative and absolute degree of these two actions may differ among drugs and drug classes. For example, the beta-blockers are known to have less ventricular antiectopic activity than the Class I antiarrhythmic agents (20). However, both the clinical trials mentioned above (16,17) and the experimental studies to be presented below stress the importance of the antifibrillatory effects of the beta-blockers, particularly in the setting of acute ischemia. Consideration of antifibrillatory effects may lead to an improved approach to risk reduction for ventricular fibrillation and sudden cardiac death.

COMPARATIVE EFFECTS OF BETA-ADRENERGIC BLOCKERS ON EXPERIMENTAL VENTRICULAR FIBRILLATION THRESHOLD

Intrigued by the prominent clinical effects on sudden cardiac death in postinfarction beta-blocker trials (17), we hypothesized that one mechanism of benefit might be on ventricular fibrillation threshold. Because little was known about the experimental antifibrillatory effects of the beta-adrenergic agents, we designed a study to assess the importance of these effects in a previously validated canine model (21). The study (22) was designed to answer several specific questions:

1. What quantitative effects on experimental ventricular fibrillation threshold do beta-blockers cause, and what is the nature of the dose response curve?
2. Do these antifibrillatory effects depend quantitatively on ancillary pharmacologic properties, such as membrane stabilizing, cardioselective, partial agonist, or alpha-adrenergic blocking characteristics?
3. Can these effects be explained and simulated by interruption of cardiac sympathetic neuronal stimulation (22)?

Methods

The study used an open chest, anesthetized dog model. Bipolar electrodes were placed in the right atrium and right ventricular outflow tract, and sequential pacing was performed after ablation of the sinus node. Internal defibrillator leads were inserted into the left ventricular apex and right atrial appendage. The midportion of the left anterior descending coronary artery was dissected free and was used for studies of the effects of temporary coronary occlusion. A stainless steel bipolar hook electrode was attached epicardially at the right ventricular septum, bordering the potential ischemic zone, for delivery of the ventricular fibrillation (VF) pulses. A left ventricular plunge electrode was used for measuring refractory peiods. The train method of determining VF threshold (VFT) was applied (21-24). During atrial pacing at a cycle length of 400 msec, 4 msec fibrillation pulses of 60 Hz frequency and 180 msec total duration were synchronized so as to scan the T wave in the vulnerable period of the heart. Current intensity was increased in increments from 5 to 100 mA or until VF developed. Stimulus trains were delivered after every ninth cycle, and three trains were delivered at each current level. The current intensity inducing sustained VF was defined as the VF threshold. When VF occurred the heart was defibrillated immediately through the internal leads and allowed to recover for at least 15 minutes. Testing was performed at baseline, both before and after 3 minutes of coronary occlusion ("ischemic threshold"), and after administration of drug or saline solution in various doses. Five beta-adrenergic blocking agents with differing accessory properties were studied: timolol [nonselective agent with excellent clinical activity (17)], pindolol (partial agonist activity), propranolol (a nonselective agent with membrane stabilizing activity), metoprolol (cardio-selective), and labetalol (additional alpha-blocking activity).

Results

Control VF Thresholds

VF thresholds (VFT) averaged 11.7 $\pm$ 1.1 mA (mean $\pm$ SE) in 46 animals during control, nonischemic testing. With ischemia, VFT was reduced to 7.0 $\pm$ 1.0 mA ($p < 0.01$ vs. nonischemic). In animals subsequently given saline alone, a flat VFT response over time was observed.

VFT Response to Intravenous Beta-Blockade

In contrast to results with saline, marked increases in VF thresholds were observed after administration of each of the five beta-blockers. A summary of the optimal VFT responses is shown in Figure 1 for nonischemic conditions and in Figure 2 for acute ischemia. The doses at which optimal

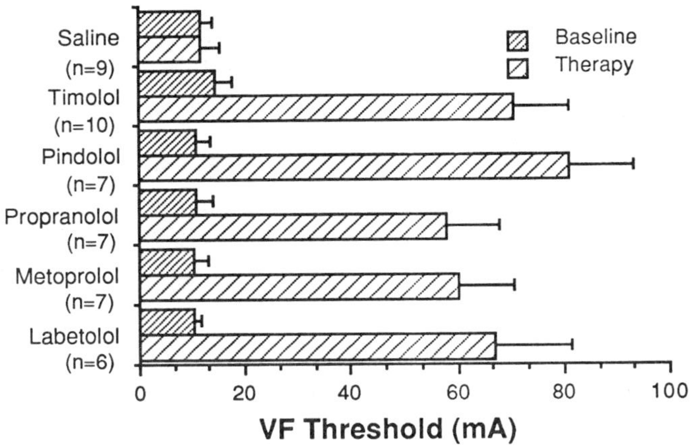

Figure 1 Optimal VFT (ventricular fibrillation threshold) responses to various IV beta-blockers in open-chest dog model under nonischemic conditions (mean ± SEM). (From Ref. 22.)

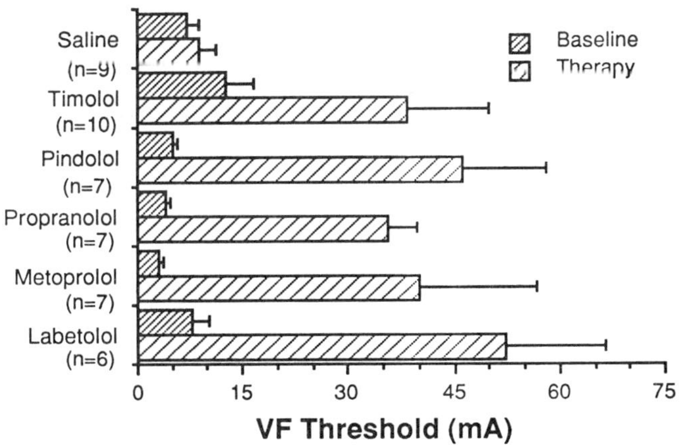

Figure 2 Optimal VFT responses to various IV beta-blockers in open-chest dog model under ischemic conditions (mean ± SEM). (From Ref. 22.)

elevations in VFT occurred are summarized in Table 1 together with reported relative beta-blocking potencies. No significant differences among agents in maximal effects on VFT were observed, although the doses at which optimal effects were achieved varied. On average, VFT was augmented to 67 ± 5 mA under nonischemic conditions and to 42 ± 5 mA during ischemia. The order of potency generally paralleled that of known beta-blocking potency, and maximal effects generally occurred at doses providing full beta-blockade. (One possible exception was that timolol appeared to cause maximal effects at lower apparent relative doses.)

Response of VFT to Stellate Ganglion Resection

In a small series of animals ($n = 3$), bilateral resection of the stellate ganglia led to variable increases in VFT, and subsequent administration of timolol caused further modest to substantial increases in VFT to levels provided by the beta-blocking drug alone.

Time-Decay in Augmentation of VFT

One hour after the final beta-blocking dose, augmented VF thresholds had declined by a mean of 14 mA for nonischemic and 11.4 mA for ischemic conditions; after 2 hours declines by means of 25 and 18 mA, respectively, had occurred.

Effects on Ventricular Refractory Periods

During incremental dosing with beta-blockers, gradual increases in refractory periods were observed, averaging 29 ± 3.3 msec under nonischemic

Table 1 Summary of Optimal Doses of Beta-Blocking Drugs

Drug	VFT (mg/kg)	Beta-blockade potency ratio
Timolol ($n = 10$)	0.01	6
Pindolol ($n = 7$)	0.1	6
Propranolol ($n = 7$)	0.3	1 (0.2 mg/kg)
Metoprolol ($n = 7$)	1.0	1
Labetolol ($n = 6$)	1.0	0.3

VFT = ventricular fibrillation threshold.
Source: Ref. 22 with permission.

and 20 ± 3.1 msec for ischemic conditions. (Baseline refractory periods were 194 ± 3.2 and 199 ± 3.3 msec, respectively.) Similar increases were induced by stellectomy, suggesting that these increases may represent antisympathetic effects.

Summary

This experimental study (22) documented a substantial antifibrillatory effect of intravenously titrated beta-adrenergic blocking agents with varying ancillary properties in an open chest, anesthetized dog model. In this model, using a pulse train for inducing VF, augmentation in VFT averaged sixfold both in the presence and absence of ischemia. Maximal effects generally paralleled known beta-blocking effects of these agents. Stellectomy alone led to increases in VFT (although variably less than full beta-blockade), suggesting the importance of this source of sympathetic stimulation in determining VFT (24).

Effects on VFT were also associated with changes in ventricular activation time (impulse conduction velocity) and ventricular refractoriness. How these and other mechanisms relate to the change in VFT is uncertain, but heterogeneity of conduction and refractoriness has been suggested to be more important than average refractory period duration (25). Perhaps beta-blockers act to "homogenize" heterogeneous sympathetic stimulation of the heart as it occurs during ischemia and neurogenic stress (26,27).

It should be noted that the stimulus-train technique requires higher current to induce VF in the absence of ischemia, but similar current strength during ischemia than the single stimulus scanning technique (27,28). In our model, drug augmentation in VFT was consistent and reproducible under both conditions, and stability in threshold in the absence of treatment was also observed. Bretylium, a drug with both early prosympathetic and later antisympathetic effects, also raises VFT in this model (21) and is known to have associated clinical antifibrillatory activity. Previous studies, using either the single stimulus technique of evaluating VFT (27) or coronary ligation (29), and testing by others of specific beta-blocking agents (27,29,30a,30b) provide additional background and support for our findings. As with other experimental studies, extrapolation from an anesthetized, open-chest canine model to the clinical situation must be made with great caution. However, the experimental association of cardiac arrhythmias with ischemia and imbalance of the autonomic nervous system (31) and these results do raise interesting hypotheses that may explain the observed clinical actions of these drugs (16,17).

COMPARATIVE EFFECTS ON VENTRICULAR FIBRILLATION THRESHOLD OF BETA-BLOCKADE AND OTHER ANTIISCHEMIC THERAPY (NITROGLYCERIN AND CALCIUM CHANNEL BLOCKADE)

Having established a marked effect of beta-blockade on VFT, we next asked whether this effect might be explained at least in part by an anti-ischemic mechanism. We studied the comparative antifibrillatory potential of representative drugs from each of the available antianginal classes: nitroglycerin (nitrate), diltiazem (calcium channel blocker), and timolol (beta-adrenoceptor blocker) in the same animal model (32). Our goal was to evaluate similarities and differences in experimental mechanisms and to formulate hypotheses for the testing and application of these classes of agents in clinical trials.

Methods

Testing for effects of drugs on VFT was performed as previously presented (22). VFT was determined in dogs assigned randomly to nitroglycerin and saline in the first set of experiments, and to diltiazem and saline in the second set of experiments. Ascending doses of each drug or saline were evaluated. In each case, determinations were made before and after the induction of acute coronary ischemia. The effect of additional beta-blockade was determined by administering timolol, 0.03 mg/kg. Nitroglycerin was infused (1) at rates sufficient to reduce main blood pressure by 15%; (2) at rates to reduce blood pressure by 30%; and (3) at the same rate as (2) but with additional phenylephrine to restore blood pressure to control levels. Diltiazem was infused at rates of 0.02, 0.04, and 0.08 mg/kg/min, each for 30 min.

Results

VFT averaged 11.8 ± 1.1 mA (n = 25) during control, nonischemic testing, and 9.4 ± 0.9 mA during ischemia. Only minor changes occurred over time with saline infusions both during nonischemic conditions (Fig. 3) and ischemia (Fig. 4). Nitroglycerin failed to increase VFT compared with the controls under either nonischemic (Fig. 3) or ischemic (Fig. 4). In contrast, diltiazem showed modest activity under each condition (Figs. 3,4). However, the addition of beta-blockade (timolol) led to a further substantial rise in VFT over the previous (diltiazem) treatment condition (Figs. 3,4).

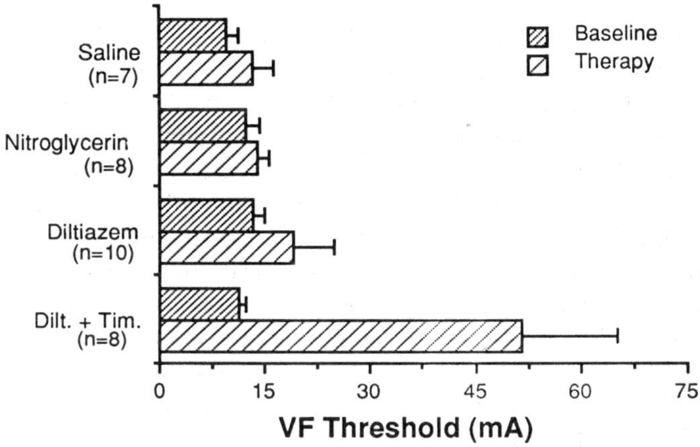

Figure 3 Comparative effects on VFT responses of various antiischemic classes in open-chest dog model under nonischemic conditions (mean ± SEM). (From Ref. 32.)

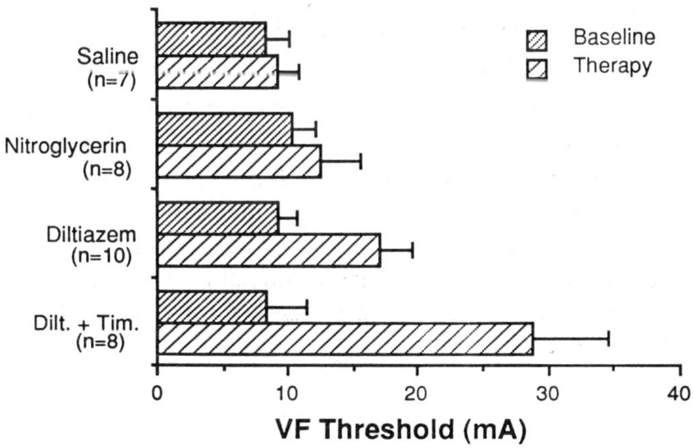

Figure 4 Comparative effects on VFT responses of various antiischemic classes in open-chest dog model under ischemic conditions (mean ± SEM). (From Ref. 32.)

Conclusion

The failure of nitroglycerin to augment VFT indicates that the effect observed is not simply a generic "anti-ischemic" effect. Calcium channel blockade showed activity in augmenting VFT which was more modest than beta-blockade. The mechanism of action of these agents was not determined, however. Antisympathetic activity or effects on intracellular calcium loading are potential mechanisms of the modest effects of diltiazem on VFT (33). Whatever the mechanisms involved, the effects of antianginal agents on experimental VFT appears to be in the order of beta-blockade (timolol) > calcium channel blockade (diltiazem) > nitroglycerin. A potential clinical correlate of this is that prophylactic therapy with beta-blockade but not calcium channel blockade has been shown to reduce the risk of mortality (including sudden death) in patients following myocardial infarction (34).

CORRELATION OF THE EFFECTS OF BETA-BLOCKADE ON EXPERIMENTAL VFT AND INDUCIBILITY OF SUSTAINED VENTRICULAR TACHYARRHYTHMIAS AFTER SUBACUTE MYOCARDIAL INFARCTION

One hypothesis to explain the protective effect of beta-blockers on ventricular fibrillation after myocardial infarction is that these drugs provide antiarrhythmic activity by means of effects on VFT and electrophysiologic inducibility of ventricular tachycardia (VT)/ventricular fibrillation in the postinfarction period. In order to test this, Gang et al. (35) used a subacute, postinfarction, closed-chest dog model of inducibile VT to examine and compare the effects of timolol and propranolol on inducible VT, and ventricular effective refractory period.

Methods

To simulate electrophysiologically guided clinical drug testing, each dog was tested on each beta-blocker on separate days and the sequence of drug administration was randomized. Experimental infarction was created by using a balloon catheter positioned in the left anterior descending coronary artery. The period of the balloon occlusion was 2 hours. Four to six days later, dogs were returned to the laboratory for retesting using a standard protocol for programmed electrical stimulation. An initial pilot study of timolol in seven dogs was followed by a randomized trial of timolol and propranolol in 15 dogs. Up to three extra stimuli (S1,S2, S3,S4) and burst ventricular pacing was used for arrhythmia induction. VF threshold was evaluated by single impulse testing (S2), delivered after a train of eight paced beats (cycle length 350 msec), and scanning diastole. Current setting of the S2 stimulus was set initially at 1 mA and then increased in increments for successive scans of diastole until VF was induced. The lowest current strength of S2 required to produce VF was defined as the VF threshold. In the pilot study, doses of timolol ranging from 0.1 to 3.0 mg/kg were administered intravenously over a 5-minute period. In the second study, doses of propranolol were 1.0, 3.0, and 10.0 mg/kg, and timolol 0.1, 0.3, and 1.0 mg/kg. Dosing was continued until VT or VF was no longer inducible or until the highest dose had been given. VF threshold was then measured.

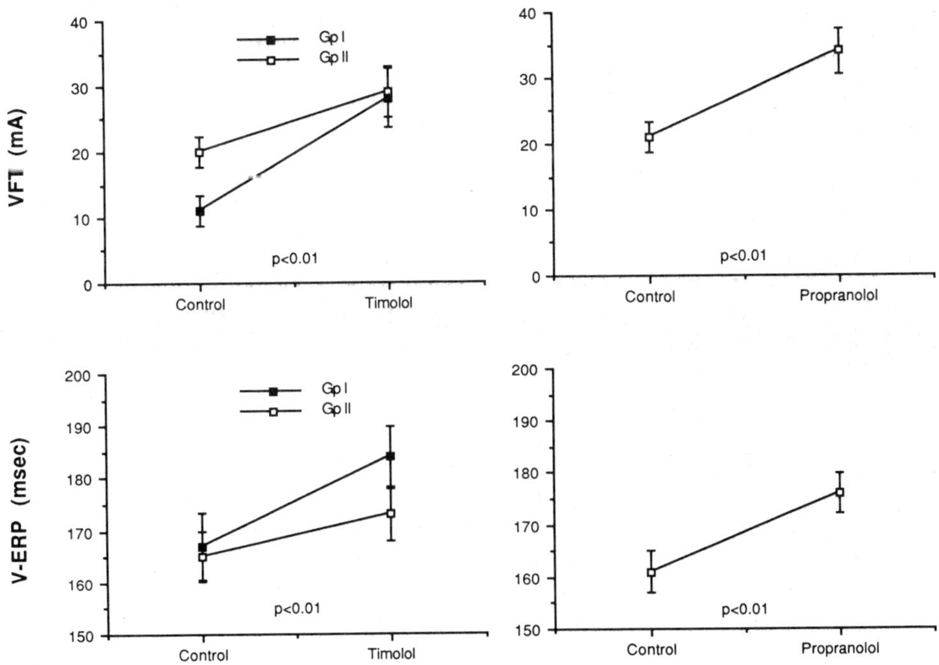

Figure 5 Effects of beta-blockade (timolol, propranolol) on experimental VFT and ventricular effective refractory period (V-ERP) in canine model of Gang et al. (mean ± SEM). (From Ref. 35.)

Results

At baseline the type of arrhythmia induced was ventricular tachycardia in four (cycle length > 200 msec) and ventricular flutter or fibrillation in 12. After both timolol and propranolol, parallel increases in VFT and ventricular effective refractory period were observed which were of similar magnitude (Fig. 5). In the pilot study of timolol, induction of sustained VT or VF was abolished in six of seven dogs. In the subsequent randomized study, one or both beta-blocking drugs prevented induction of VT/VF in 11 of 15 dogs (73%). Timolol was effective in 7 of 15 and in 2 of these was the only effective beta-blocker. Propranolol was effective in 9 of 15 and was the only effective drug in 4 dogs. Differences between drugs were not significant. When effective, the first dose of each drug was usually (70%) adequate to demonstrate a response. A correlation between changes in VFT and a response to programmed stimulation was observed. The increase in VFT was significantly greater in the 22 dogs responding to at least one beta-blocker than in the 13 nonresponders (15 ± 9 vs. 8 ± 9 mA, $p < 0.05$). No difference between the elevation of VFT was observed among responders between the two drugs (15 mA average increment for each).

These more recent studies of the effects of beta-blockade on VFT (22, 32,35) are consistent with the majority of earlier studies of VFT using these and other agents (27,29,30a,30b,36-40).

EFFECTS OF SYMPATHETIC GANGLION RESECTION IN PREVENTION OF VENTRICULAR FIBRILLATION CAUSED BY ACUTE MYOCARDIAL ISCHEMIA

Introduction

If beta-blockers affect the VFT primarily by interrupting sympathetic neuronal traffic to the heart, then interruption of such traffic would be expected to beneficially influence effects both on experimentally determined VFT and, perhaps, spontaneously occurring VFT in response to acute myocardial ischemia. The beneficial effects on ischemic VFT by resection of the stellate ganglia have previously been shown in our laboratory (22,24).

Effect of Stellectomy on VF in Canine Model of Schwartz and Stone

The ability of selective stellectomy to prevent VF caused by myocardial ischemia has also been shown in a conscious dog model with anterior myocardial infarction by Schwartz and Stone (41). In this study, 32 dogs had anterior myocardial infarction produced by ligation of the left anterior descending coronary artery. One week later, they were randomly allocated to a control group or an experimental group that underwent left stellectomy. One month later, acute ischemia was induced in these dogs (while conscious) by inflation of a balloon occluder previously positioned around the circumflex coronary artery for 10 minutes. Ventricular fibrillation occurred in 11 (65%) of 17 control dogs, but only five (33%) of 15 dogs who had undergone left stellectomy ($p < 0.05$). Parallel reductions in overall mortality were also observed, from 12 (71%) among controls to 6 (40%) among the sympathectomy group ($p < 0.05$). Further, the incidence of arrhythmias was less in survivors in the treated group compared to the control group.

Summary and Conclusion

Schwartz and Stone (41) concluded that interruption of the major neuonal route of sympathetic stimulation to the left ventricle via the left stellate ganglion exerted a major protective effect against the occurrence of VF when conscious dogs with previous myocardial injury (old anterior myocardial infarction) underwent acute myocardial ischemia in a distant zone of vascular supply.

Experimental results must be interpreted cautiously when applied to the clinical setting, but this study involved a more direct measure of the propensity toward VF in the setting of acute ischemia than determinations of the effects on VF threshold alone. Results of the study were consistent with the hypothesis that blockade of sympathetic nervous traffic to the heart during ischemia increases the threshold both for experimental induction of VF as well as spontaneous occurrence of VF.

THE EFFECT OF BETA-BLOCKERS AND OTHER ANTIARRHYTHMIC DRUGS ON VF AND OTHER LIFE-THREATENING ARRHYTHMIAS INDUCED BY ACUTE MYOCARDIAL ISCHEMIA AND SYMPATHETIC HYPERACTIVITY

Introduction

Testing of beta-blockers and other antiarrhythmic medications in a more physiologic, clinically relevant model of ischemic ventricular fibrillation was evaluated by Schwartz et al. in a feline model (42). Their model was developed based on evidence strongly supporting the concept that elevated sympathetic activity and transient myocardial ischemia may act in concert as a precipitant mechanism of many clinical episodes of VF. Acute myocardial ischemia activates afferent cardiac sympathetic fibers and elicits a reflex excitatory cardiac sympathetic response that is channeled preferentially through left-sided sympathetic nerves. Because anesthesia reduces pain and fear associated with ischemia and interferes with reflex autonomic responses, models using anesthetized animals may also underestimate the role of sympathetic hyperactivity in triggering VF and related arrhythmias. The model of Schwartz et al. (42) was designed to solve these problems and allow more physiologically relevant testing of antiarrhythmic agents.

Methods

Open chest anesthetized cats were prepared by right stellectomy, to decrease cardiac electrical stability, and isolation of the proximal left anterior descending coronary artery to allow transient occlusion. The left stellate ganglion was isolated and prepared for electrical stimulation.

During each experimental trial, a 2-3 minute coronary occlusion was performed. The left stellate ganglion was electrically stimulated for 30 seconds at the beginning of the last minute of occlusion. Animals with reproducible arrhythmias were used for subsequent drug trials ($n = 93/148$). Drugs tested included: lidocaine 2 mg/kg, mexiletine 3.6 mg/kg, propafenone 2 mg/kg, prazosin 0.1 mg/kg, propranolol 0.2 mg/kg, amiodarone 1.5-3.0 mg/kg, and verapamil 0.2 mg/kg.

A quantitative analysis was performed on ventricular arrthythmias occurring during and until 60 minutes after coronary occlusion and graded as: 0 = no premature ventricular complexes (PVC's); 1 = 1-10 PVCs; 2 = 11-50 PVCs; 3 = VT (≥ 5 PVCs in a row); 4 = VF.

Results

Effects of representative antiarrhythmic drugs from classes I-B (lidocaine, mexiletine), I-C (propafenone), II (propranolol), III (amiodarone), and IV (verapamil), as well as the alpha-adrenergic blocker prazosin, are presented in Figure 6. Highly significant reductions in arrhythmias were noted after propranolol, but not after the Class I antiarrhythmic agents. Reductions were also caused by amiodarone and verapamil as well as prazosin.

Specifically for VF, combined experience with the three Class I agents showed that a total of 12 animals (34%) had VF at the baseline control study, and, similarly, 12 of 35 (34%) animals experienced VF after therapy. In contrast, propranolol was associated with marked reductions in the

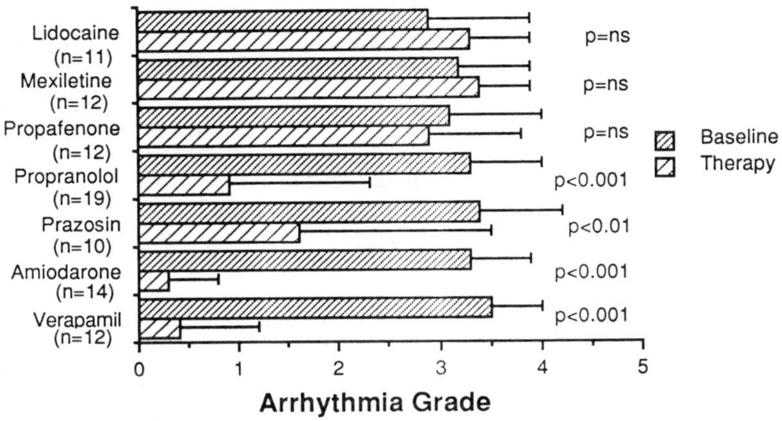

Figure 6 Effects of beta-blocker and other antiarrhythmic drugs on ventricular arrhythmias induced by acute myocardial ischemia and sympathetic hyperactivity in a feline model (mean ± SEM). (From Ref. 42.)

number of animals experiencing VF, from 8 of 19 (42%) to one (5%). Similarly, amiodarone and verapamil prevented VF, and prazosin reduced the incidence of VF from 6/10 to 3/10.

Conclusions

The failure of Class I antiarrhythmic agents in this model may appear surprising, given their widespread clinical use to treat life-threatening arrhythmias. However, results of previous clinical trials (15) and the recent CAST study (14) emphasize the failure of these agents to prevent sudden death and mortality in the setting of ischemic heart disease. In view of these trials, the results of this model are consistent. Blockade of sympathetic alpha- and beta-adrenergic receptors afforded protection in about 60% and 80% of animals, respectively. Of these two, beta-blockade (propranolol) appeared to provide more effective prevention.

These results are consistent with both experimental effects on VFT, previously reviewed (22,35), as well as clinical trials of beta-blockers (16). Amiodarone, a drug with Class III activity, is also a noncompetitive antagonist of both alpha- and beta-adrenergic stimulation as well as a coronary vasodilator. Its clinical use, however, is limited by its organ toxic potential (20). Verapamil has multiple effects, which may be of potential benefit in acute ischemia, including a noncompetitive antiadrenergic effect and a salutary action on coronary flow. Calcium channel blockers, as noted, may also increase the threshold for experimental VF (32,33), and clinically, in patients with preserved (but not reduced) left ventricular function, reduce mortality (43).

ANTIFIBRILLATORY ACTIVITY OF BETA-ADRENERGIC BLOCKADE IN A CONSCIOUS CANINE MODEL OF SUDDEN CORONARY DEATH

Introduction

A further step in the development of relevant pathophysiologic models of clinical sudden coronary death has been taken by Patterson et al. (44). This model superimposes acute ischemia on top of previous distant ischemic injury in a conscious dog model with intact sympathetic innervation and reflex response. This model has allowed important testing of pharmacologic agents potentially useful in sudden death prevention, including the beta-adrenergic blocking agents.

Methods

In anesthetized mongrel dogs, a left thoracotomy was performed and occlusion of the left descending coronary artery made after a critical stenosis was produced to limit the hyperemic response. After 90 minutes of occlusion, flow was restored through the stenosed artery. The left circumflex coronary artery was next isolated near its origin and a 30-gauge insulated silver wire inserted into the lumen. The wire was then secured to the surface of the heart and directed to the body surface. Plunge electrodes were also placed in the interventricular septum and right ventricular outflow tract and electrical leads tracked from these wires to the body surface. On the third day after myocardial infarction, animals were randomly allocated to treatment groups including saline and three doses of nadolol (45). Low-dose d,l-nadolol was given as 1 mg/kg every 12 hours, high dose as 8 mg/kg every 8 hours, and the non-beta-adrenergic receptor blocking isomer, d-nadolol (as a further control), 1 mg/kg every 12 hours. After 24 hours of treatment (two doses), programmed electrical stimulation was performed with the animal conscious and resting comfortably in a sling. After administration of the third treatment dose, a thrombus-generating anodal current of 150 microamps was applied to the intimal surface of the left circumflex coronary artery. Twelve hours later the fourth treatment dose was given and the electrical current discontinued. Continuous electrocardiographic monitoring of the conscious ambulatory dog was transmitted via telemetry and recorded on magnetic tape for 6-8 hours, followed by intermittent sampling until the end of 24 hours.

Results

The occurrence of death from VF in animals treated with saline and the three regimens of nadolol is presented in Figure 7. In saline-treated animals, anodal current stimulation was followed by coronary thrombosis (confirmed postmortem), ST segment changes, sinus tachycardia and QT segment prolongation, appearance of ventricular premature beats, and finally, ventricular fibrillation, in 14 (93%) of 15 animals. Pretreatment with d-nadolol, the non-beta-adrenergic blocking isomer, failed to prevent these changes, and VF developed in all eight animals (100%). However, both low- and high-dose d,l-nadolol, while having no effect on coronary artery thrombosis or ischemic ST segment changes, decreased the incidence of VF and increased survival at 24 hours to 56% (5 or 9) in the low-dose and 63% (8 of 13) in the high-dose groups. The survival rate was significantly greater than that observed with saline treatment (7%) for both groups ($p < 0.01$). Further, The major mode of death in nadolol-treated animals was not VF but complete heart block.

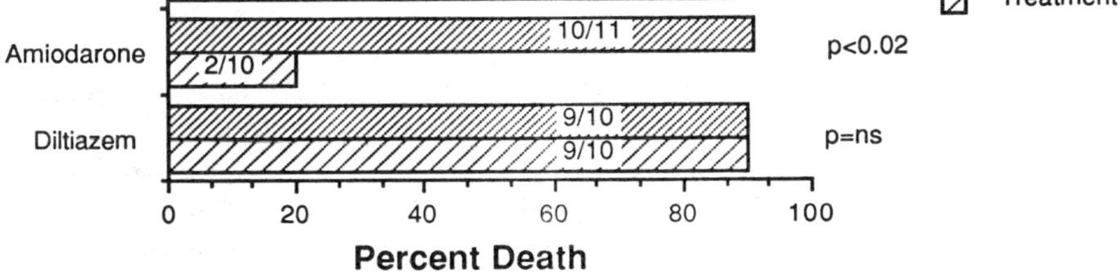

Figure 7 Effects of beta-blockers and other antiarrhythmic drugs on ischemic ventricular fibrillation in a conscious canine model of sudden cardiac death. (From Refs. 44-51.)

Conclusion

Thus, this study in a conscious sudden death model of VF suggests that nadolol, a noncardioselective beta-adrenoceptor blocker without membrane effects, is effective in reducing the incidence of VF due to sudden coronary occlusion in the setting of previous infarction. Although extrapolation of experimental results to the clinical setting should be done cautiously, the many similarities between this model and the clinical mechanisms of VF suggest the hypothesis that results in this model may predict clinical activity of pharmacologic agents.

ANTIFIBRILLATORY EFFECTS OF OTHER ANTI-ARRHYTHMIC AGENTS IN A CONSCIOUS CANINE MODEL OF SUDDEN DEATH DUE TO VF

Summary of Studies

Lucchesi and colleagues have evaluated several other agents potentially effective in reducing ischemic VF in the conscious canine model. These studies have included evaluations of Class I antiarrhythmic therapy (flecainide) (46), Class III antiarrhythmic therapy (bretylium, amiodarone, d-sotalol) (47-49), combined Class II and III therapy (d-l-sotalol) (50), and Class IV therapy (diltiazem) (51). Results for these studies are presented in Figure 7. In this model, Class I antiarrhythmic therapy (flecainide) was ineffective, and Class III therapy with bretylium, a sympathetic ganglionic blocking agent, and amiodarone, which possesses noncompetitive sympathetic blocking activity, were effective. Similarly, both d-sotalol and d,l-sotalol reduced ischemic VF. Calcium channel blockade (diltiazem) delayed, but did not prevent, eventual mortality.

SUMMARY

The series of studies reviewed above demonstrates the effective antifibrillatory potential of beta-adrenergic blocking drugs tested alone and in comparison with other agents, in experimental models of increasing degrees of sophistication, from direct measurements of electrical VF threshold in anesthetized animals to activity against spontaneous VF in conscious animals with acute ischemia occurring in the setting of distant myocardial injury. In each of these models, beta-adrenergic blockade, pharmacologically and, in some cases, via stellectomy, resulted in an increase in the threshold for VF and a reduction in the spontaneous occurrence of VT/VF.

In contrast, Class I antiarrhythmic agents were not shown to be of significant benefit in these models. Other agents sharing antiadrenergic effects, including amiodarone, bretylium, and calcium channel blockers, were also effective in some of these models, although the mechanisms for their action may be more complex and include actions other than sympathetic blockade alone.

CONCLUSIONS

Given the safety and widespread clinical experience with, and understanding of the mechanisms of beta blockade, these drugs would appear to be prototypes for testing of antifibrillatory effects in experimental models and preferential agents for clinical trials.

Although known to exert cardioprotective effects following myocardial infarction (16), beta-blockers are currently less utilized than in the past (14). The discrepancy between antiectopic effects of Class I agents and clinical as well as experimental occurrence of ventricular fibrillation (14, 15,46), as opposed to the close, consistent correlation between VF threshold, inducibility of ventricular arrhythmias and infarct size (52), and effects of pharmacologic intervention (16,22,42,45,) suggest that VF threshold effects may be a better predictor of clinical outcome and a better basis for future pharmacologic and other interventional trials aimed at reducing the incidence of sudden coronary death than traditional measures of antiectopic activity.

REFERENCES

1. Lown B. Sudden cardiac death: the major challenge confronting contemporary cardiology. Am J Cardiol 1979; 43:313-28.
2. Kempf FC, Josephson ME. Cardiac arrest recorded on ambulatory electrocardiograms. Am J Cardiol 1984; 53:1577-82.
3. Panidis IP, Morganroth J. Sudden death in hospitalized patients: cardiac rhythm disturbances detected by ambulatory electrocardiographic monitoring. J Am Coll Cardiol 1983; 2:798-805.
4. Pratt CM, Francis MJ, Luck JC, Wyndham CR, Miller RR, Quinones MA. Analysis of ambulatory electrocardiograms in 15 patients during spontaneous ventricular fibrillation with special reference to preceding arrhythmic events. J Am Coll Cardiol 1983; 2:789-97.
5. Ruberman W, Weinblatt AB, Goldberg JD, Frank CW, Shapiro S. Ventricular premature beats and mortality after myocardial infarction. N Engl J Med 1977; 297:750-7.

6. Moss AJ, Davis HT, DeCamilla J, Bayer LW. Ventricular ectopic beats and their relation to sudden and non-sudden cardiac death after myocardial infarction. Circulation 1979; 60:998-1003.
7. Bigger JT, Jr., Fleiss JL, Kleiger R, Miller JP, Rolnitzky LM, and the Multicenter Post-Infarction Group. The relationship between ventricular arrhythmias, left ventricular dysfunction, and mortality in the 2 years after myocardial infarction. Circulation 1984; 69:250-8.
8. Mukharji J, Rude RE, Poole WK, Gustafson N, Thomas LH, Jr., Strauss HW, Jaffe AS, Muller JE, Roberts R, Raabe DS, Jr., Croft CH, Passamani E, Braunwald E, Willerson JT and the MILIS Study Group. Risk factors for sudden death following acute myocardial infarction: two-year follow-up. Am J Cardiol 1984; 54:31-6.
9. Kostis JB, Byington R, Friedman LM, Goldstein S, Furberg C. Prognostic significance of ventricular ectopic activity in survivors of acute myocardial infarction. J Am Coll Cardiol 1987; 10:231-42.
10. Bigger JT, Jr. Identification of patients at high risk for sudden cardiac death. Am J Cardiol 1984; 54:3D-8D.
11. Bigger JT, Jr. Definition of benign versus malignant ventricular arrhythmias: targets for treatment. Am J Cardiol 1983; 52:47C-54C.
12. The Cardiac Arrhythmia Pilot Study (CAPS) Investigators. Effects of encainide, flecainide, imipramine and moricizine on ventricular arrhythmic during the first year after myocardial infarction: the CAPS. Am J Cardiol 1988; 61:501-9.
13. Woosley RW. Indications for antiarrhythmic therapy: a wealth of controversy, a dearth of data. Ann Intern Med 1988; 108:450-2.
14. The Cardiac Arrhythmia Suppression Trial (CAST) Investigators. Preliminary report: effect of encainide or flecainide on mortality in a randomized trial of arrhythmia suppression after myocardial infarction. N Engl J Med 1989; 321:406-12.
15. Furberg CD. Effect of antiarrhythmic drugs on mortality after myocardial infarction. Am J Cardiol 1983; 52:32C-36C.
16. Yusuf S, Peto R, Lewis J, Collins R, Sleight P. Beta-blockade during and after myocardial infarction: an overview of the randomized trials. Prog Cardiovasc Dis 1985; 27:336-67.
17. The Norwegian Multicenter Study Group. Timolol-induced reduction in mortality and reinfarction in patients surviving acute myocardial infarction. N Engl J Med 1981; 304:801-7.
18. Anderson JL. Antifibrillatory versus antiectopic therapy. Am J Cardiol 1984; 54:7A-13A.
19. Rosenthal ME, Oseran DS, Gang E, Peter T. Sudden cardiac death following acute myocardial infarction. Am Heart J 1985; 109:865-75.
20. Anderson JL. Current clinical perspectives on antiarrhythmic drug therapy. Federation Proc 1986; 45:2213-19.

21. Anderson JL, Patterson E, Conlon M, Pasyk S, Pitt B, Lucchesi BR. Kinetics of antifibrillatory effects of bretylium: correlation with myocardial drug concentrations. Am J Cardiol 1980; 46:583-92.
22. Anderson JL, Rodier HE, Green LS. Comparative effects of beta-adrenergic blocking drugs on experimental ventricular fibrillation threshold. Am J Cardiol 1983; 51:1196-202.
23. Kniffen FJ, Lomas TE, Counsell RE, Lucchesi BR. The antiarrhythmic and antifibrillatory action of bretylium and its o-iodobenzyl trimethylammonium analog, UM-360. J Pharmacol Exp Ther 1975; 192:120-8.
24. Kliks BR, Burgess MJ, Abildskov JA. Influence of sympathetic tone on ventricular fibrillation threshold during experimental coronary occlusion. Am J Cardiol 1975; 36:45-9.
25. Cardinal K, Sasyniuk B. Electrophysiologic effects of bretylium tosylate on subendocardial Purkinje fibers in infarcted canine hearts. J Pharmacol Exp Ther 1977; 204:159-74.
26. Kralios FA, Martin L, Burgess MJ, Millar K. Local ventricular repolarization changes due to sympathetic nerve-branch stimulation. Am J Physiol 1975; 228:1621-6.
27. Bacaner MB. Quantitative comparison of drugs used in the treatment of ventricular arrhythmias. Am J Cardiol 1968; 21:504-12.
28. Axelrod PJ, Verrier RL, Lown B. Vulnerability to ventricular fibrillation during acute coronary arterial occlusion and release. Am J Cardiol 1975; 36: 776-82.
29. Kauman AJ, Aramendia P. Prevention of ventricular fibrillation induced by coronary ligation. J Pharmacol Exp Ther 1968; 164:326-32.
30a. Khan MI, Hamilton JT, Manning GW. Protective effect of beta-adrenoceptor blockade in experimental coronary artery occlusion in conscious dogs. Am J Cardiol 1972; 30:832-7.
30b. Patterson E, Lucchesi BR. Antifibrillatory properties of the beta-adrenergic receptor antagonists, nadolol, sotalol, atenolol, and propranolol, in the anesthetized dog. Pharmacol 1984; 28:121-9.
31. Randall WC, Thomas JX, Euler DE, Rozanski GJ. Cardiac dysrhythmias associated with autonomic nervous system imbalance in the conscious dog. In: Schwartz PJ, Brown AM, Malliani A, Zanchetti A, eds. Neural mechanisms in cardiac arrhythmias. New York: Raven Press, 1978:123-38.
32. Anastasiou-Nana M, Nanas J, Menlove RL, Anderson JL. Experimental antifibrillatory effects of calcium channel blockade with diltiazem: comparison with beta-blockade and nitroglycerin. J Cardiovasc Pharmacol 1984; 6:780-7.
33. Clusin WT, Buchbiner M, Harrison DC. Calcium overload, "injury" current, and early ischemic cardiac arrhythmias—a direct connection. Lancet 1983; 1:272-3.
34. Yusuf S, Wittes J, Friedman L. Overview of results of randomized clinical trials in heart disease: 1. Treatments following myocardial infarction. JAMA 1988; 260:2088-93.

35. Gang ES, Bigger JT, Uhl EW. Effects of timolol and propranolol on inducible sustained ventricular tachyarrhythmias in dogs with subacute myocardial infarction. Am J Cardiol 1984; 53:275-81.
36. Rosati RA, Alexander JA, Wallace AG, Sealy WC, Young WC. Failure of beta-adrenergic blockade to alter ventricular fibrillation threshold in the dog. Circ Res 1966; 19:721-5.
37. Spear JR, Moore EN, Riccintti M. The effect of d- and l-optical isomers of propranolol on the ventricular fibrillation threshold. Eur J Cardiol 1978; 7: 117-23.
38. Wellens D, Wauters E. Modification of ventricular fibrillation threshold after sympatholytic drugs in the dog. Arch Int Pharmacodyn 1972; 198:355-71.
39. Jaillon P, Schnittger I, Griffin JC, Winkle RA. The relationship between the repetitive extrasystole threshold and the ventricular fibrillation threshold in the dog. Circ Res 1980; 46:599-605.
40. Hodess AB, Spear JF, Moore EN. Effects of timolol on the ventricular fibrillation threshold (abstr). Clin Res 1979; 27:175A.
41. Schwartz PJ, Stone HL. Left stellectomy in the prevention of ventricular fibrillation caused by acute myocardial infarction. Circulation 1980; 62:1256-65.
42. Schwartz PJ, Vanoli E, Zaza A, Zuanetti G. The effect of antiarrhythmic drugs on life-threatening arrhythmias induced by the interaction between acute myocardial ischemia and sympathetic hyperactivity. Am Heart J 1985; 109:937-48.
43. The Multicenter Diltiazem Post Infarction Trial Research Group. The effect of diltiazem on mortality and reinfarction after myocardial infarction. N Engl J Med 1988; 319:385-92.
44. Patterson E, Holland K, Eller BT, Lucchesi BR. Ventricular fibrillation resulting from ischemia at a site remote from previous myocardial infarction. A conscious canine model of sudden coronary death. Am J Cardiol 1982; 50:1414-23.
45. Patterson E, Lucchesi BR. Antifibrillatory action of d,1 nadolol in a conscious canine model of sudden coronary death. J Cardiovasc Pharm 1983; 5:737-44.
46. Kou WH, Nelson SD, Lynch JJ, Montgomery DG, DiCarlo L, Lucchesi BR. Effect of flecainide acetate on prevention of electrical induction of ventricular tachycardia and occurrence of ischemic ventricular fibrillation during the early postmyocardial infarction period: evaluation in a conscious canine model of sudden death. J Am Coll Cardiol 1987; 9:359-65.
47. Holland K, Patterson E, Lucchesi BR. Prevention of ventricular fibrillation by bretylium in a conscious canine model of sudden coronary death. Am Heart J 1983; 105:711-16.
48. Patterson E, Eller B, Abrams G, Vasiliades J, Lucchesi B. Ventricular fibrillation in a conscious canine model of sudden coronary death: prevention by acute and chronic amiodarone administration. Circulation 1983; 68:857-64.

49. Lynch JJ, Coskey LA, Montgomery DG, Lucchesi BR. Prevention of ventricular fibrillation by dextrorotatory sotalol in a conscious canine model of sudden coronary death. Am Heart J 1985; 109:949-58.
50. Lynch JJ, Wilbur DJ, Montgomery DG, Hsieh TM, Patterson E, Lucchesi BR. Antiarrhythmic and antifibrillatory actions of the levo and dextro rotatory isomers of sotalol. J Cardiovasc Pharmacol 1984; 6:1132-41.
51. Patterson E, Eller BT, Lucchesi BR. Effects of diltiazem upon experimental ventricular dysrhythmias. J Pharmacol Exp Ther 1983; 225:224-32.
52. Gang ES, Bigger JT, Jr., Livelli FD, Jr. A model of chronic ischemic arrhythmias: the relation between electrically inducible ventricular tachycardia, ventricular fibrillation threshold and myocardial infarct size. Am J Cardiol 1982; 50:469-77.

3

Rationale for Antiarrhythmic Actions of Beta-Blockers

Philippe Coumel
Hôpital Lariboisière, Paris, France

INTRODUCTION

Beta-blockers form the second of the Vaughan-Williams's four classes of antiarrhythmic drugs (1). Numerous trials have in recent years demonstrated their beneficial effects in the prevention of sudden death (2,3). At the same time an increasing amount of experimental and clinical information was obtained about the nature and the mechanisms of cardiac arrhythmias in general, and during sudden death in particular. Thus, formulating the rationale for antiarrhythmic actions of beta-blockers should not be in principle a difficult task. In fact, this is not so easy if one takes into account several other considerations. For instance, it must be recalled that the rationale for beta-blocker use in therapeutic trials was principally their antiischemic rather than antiarrhythmic properties, and their cardiac "protective effect" is still mainly interpreted in these terms in the literature. There is a striking contrast between the ever-greater clinical use of beta-blockers as antiarrhythmics and the fact that practically none of them is officially accepted and marketed as such. Finally, the contrast is not less striking between the efficacy of type I antiarrhythmics in trivial arrhythmias and their absence of action (4,5), recently documented as indeed a deleterious effect (6) on cardiac death. In this chapter, we shall try to unearth the reasons for such apparent contradictions or paradoxical situations.

Clinical-Pharmacological Characteristics of Beta-Blockers

Pharmacological Characteristics

There are now some 20 beta-blockers available clinically, at least in countries the regulations of which do not dramatically limit the therapeutic armamentorium. Propranolol has been the reference drug since the 1960s. Pindolol, oxprenolol, acebutolol, alprenolol, sotalol, atenolol, and timolol were developed in the 1970s. Since 1980 labetalol, metoprolol, butofilolol, nadolol, betaxolol, pentobutolol, and more recently tertatolol, cycloprolol, and celiprolol have been marketed. All these drugs can be individualized in pharmacological terms.

Cardioselectivity was originally important in terms of tolerance (bronchospasm). Now that the presence of $beta_1$ rather than $beta_2$ receptors in the heart is viewed as a matter of predominance instead of exclusivity (7), this aspect may have some importance in other domains. The presence of $beta_2$ receptors in the heart is marked in the sinus node region: The sinus rate is the easiest variable to study for evaluation of beta-blockade, but we do not have information on the proportion of $beta_1$ and $beta_2$ receptors in potential arrhythmogenic areas, so that arrhythmias and heart rate may not respond in the same way to drugs. Biases can be generated when comparing more or less cardioselective agents (acebutolol, atenolol, betaxolol, metoprolol, practolol) to others through the sinus rhythm. The problem becomes even more complicated if one considers the partial agonist activity of acebutolol, pentobutolol, alprenolol, oxprenolol, pindolol, and xamoterol (in an increasing order of intrinsic adrenergic effect) and the different action on $beta_1$ and $beta_2$ receptors of the recently introduced cycloprolol, celiprolol, or dilevalol, not to speak of the possible alpha-adrenoceptor blocking activity of labetalol.

Clinical Implications

The impact of such characteristics is not simply a matter of pharmacological classification. It is not correct to amalgamate the antiischemic and the antiarrhythmic effects of drugs, and to restrict their particularities to problems of tolerance in heart failure (in which context their possible efficacy will also have to be discussed). The possible direct antiarrhythmic effects have been overemphasized for some drugs like propranolol, and it is now clear that the concentrations required for membrane activity to become prominent are outside the range used in clinical practice. On the other hand, a marked and uniform prolongation of the action potential at any given heart rate has been pointed out by Vaughan-Williams (1) as well as results from the permanent interference with the normal sympathetic control of the heart. It thus constitutes a Class III effect that is permanently ignored, with the exception of sotalol (8), the beta-blocking potency of which can be, in turn, overevaluated if judged from the degree of bradycardia it induces. Otherwise, there is more and more evidence that the type III effect and amiodazone-like effect are by no means synonymous as far as their antiarrhythmic effects are concerned.

Such considerations should prepare the clinician to observe differences in the results obtained with this or that beta-blocker. It is indeed our experience that an arrhythmia may be qualified as resistant to beta-blockers, and not actually resistant to a more powerful agent like nadolol (9,10) or to a drug with different properties like sotalol. It is even more important to realize that the intensity of the observed effect depends to a large extent on the patient's status. Pindolol or xamoterol may actually increase or decrease the 24-hour mean heart rate when used in normal subjects or in patients with heart failure, respectively. Action of beta agonists or antagonists essentially depends on the level of the patient's adrenergic tone. More commonly, we recently saw that acebutolol at the same dosage decreased the heart rate of 15 subjects by an average of 10%, whereas in 13 patients with a left ventricular hypertrophy and in 13 patients with heart failure a 20% decrease was observed (11).

How to Approach the Rationale for Beta-Blocking Therapy

The rationale for using beta-blockers in arrhythmias can be considered in two ways, which we can label as "direct" and "indirect." The direct approach simply consists of collecting the experimental data that demonstrate the arrhythmogenic effects of catecholamines, so that the use of beta-blockers appears logical. The clinical evaluation is then carried out according to the standards established for type I antiarrhythmic drugs, and thus essentially based on the quantification of trivial arrhythmias. This straightforward approach has in fact many practical biases and drawbacks that explain in large part why beta-blockers are underevaluated as major antiarrhythmic agents. The indirect approach consists of starting from the demonstrated favorable effect of beta-blockers in sudden death prevention and examining the extent to which this is due to the antiarrhythmic effect of these drugs in particular circumstances not adequately explored in routinely observed arrhythmias.

THE DIRECT APPROACH

Electrophysiological Properties of Beta-Blockers

Electrophysiological properties of beta-blockers have been extensively studied experimentally and in humans, and it is not our aim to review them in detail (12). Beta-blockers reduce sinus node automaticity, prolong the sinoatrial, intraatrial, and atrioventricular conduction times, and increase refractoriness of the atrioventricular node. His-Purkinje system automaticity, refractoriness, and conduction are depressed to a variable extent, and the same applies to atrial and ventricular myocardial tissues. Blocking the agonistic effect of circulating or neurally released catecholamines is the mode of action on the cardiac cells common to all these drugs. Though obvious in principle, this fundamentally indirect mode of action must always be kept in mind. It implies that the magnitude of the changes directly depends on the existing vago-sympathetic balance and can never be accurately predicted.

The Role of Adrenergic Stimulation in Arrhythmias

The real question is not whether or not adrenergic stimulation is involved in this or that arrhythmia, but to what extent: Its presence can always be detected, but its role may be more or less easy to detect. Experimentally, it is well established that catecholamines make more active any electrophysiological mechanism, and often simply conditions its presence or its absence. This goes for normal and abnormal automaticity, triggered activity related to early or delayed afterdepolarizations, and also reentry if one considers that an adequate balance between various factors (conduction speed, unidirectional block, and refractory period duration) is essential.

Cellular Electrophysiological Mechanism

Referring particularly to coronary artery disease, all types of electrophysiological mechanisms possibly involved in arrhyhmias are exacerbated by adrenergic stimulation. Among many studies, this was shown by Kimura (13): Purkinje fibers overlying healed infarct scars have altered physiology of spontaneous automaticity, enhanced responses to alpha-adrenergic interventions, and a tendency to triggered activity. Both alpha- and beta-adrenergic effects may result in worsening of arrhythmias by augmentation of afterpotentials in healed myocardial infarction. Vincent (14) otherwise shows that activation of $beta_2$-adrenoceptors causes a dose-dependent decrease in plasma potassium, probably by shifting potassium into the cell, a phenomenon that can be rapid, observed during exercise (15). By this mechanism (16) epinephrine may cause hypokaliemia and predispose to arrhythmias. Thus, preventing the sympathetically induced ionic changes and their arrhythmogenic effects may be another modality of the cardioprotective action of beta-blockers.

Arrhythmia Components and their Evaluation

In the experimental models of ischemia (17,18), adrenergic stimulation is always essential for obtaining arrhythmias, and particularly the most severe ones like ventricular fibrillation. Usually, however, the adrenergic stimulation intervenes in the setting of an acute ischemia, whereas its role is less evident in models of chronically infarcted animals in which the ventricular tachyarrhythmias are induced by programmed stimulation. Even in such a case where in theory the role of the arrhythmogenic substrate is largely predominant, the two other components of the arrhythmia triangle (19) cannot be ignored (Fig. 1). A triggering factor, usually a

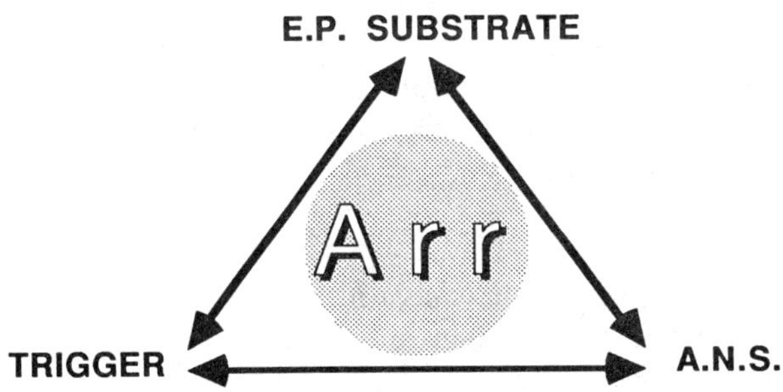

Figure 1 The "arrhythmia" triangle. Three components are necessary for an arrhythmia to appear. The electrophysiological substrate is usually responsible for the repetitive activity of the clinical tachyarrhythmia. It is not permanently active, and a trigger is necessary to induce it. Not just any extrasystole can fire any potential substrate, and the combination of the two is modulated by the autonomic nervous system (ANS).

premature beat, is necessary in the natural conditions. We know from programmed stimulation studies that its characteristics of prematurity and area of origin are essential to initiate the substrate and can depend on the degree of adrenergic stimulation. The substrate also depends on the adrenergic drive and can be more or less easily activated with a more or less sustained repetitive response. All these aspects are easy to verify in vitro where the adrenergic stimulation is under control. In the clinical situation, however, it may be more difficult. Isoprenaline infusion does reproduce a humoral adrenergic stimulation, but neurally mediated sympathetic actions have inhomogeneous effects in the myocardial tissues, which can be much more arrhythmogenic and are difficult to mimic in experimental models.

The best tool to evaluate the relationships between the autonomic nervous system and arrhythmias is certainly ambulatory monitoring, on the condition to pay attention to the behavior of arrhythmias as a function of their environment. For instance, the absence or the presence, and the duration of the repetitive response following a ventricular premature beat is strongly correlated with the mean heart rate in the minutes that precede the events (20). As the sinus rate itself reflects the balance of the vagosympathetic influences, the relationship with arrhythmias is then in principle easy to establish. Nagasawa's anecdotal case report (21) of a rebound effect induced by clonidine withdrawal, with the development of a ventricular tachycardia is through a pharmacological approach quite illustrative of the sympathetic influence on the repetitive activity of arrhythmogenic substrates. A syndrome of excessive efferent sympathetic activity is well-known in this setting that includes elevated serum catecholamine concentrations. Withdrawal phenomena following beta-blocking drugs have different expressions (22) and provide informations about the pathophysiology of the autonomic nervous system.

Limitations of Our Investigations

Two major difficulties must be taken into account in order to properly use Holter recordings as a mode of investigation of the relationships between arrhythmias and the autonomic nervous system. One is that isolated premature beats, the usual trigger of tachyarrhythmias, are often rate-dependent as well as adrenergic-dependent. Due to their electrophysiological mechanism, e.g., parasystole, they tend to disappear as the heart rate accelerates, whereas at the same time the mechanism responsible for the sustained tachyarrhythmia, e.g., triggered activity, may be enhanced. This is why the exercise test is not always reliable (23,24): Though largely and logically utilized for detecting catecholamine-related arrhythmias, it may provoke or suppress them in a rather unpredictable way.

The second difficulty is caused by the "adrenergic paradox" (19), according to which the greater the arrhythmia dependence on the sympathetics, the more difficult its detection through the usual markers: If an arrhythmia is indeed very sensitive to catecholamines, a tiny acceleration of the heart rate corresponding to a limited adrenergic predominance may be easily missed as heralding a sympathetic stimulation. It results from this quite logical state of things that if the arrhythmias provoked by a exercise test are indeed an indication for beta-blockers, the latter do not necessarily provide the most effective protection in the long term. Therefore, in patients with unaltered myocardial function, no modifications of the autonomic nervous system, the relationships between ventricular arrhythmias, and their environment of sinus rhythm are easy to evidence in Holter recordings (20). As a consequence of the adrenergic paradox, these correlations tend to become less significant as the degree of heart failure increases (25) though arrhythmias are becoming at the same time even more adrenergic dependent. Another problem may be to interpret the adrenergic paradox itself, in the sense that the marker used, i.e., the sinus rhythm, may become unreliable: This should be suspected every time some degree of downregulation of the beta receptors is present.

Interactions Between Arrhythmias and the Autonomic Nervous System

Arrhythmias themselves have feedback effects on the autonomic nervous system through their hemodynamic consequences. Even if it is difficult to detect an appreciable rise in catecholamine levels just after the onset of a ventricular tachyarrhythmia, Morady (26) observed a threefold increase after conversion of electrically induced tachyarrhythmias in humans. Of course, a proper effect of the 1000 joule countershocks was possibly included in this evaluation, but there is little doubt that hemodynamic consequences of arrhythmias can induce a baroreflex-mediated reaction. One of the mechanisms of severe tachyarrhythmias is the deterioration of one form of ventricular tachycardia into another form, more rapid and/or regular and polymorphic, finally degenerating into ventricular fibrillation (27). A sort of vicious circle conceivably exists between the tachyarrhythmia, its hemodynamic consequences, and the adrenergic reaction, where an explanation for the protective role of beta-blockers may be proposed. It has been shown that even isolated extrasystoles provoke fluxes of muscle sympathetic nerve activity in humans, comprising surges of sympathetic activity larger than those occuring during sinus rhythm (28, 29). The shorter the coupling interval of the premature beats, the greater the magnitude of the bursts of sympathetic activity (30).

Conclusion

Numerous observations lead one to conclude that adrenergic stimulation is indeed an important component of arrhythmias. Evaluating the degree of dependence and interaction remains difficult, and none of the usual techniques of clinical investigation is easy to use and reliable in all circumstances. Invasive explorations are not designed for this approach, and the preference that was given for a long time to this technique for investigating arrhythmia mechanisms partly explains why this aspect has been neglected. The exercise test has its limitations in terms of reliability, reproducibility, or simply possibility for the patient to perform. In any case it is an unusual provocative maneuver that by no means reflects the reality of daily life: The best evidence of which is that exercise-induced sudden deaths represent only a small minority of fatalities.

Ambulatory monitoring certainly is a better tool, but it is difficult to exploit. Just quantifying arrhythmias does not allow one to assess their adrenergic dependence, especially if one considers that the most adrenergic-dependent ones are not the most abundant but the most severe (31), which is totally different and culminates in the phenomenon of ventricular fibrillation and sudden death. Obviously there is no way to evaluate exactly the probability of occurrence or the adrenergic dependence of lethal arrhythmias that by definition occur only once in the patient's life and then terminate it. A too-large emphasis has been put on "life-threatening" arrhythmias, probably at the expense of really lethal arrhythmias: This trend is pernicious because it implies that the determinants, hence the treatments of life-threatening and lethal arrhythmias are identical, which is probably not true.

Documented Antiarrhythmic Actions of Beta-Blockers

Experimental Data

Using the ventricular fibrillation threshold to determine the antifibrillatory potency of beta-blockers, Anderson et al. (32) showed that it generally paralleled the known ratios of beta-blocking efficacy for pindolol, propranolol, metoprolol, and labetalol. Timolol had an apparently greater potency. All five beta-blocking drugs caused substantial (average sixfold) increases in the ventricular fibrillation threshold under both nonischemic and ischemic conditions. For Gang et al. (33), timolol and propranolol were equally effective in abolishing inducible ventricular tachycardia of fibrillation in the dog in the subacute phase of myocardial infarction. Sotalol was compared to metoprolol (8) on reentrant-inducible ventricular tachyarrhythmias in conscious dogs 3-8 days after myocardial infarction. Sotalol was apparently much more potent than metoprolol in preventing or slowing the tachyarrhythmias (56% vs. 7%) in these particular conditions. This was apparently related to a significantly greater effect on the effective refractory periods in the normal myocardium, the difference being even greater in the infarct zone.

The most convincing and comprehensive model for studying the effect of beta-blockers was proposed by Patterson et al. (34), who made clear the distinction between the control of the substrate and of the trigger after myocardial infarction. In the subacute period of 6-24 hours after coronary ligation in dogs, the spontaneous triplets that ordinarily triggered the sustained ventricular tachycardias disappeared on nadolol, whereas artificial induction of the latter remained possible.

Clinical Data

Large discrepancies can be found in the literature concerning the antiarrhythmic efficacy of propranolol, with evaluations ranging from 20% (35) to 70% (36). The possible causes for such differences are numerous. They include the comparison of oral and intravenous administrations, the mode of assessment (suppression of ventricular tachycardia artificial induction or counts of ventricular premature beats at Holter), and overall the patients' conditions and the regimens used. In an experiment (37) with 25 patients (11 with a healed myocardial infarction) the suppression of arrhythmias of simple and complex types by atenolol (50-200 mg/day) was on the order of 70%. For Glasser et al. (38), who compared propranolol and acebutolol with placebo, the mean number of extrasystoles/hour were 87, 119, and 267, respectively, a significant difference between beta-blockers and placebo but not between the two drugs, and the clinical diagnosis was not precise. The mean efficacy of acebutolol (39) is on the order of 50%, a proportion that is frequently found by other investigators using other drugs, from pindolol (40) to nadolol (41).

The experience recently reported by Brodsky et al. (42) in sustained ventricular tachyarrhythmias concludes that beta-blockade was effective on the long-term (>2 years) in 75% of the cases, and that a left ventricular ejection fraction over 45%, the absence of coronary disease, and age >60 years were predictors of good efficacy. This is in apparent contradiction with our own experience (43) in patients with resistant ventricular tachyarrhythmias also followed on the long term, but in the setting of heart failure: In our cohort the greater benefit was observed in the most severely diseased patients. But looking at the baseline characteristics shows that the two series are not comparable, with a mean ejection fraction of 30% in our patients, whereas only three patients had less than 30% in Brodsky's series (mean value 52%). Half of the patients in this study had no detectable heart disease and arrhythmias were exercise-induced in 50%, whereas all our patients had either old myocardial infarctions or congestive cardiomyopathies and very few of them were capable of performing an exercise test. The discrepancies between the two series are in fact quite illustrative of the implications of the adrenergic paradox.

Conclusion: The Limited Value of the Direct Approach

It is of utmost importance to realize that we must not evaluate the antiarrhythmic effects of beta-blockers using the standards that have been adopted for type I antiarrhythmic drugs: This is the fundamental reason why their effective and useful antiarrhythmic action is largely missed. The real problem is to determine whether the clinically relevant effect of beta-blockers is to reduce the number of extrasystoles or to prevent the ventricular tachycardia or the ventricular fibrillation they can announce. These severe tachyarrhythmias are indeed dependent on the adrenergic stimulation, whereas this evidence is much less clear for isolated premature beats, so that one should not be surprised that a possible efficacy on the tachyarrhythmias does not necessarily coincide with the suppression of trivial extrasystoles. Another important issue, and a general rule, is that diseased patients are more hyperadrenergic than subjects with idiopathic arrhythmias: The greater sensitivity of their sinus rate also tends to apply to tachyarrhythmias. The present "direct approach" to the rationale, that refers to the general methods of evaluation of antiarrhythmics, does not really fit with the particular mode of action of these drugs, and may not provide the most convincing arguments for their use.

A further illustration of this situation can be found in the now demonstrated beneficial effect of beta-blockers on tachyarrhythmias of the congenital long QT syndrome (44): The antiarrhythmic efficacy of beta-blockers on lethal tachyarrhythmias is not approachable through the quantification of any routinely observed simple cardiac arrhythmia in these candidates to sudden death, but only through epidemiological surveys.

For a large part, the same applies to many arrhythmias that are amenable to beta-blockers, thus justifying the "indirect approach."

THE INDIRECT APPROACH

The indirect approach consists of exploring to what extent the established beneficial effect of beta-blockers on sudden death prevention is related to the effects of these drugs on cardiac arrhythmias. This implies that what is known of the mechanisms of sudden death should be confronted with the effect of beta-blockers.

Three main parameters are involved in the mechanisms of sudden death: ischemia as the main causal disease of cardiac mortality, heart failure, whatever its cause, and ventricular tachyarrhythmias. It is established that they are the predictors of sudden death and cardiac death. The distinction between cardiac death and sudden death is often essentially considered a matter of definition, but it appears that any influence, notwithstanding its beneficial or detrimental character, applies to both. Another fact that progressively emerges from numerous therapeutic trials is that addressing individually one of the three factors does not significantly improve the duration of life, whereas beta-blocking therapy does. This seems to be the key problem, because it implies that the three factors necessarily interact (Fig. 2) and that any beneficial action of any drug cannot be explained in a single and simple way.

Beta-Blockers and Cardiac Mortality

Modalities of Sudden Death

With the development of the Holter technique, more and more cases of sudden death have been recorded during ambulatory monitoring, so that their modalities if not their mechanisms are better known, and ventricular tachyarrhythmias are largely predominant. In the 157 cases we collected with Bayès et al. (45), only 26 (16.5%) were due to bradyarrhythmias. Admittedly the data collection is biased since by definition the tracings were obtained in patients who were on ambulatory recording for some reason, particularly the evaluation of arrhythmic events or antiarrhythmic treatments. This may explain, for instance, the rather large proportion of torsades de pointes (20 cases, 12.7%) that, on the other hand, often tends to be minimized due to the difficulty of establishing this diagnosis from the published data. By and large, 70% of the cases of recorded sudden death were ventricular tachyarrhythmias. Among them, only 13

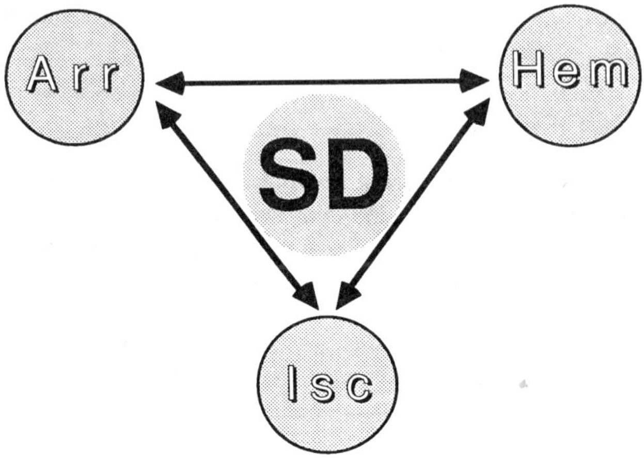

Figure 2 The "sudden death" triangle. Sudden death (SD) likely results from the interaction between arrhythmic (Arr) and hemodynamic (Hem) factors, the causal disease being most often of ischemic (Isc) nature.

cases were primary ventricular fibrillations, whereas the vast majority (98 cases) were ventricular tachycardias degenerating into ventricular fibrillation. Whatever the biases that can be expected in this type of survey, it is not surprising to find a large proportion of ventricular tachyarrhythmias in people who die within 1 hour after the onset of symptoms. There are no such data referring to "cardiac death" rather than "sudden death," and the proportion of "agonic" tracings must be higher in this setting, including cardiac standstill, electromechanical dissociation, and "slow" ventricular tachycardias with very wide QRS complexes. In such cases the distinction between cardiac death and sudden death is artificial in a number of cases. On the other hand, the really instantaneous death, due to primary ventricular fibrillation, represents a very limited number of cases to which the discussion should not be limited. The fact is that sudden death has to do with ventricular tachyarrhythmias, but the real problem is to determine whether they really cause it or in some cases may represent only the final marker that something disastrous happened in the heart.

Beta-Blockade and the Prevention of Cardiac Death

Excellent reviews covering a number of smaller or larger therapeutic trials, the total number of which now exceeds two dozen, can be found in the literature. Their consistent results explain why we do not expect many more secondary prevention trials of sudden death or cardiac death, as it has become unethical to propose a protocol including a control group of patients not receiving beta-blockers.

Secondary Prevention Trials The analysis of Yusuf et al. (2) including 26 published clinical trials, extended with the data from Isis 1 covers over 28,000 patients: Mortality was reduced by an overall mean of 13%. The Beta-Blocker Pooling Project (3) considered data from nine major trials (more than 200 patients enrolled 1-45 days after acute MI and followed during at least 1 year) involving half this number of patients (exactly 13,679) and demonstrates a 24% mortality reduction in the treated groups. Importantly, the benefit is shown as higher (up to 50%) in subgroups having a higher placebo group mortality. They are characterized by the existence of a previous infarction, angina pectoris, or mechanical or electrical complications. Groups with a smaller mortality also benefit, but to a lesser extent, which is not consistent among the trials. Gender, baseline level of heart rate or blood pressure, and time of initiation of treatment do not seem to play an important role. Curiously, age subgroups between 50 and 59 experience the largest reduction in mortality (37%), a highly significant result that seemed homogeneous among the trials. No significant adverse effect could be detected for any of the 36 subgroups considered in the Beta-Blocker Pooling Project.

Other Trials The beneficial effect of beta-blockers seems to extend to postintervention trial mortality: Studying the 2- to 7-year period following the initial 3-year metoprolol trial, Olsson et al. (46), using a Cox regression analysis taking 13 different variables into account, constructed a model describing the risk for subsequent death. The model identified the following important variables: male gender (relative risk = 2.4), beta-blocker withdrawal (= 2.1), and ongoing treatment with digitalis (= 2.3). On the other hand, in primary prevention studies reviewed by Dollery (47) in hypertensives, beta-blockers have not been demonstrated as beneficial: Reduction in stroke may reach 45%, whereas reduction in myocardial infarction was about 8%, a proportion that reached significance only by pooling the data. A similar reduction was reached in hypertension trials before beta-blockers came into general use.

Particular Aspects

Cardiac death and sudden death. Our purpose is not to review in detail these important trials, but simply to point out some aspects that deal with the general problem of cardiac death and sudden death, or shed some light on the particular mechanism of action of beta-blockers. For instance, it should be noted that in the Beta-Blocker Heart Attack Trial (48), patients with congestive heart failure in the propranolol group experienced a similar decrease in the total mortality (27%) compared with those without congestive heart failure (25%), whereas propranolol decreased the occurrence of sudden death by 47% in the patients with prior heart failure compared with 13% without congestive heart failure. Metoprolol has also been shown to be more beneficial to patients with an altered left ventricular function in the acute stage, in terms of mortality (49). These observations are consistent with the discrepancies we noted between Brodsky et al.'s experience (42) and ours (43) about the beta-blockers' efficacy in the long-term treatment of sustained ventricular tachycardias, and the bias introduced by the presence or the absence of myocardial dysfunction.

Diabetics and beta-blockers. The beneficial effect of beta-blockers on mortality is particularly marked in diabetics, and this is quite apparent from the two largest studies with metoprolol pooled by Malmberg et al. (50). In the MIAMI trial mortality was decreased from 11.3 to 5.7%, and the occurrence of late infarction from 4.5 to 3.1% during 15-day follow-up. In the Göteborg Metoprolol trial the mortality at 3 months was reduced from 17.9 to 7.5%, and late infarction was reduced from 16.4 to 3.8%. In addition, very interestingly, the mean heart rate before randomization was significantly higher in diabetic than in nondiabetic patients in both studies: 79.6 beats/min vs. 72.4 ($p < 0.0001$) in the Göteborg trial, 85.2 beats/min vs. 82.6 ($p < 0.001$) in the MIAMI trial. The neuropathy primarily involving the vagal innervation, the dramatic increase of catecholamine and other insulin antagonists during the acute phase of myocardial infarction, and the concomitant increase in arterial free fatty acids related to the diminished glucose utilization may be especially deleterious in diabetics with a diminished capability to produce or utilize insulin.

Sinus rate and beta-blockers. Not all the trials have demonstrated significant effect on mortality. In the pindolol trial (51) involving a total of 529 patients, the 2-year mortality of 17% was equal in the treated patients and in the placebo group. The same applies to the oxprenolol study (52), in which one can note that no difference in heart rate was found at night between treated and untreated patients, whereas the daytime heart rate was significantly lower in treated patients. Such an observation suggests that patients in this trial were not very sensitive to the beta-blocking treatment, or that the drug did not produce a strong enough beta-blockade, or that the beta-agonistic activity blunted to some extent the favorable effect of the antagonist properties. Kjekshus (53) has nicely shown the correlation between the reduction of mortality and the reduction in heart rate during the trials. Although we do not share the interpretation he proposes of a cause-and-effect relationship between the two phenomena, the fact is that the correlation exists. As already alluded to, there is theoretical and practical evidence that the effects of beta-blockers depend on the patient's adrenergic state and on the power of the drug, so that adrenergic-dependent mechanisms of death (arrhythmias, etc.) may be more or less favorably influenced by the treatment, with the sinus rate as a marker of this influence but not its mechanism.

Beta-Blockers and Ischemia

Ischemia, Tachyarrhythmias, and Sudden Death

The incidence of ischemic ST changes in patients developing lethal tachyarrhythmias while bearing an ambulatory recorder is surprisingly low (45), of the order of 15%. Several explanations can be proposed including technical reasons that would not, however, explain why the incidence of ST changes coinciding with bradyarrhythmias is much higher. It is established (54) that ischemia is present in one third of myocardial infarctions that have no complication and are suitable for exercise testing, that 50% of them have only silent ischemia (type 2), and that 75% of all episodes of myocardial ischemia are silent. Ischemia as the cause of the disease that finally leads to death is not in question. What is very unclear is to what extent acute ischemia is the mechanism immediately inducing the lethal arrhythmia, once acute coronary thrombosis is of course discounted (55).

Quyyumi et al. (56) stresses the rarity of ischemic ventricular tachycardias in 24-hour recordings of 74 coronary patients analyzed in terms of ST-segment changes and ventricular tachycardia. One of 22 patients with single-vessel disease, 1 of the 22 patients with double-vessel disease, and 4 of the 30 patients with triple-vessel disease had nonsustained ventricular tachycardias. Four of the 6 patients also had episodes of reversible ST-segment changes, but ventricular tachycardia was related to these episodes in only two patients, an overall very low incidence.

Antiischemic Procedures and the Prevention of Sudden Death

Medical Treatment of Ischemia Relief of ischemia has not demonstrated so far any significant benefit in the prevention of cardiac death. This applies to surgical as well as medical approach through vasodilators and calcium antagonists, and tends to confirm that ischemia is rarely the direct cause of sudden death. In the diltiazem trial (57) no overall impact on mortality or cardiac events was observed, a neutral effect that reflected a diltiazem-related reduction in cardiac events in the majority of patients without left ventricular dysfunction and an increase of such events in the minority of patients with left ventricular dysfunction. In the nifedipine trial (58), mortality and occurrence of cardiac event were quite identical in the placebo and in the treated group. In the Trent study (59) a nonsignificant (+6.9%) increase of mortality was observed with nifedipine. Verapamil (60) gave more encouraging (−7.8%) though not significant results.

This is in sharp contrast to the experimental situation (18) in which Schwartz et al. observed a striking protective effect of diltiazem against the malignant arrhythmias induced in cats by the combination of acute myocardial ischemia and sympathetic hyperactivity. Diltiazem was also effective in reducing the incidence of reperfusion arrhythmias. Thus these encouraging experimental data not confirmed in the clinical situation suggest that the latter is different, and suggest that ischemia does not often play a direct role in the genesis of sudden death, whereas sympathetic hyperactivity does.

Even the effects of agents not supposed to address one particular mechanism can in fact have unclear modes of action. For instance, sulfinpyrazone, a platelet aggregation inhibitor, was credited by Raeder et al. (61) with attenuating the reduction of the ventricular fibrillation threshold during sympathetic humoral stimulation, added to its effect on the beta-adrenergic blockade with practolol, and membrane stabilization with lidocaine.

Surgical Treatment When one considers the prevalence of ventricular arrhythmias in coronary patients and the large proportion of them who undergo coronary bypass surgery, the number of reports dealing with successful cure of tachyarrhythmias by revascularization surgery is surprisingly low: 9 patients reported by Rasmussen et al. (62) among 400 consecutive patients undergoing surgery have a convincing history because they were selected on strict criteria including severe coronary artery lesions at angiography, severe exercise-induced angina and corresponding ECG changes, normal or near-normal left ventricular function without previous infarction, and overall a reproducible ventricular tachyarrhythmia occuring during exercise in the presence of angina and ST-segment depression, with no tendency to arrhythmias in the resting state. Similar positive, carefully selected cases are occasional and anecdotal (63), but important in essence: They demonstrate that directly ischemia-dependent tachyarrhythmias do exist, and at the same time they show how rare they are. If it is established that bypass surgery reduces mortality at least in subgroups with lesions of the main left coronary artery (64), it does not reduce the incidence of infarct recurrence (65), and one could argue that, in addition to reducing ischemia, the bypass procedure could well influence cardiac arrhythmias through a reduction of the sympathetic discharge due to some degree of denervation.

Conclusion

Relief of ischemia seems to provide a cardioprotective effect by reequilibrating the balance between oxygen supply and demand. This balance is not stable, and the role of small vessel vasospastic changes (Fig. 3) has been emphasized. A number of secondary prevention trials have been undertaken according to this rationale. If the decrease of the oxygen demand, particularly through a relative bradycardia when beta-blockers are used, is not debatable and certainly contributes to a better supply-demand balance, it is well established in clinical practice that symptomatic angina is better controlled by vasodilators, calcium antagonists, and surgery than by beta-blockers. Thus, there is ample evidence that if the relief of ischemia may certainly contribute to the beneficial effect of beta-blockers, it does not explain the very mechanism by which this benefit is obtained. Needless to say, the occasional benefit of ischemia relief would not apply

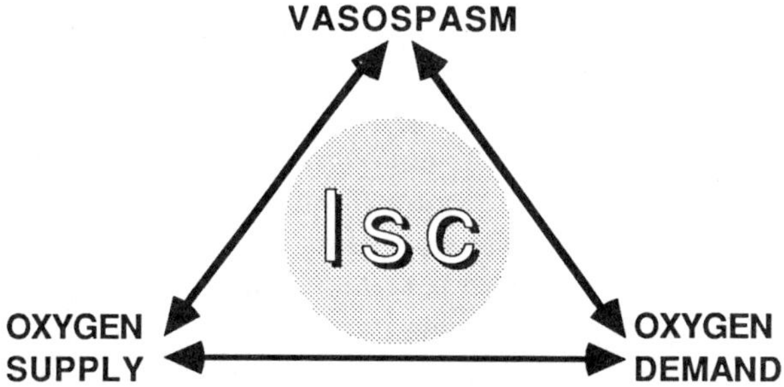

Figure 3 The "ischemia" triangle. Ischemia classically results from the imbalance between oxygen supply and oxygen demand. But vasospastic phenomena, particularly in small coronary vessels, may be modulated by various factors including the autonomic nervous system, and can play an intermittent role.

to cases where beta-blockers are also beneficial but where ischemia is certainly not in cause, i.e., in cardiomyopathies. Influences on heart failure and arrhythmias are the two other possible mechanisms of benefit.

Beta-Blockers and Heart Failure

Beta-Adrenoceptor Function in Heart Failure

The failing heart causes activation of the sympathetic system through baroreceptor perception of decreased ventricular performance. Plasma levels of catecholamines are increased, but myocardial stores of catecholamines are decreased (66). This apparent paradox results from decreased reuptake (67) or increased release of norepinephrine from myocardial sympathetic nerve endings, or both. Heart failure is well compensated initially thanks to the support of the increased sympathetic tone that with no doubt is beneficial at first. However, subsensitivity to beta-adrenergic stimulation develops with advancing heart failure. Even in the absence of heart failure, a decreased beta-adrenergic receptor density and an impaired inotropic response to isoproterenol can be seen in the uninvolved right ventricle 3 days after left ventricular infarction in guinea pigs (68), which can be prevented by beta-blockers. Upregulation of beta-adrenergic receptor density in infarcted areas can also be obtained by beta-blockers (69).

Of interest might be the observation that if the $beta_1$-adrenoceptors are reduced whatever the cause of the cardiac failure, the $beta_2$-adrenoceptor function is nearly normal in patients with congestive cardiomyopathy (70) but equally reduced in patients with mitral valve disease (71). And one can remark that ventricular tachyarrhythmias are more frequent in the former but often coexist with heart failure, whereas sudden death is not unusual in the latter even in the absence of heart failure. Differences in substrates might not be the only cause. Catecholamines are affected differently in the two diseases. Norepinephrine is a rather selective $beta_1$-adrenoceptor agonist, whereas the second endogenous catecholamine, epinephrine, is a nonselective beta-adrenoceptor agonist having an equal affinity to $beta_1$- and $beta_2$-adrenoceptors: Accordingly it could lead to a concomitant downregulation of $beta_1$- and $beta_2$-adrenoceptors. Brodde et al. (71) found some preliminary data to suggest that the level of both types of catecholamines could be different in the two forms of cardiopathy; this remains to be firmly established.

Clinical Correlations and Arrhythmia Behavior in Heart Failure

Exploration of the Autonomic Nervous System The clinical correlates of these complex phenomena can be found in the changes of heart rate variability, which reflects at the sinus node level the status of the autonomic nervous system. An increasing interest is presently paid to investigating the physiology of the system through the evaluation of the heart rate variability by spectral (72) or nonspectral (73) methods. A decreased heart rate variability, which reflects the loss of flexibility of the physiological vago-sympathetic interactions, is detected in pathological situations that are not restricted to heart failure (74) and do have prognostic implications (75). Investigations of the system through baroreflex sensitivity (17,76) suggest similar conclusions.

The decreased possibilities of the heart rate adaptation to the patient's activity have an important implication: the concomitant loss of sensitivity of the heart frequency as a marker of the vagal or sympathetic predominance at the sino-atrial level. This is a possible mechanism involved in the adrenergic paradox (19): In the presence of an apparently weak relationship between heart rate acceleration and arrhythmia occurrence, there is no way to distinguish between an increased sensitivity of the arrhythmogenic substrate to adrenergic stimulation, and a decreased sensitivity of the marker of this stimulation at the sinus node level.

Arrhythmias in Heart Failure Arrhythmia behavior cannot be indifferent to the considerable changes of the autonomic nervous system balance in the presence of patent or latent heart failure, and one cannot expect that the impact of these changes may be beneficial. In fact, the anatomical substrate responsible for heart failure creates the conditions in which an increased adrenergic stimulation occurs in the presence of diseased tissues that are most susceptible to constitute arrhythmogenic substrates (Fig. 4): Any therapeutic intervention capable of disrupting this vicious circle should decrease the incidence of potentially lethal tachyarrhythmias.

Glover and Littler's experience (77) over a series of 50 patients with severe ischemic chronic heart failure and a 62% 2-year mortality shows that sudden and nonsudden deaths are equally common and that there is an inverse relation between left ventricular ejection fraction and Lown grade of arrhythmias. Severe ventricular arrhythmias thus appear to be a marker for severe left ventricular damage, an opinion that is shared by Gottlieb et al. (5) in a rather comparable series of seriously diseased patients.

From 43 patients with chronic heart failure from dilated cardiomyopathy (28 ischemic, 15 idiopathic) studied by Chakko and Gheorghiades (78), 88% had complex arrhythmias (multiform, repetitive) and 51% had nonsustained ventricular tachycardias. They were randomized to either placebo or antiarrhythmic therapy (quinidine and procainamide), and at a mean follow-up period of 16 months there were 16 deaths, 10 of which

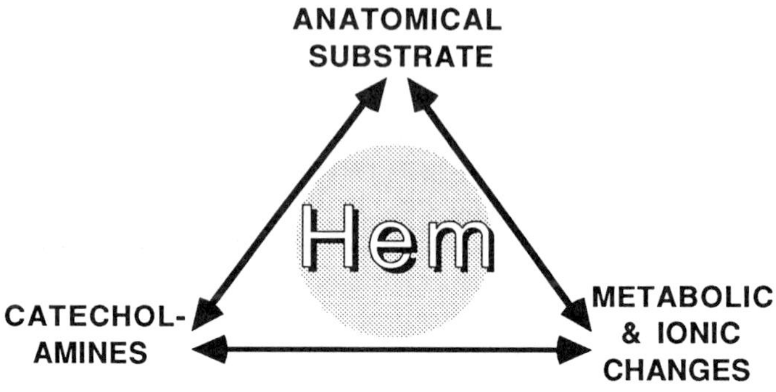

Figure 4 The "hemodynamic" triangle. The failure of hemodynamic functions (Hem) depends on the importance of the anatomical substrate and of the metabolic and ionic changes, and is responsible for the increased level of catecholamines.

were sudden and unexpected. No significant differences in the incidence of sudden death and overall mortality were noted between the patients treated and not treated by type I antiarrhythmics. Among patients with nonsustained ventricular tachycardias, those who died suddenly had a significantly lower ejection fraction (0.15% ± 0.01) than those who survived (0.23 ± 0.02; $p < 0.01$).

Treatment of Heart Failure and Prevention of Death

Treatment of Symptoms Treatments directly addressing the symptoms of heart failure have not demonstrated so far any benefit in terms of reduced mortality in the long term. This applies in particular to drugs with a beta-adrenoceptor agonist activity. Orally active phosphodiesterase inhibitors (amrinone, milrinone) that retard the degradation of catecholamines seem to be arrhythmogenic if one considers the high frequency of sudden death in the treated patients (79). Digitalis itself has been frequently suspected to be an independent factor of increased mortality, but Byington et al.'s (80) careful analysis of the Beta-Blocker Heart Attack Trial patients taking digitalis indicates that the higher mortality rate was probably related to more extensive cardiovascular damage rather than to digitalis therapy per se: Age, prior history of heart failure, angina pectoris, and complex arrhythmias were the factors of severity. Recently, Fergusson et al. (81) brought direct evidence, from sympathetic neural recordings in heart failure patients, that intravenous administration of digitalis glycosides produced a marked sympathoinhibitory response: In theory this would have a beneficial effect but does not exclude of course a possible direct arrhythmogenic effect of digitalis.

Beta-Blockers Swedberg et al. were the first in the 1970s (82) to report on the beneficial effects of beta-blockers in patients with idiopathic dilated cardiomyopathy. Since that time studies have become more frequent, with consistent results. For Heilbrunn et al. (83) long-term (6 months) metoprolol therapy in heart failure from dilated cardiomyopathy is associated with an increase in myocardial beta-receptor density, a significant improvement in resting hemodynamic output, and an improved response to catecholamine stimulation. These changes indicate a restoration of beta-adrenergic sensitivity possibly related to the observed upregulation of beta-adrenergic receptors.

Vasodilators The consensus trial (84) has demonstrated that enalapril, an angiotensin converting enzyme inhibitor, prolongs life. Webster et al. (85) had shown the effect of enalapril in heart failure patients ($n = 10$, NYHA classes II-III) with ventricular extrasystoles, couplets, and ventricular tachycardia. Compared with placebo patients the frequency of arrhythmias was significantly decreased (about 80%) with the exception of one patient. An increase in plasma potassium levels of 0.33 mmol/liter in the treated patients may have played a role. Ace inhibitors have been reported to lower the plasma norepinephrine levels at least in the short-term period (86,87), a finding that was not confirmed by Webster et al. (85). But peripheral plasma norepinephrine levels are a poor index of sympathetic outflow to the heart (88), and in the absence of any direct antiarrhythmic effect of enalapril one is forced to assume that this action is exerted through the effect on heart failure itself. A consistent finding on extrasystoles was also done by Cleland et al. (89). In this situation of a very severe prognosis (90,91) with an incidence of sudden death that ranges from 39 to 60% in the series reviewed by Packer (92), the mechanisms of cation repletion, and reduction of circulating levels of neurohormones (catecholamines, angiotensin II) may help explain the reduction of mortality (93). From animal experiments, Maisel et al. (94) concluded that captopril may increase the number and responsiveness of postsynaptic cardiac beta-adrenoceptors, most likely by preventing downregulation.

Conclusion

Heart failure obviously sets the stage for severe ventricular arrhythmias by enhancing the level of adrenergic stimulation that facilitates all arrhythmogenic mechanisms. Any further increase of sympathetic activity with the aim of correcting the symptoms of pump failure at best does not influence the incidence of sudden death and is in fact suspected to increase it. The contrary applies to beta-blockers, and seems to also be the mechanism of efficacy of ace inhibitors. Prognostic information from myocardial function, autonomic nervous system, and arrhythmia is obviously closely linked, which does not mean that it is redundant but implicates that any therapeutic action that decreases the sympathetic activity must have beneficial effect through the adrenergic-dependent tachyarrhythmias.

Beta-Blockers and Arrhythmias

Arrhythmias and the Secondary Prevention Trials with Antiarrhythmics

Our purpose is not to review the various trials that have failed to demonstrate any reduction of mortality by suppressing arrhythmias with type I antiarrhythmic drugs. The consistent trends of an increased mortality rate, already observed in particular in the impact study with mexiletine (4), was recently confirmed for encainide and flecainide in the CAST study (6), probably because of the use of more powerful drugs in an increased number of better-targeted patients. This absence of overall statistical benefit does not exclude any possible benefit in limited subgroups of patients using other drugs. This was, for instance, suggested in two trials involving aprindine (5,95), and, not inconceivably, this can apply to other type I antiarrhythmics. Simply, after the significant results of the CAST study, undertaking other sudden death prevention trials with type I antiarrhythmics will become as difficult as performing the same studies with beta-blockers, though for exactly opposite reasons. Among the problems recently introduced by the results of the CAST study, the most difficult is not to understand the reasons for the very low mortality rate of the placebo group, but to explain the increased mortality of the treated group (96).

Arrhythmias and the Secondary Prevention Trials with Beta-Blockers

A good indication that arrhythmia suppression was not the target for treatment in practically any of these sudden death prevention trials is that in many of them valuable information is simply lacking. The Beta-Blocker Pooling Project (3) mentions that information on arrhythmias was available in approximately one third of the patients. In the BHAT trial (97,98) ventricular arrhythmias were studied in a random sample of 25% of the study population. The increased prevalence of ventricular arrhythmias at 6 weeks was blunted by propranolol therapy. Patients benefited from propranolol to the same relative degree whether they had no or complex arrhythmias, a criterion that however conditioned a different prognosis. In other works, the effects of beta-blockade on ventricular premature beats, while present, does not reflect by itself the drug's beneficial effects, thus suggesting that the mechanism should be different, involving in particular the prevention of ventricular fibrillation.

In the metoprolol study including a 3-year follow-up (99), arrhythmias were monitored at baseline and after 1, 6, 12, 24, and 36 months (6-hour recordings, about 150 patients treated or with placebo in each group). The increase in both the complexity of arrhythmias and the frequency of extrasystoles observed in the placebo group was blunted by metoprolol. Treatment effect on mortality was similar in patients both with and without complex arrhythmias before treatment. In a retrospective analysis, the outcome of metoprolol-treated patients was evaluated. In patients in whom the arrhythmia frequency was reduced by >75% after 3 days of treatment, mortality was lower as compared to those who did not show this treatment response. In the acute phase, the arrhythmia analysis performed by Rydén et al. (100) in the metoprolol study showed no effect on the occurrence of ventricular premature beats or short bursts of ventricular tachycardia. However, a striking and important finding was an effect on ventricular fibrillation.

Experimental Data

Experimentally, transmural myocardial infarction produces areas of both sympathetic and vagal afferent denervation in infarcted and in noninfarcted myocardium apical to the region of infarction. This afferent denervation is not homogeneous in all areas, thereby possibly favoring the occurrence of arrhythmias (101). The development of a postdenervation supersensitivity suggests at the same time possible therapeutic approaches (102) but also the notion of a great complexity.

Actually, the complexity of the relationships between ischemia, autonomic nervous system, and arrhythmias is illustrated in Janse et al.'s study (103) exploring comparative effects of right and left stellate ganglion stimulation and removal. The authors cannot determine whether the arrhythmogenic effects of left stellate stimulation and right stellectomy resulted from an increased likelyhood for reentry in the epicardium of the ischemic zone. But they demonstrated that left stellate stimulation as well as right stellectomy increased the degree of TQ-segment depression in the extracellular electrograms and increased the area showing negative TQ potentials indicating decreased resting membrane potentials. The opposite effects were obtained by left stellectomy. No differences were found according to the site of ischemia by occluding the left anterior coronary artery or the circumflex branch.

The possible beneficial effect of interventions on the innervation of the heart is presently being tested (104), and there are indeed theoretical bases for such an approach. Selective block of the right and left stellate ganglia in humans (105) confirms the dominance of the left side, though the influence on myocardial refractoriness was less apparent in this study than the influence on normal and abnormal (Kent bundle) conduction systems, and a prolongation of the QT interval was obtained by right rather than left stellate ganglion block.

Conclusion: Arrhythmia Suppression and Mortality

The impression that emerges from comparing clinical and experimental data from secondary prevention trials involving either antiarrhythmics or beta-blockers is that arrhythmias that provoke sudden death are not the ones that were routinely observed during the patients' follow-up. A corollary of this statement may be that most probably arrhythmogenic phenomena that provoke an increased mortality of patients on antiarrhythmics are not the drug-induced arrhythmias that are usually categorized in the conventional studies. Referring again to the experience of recorded sudden death (27) clearly implicates the role of adrenergic stimulation when one considers the significant heart rate acceleration that often precedes the terminal event. What is also striking is that the terminal event may be totally different from any previously observed arrhythmia, for instance, in the case of a primary ventricular fibrillation. It may also recall the previous arrhythmia, but with a modified pattern including a different morphology of the ventricular tachycardia, shorter coupling intervals, longer and faster runs of tachycardia that all suggest an adrenergic origin of the modifications. When an iatrogenic arrhythmia is the cause (torsade de pointes, wide QRS tachycardia), it is also different from the simple increase of basic arrhythmias.

Suppressing more or less drastically the arrhythmias routinely observed in the postmyocardial infarction period has no direct relationship to long-term survival. Eradication is more easily obtained with class I than with class II antiarrhythmic agents, but the fact that the former increases, and the latter decreases the mortality rate obviously demonstrates the lack of correlation between appearance and reality. This does not mean, of course, that arrhythmias have nothing to do with either the prevention or the provocation of sudden death. In short, the quantity and the complexity of routinely recorded arrhythmias do have a prognostic value that is partly independent of other important factors like ischemia and heart failure. However, a serious failure in the rationale for the prevention of sudden death is to take trivial arrhythmias not only as markers for prognosis but as targets for treatment. In other words, the arrhythmias that kill are not the ones that are routinely recorded.

CONCLUSIONS

The rationale for using beta-blockers as antiarrhythmics is based on numerous direct as well as indirect arguments that additively form a solid body of evidence. The indirect arguments we have drawn from the sudden death data and preventive therapy are for us more convincing than direct arguments based on conventional approaches. The rationale for using beta-blockers is essentially based on the established relationships between the autonomic nervous system and arrhythmias. However, the problem is that these relationships are often characterized by paradoxical behaviors, occurring in situations that are difficult to reproduce experimentally and are clinically exceptional enough to happen only once if they lead to sudden death. A example of this situation is formed by the long QT syndrome, which is the best example of arrhythmias amenable to beta-blockers with no experimental model and a very few anecdotical examples demonstrating clinically the intervention of a neurally mediated adrenergic stimulation (106,107).

The important problem of sudden death prevention is even more intriguing. On the one hand, we have many data on the determinants of sudden death, the prognostic factors that are tempting to consider for therapeutic strategy, and on the other hand, taking them individually as therapeutic targets is disappointing or even detremental for the patient: This applies to the individual treatments of ischemia, heart failure, and arrhythmias. Figure 5 proposes an explanation for such a curious situation: If ischemia, heart failure, and arrhythmias are supposed to be interactive in the determinism of sudden death, one can conceive that addressing only one of them may finally be ineffective or even deleterious by destabilizing the delicate equilibrium that keeps the patient alive. On the contrary, one must realize that each of these factors has to do in some way with the

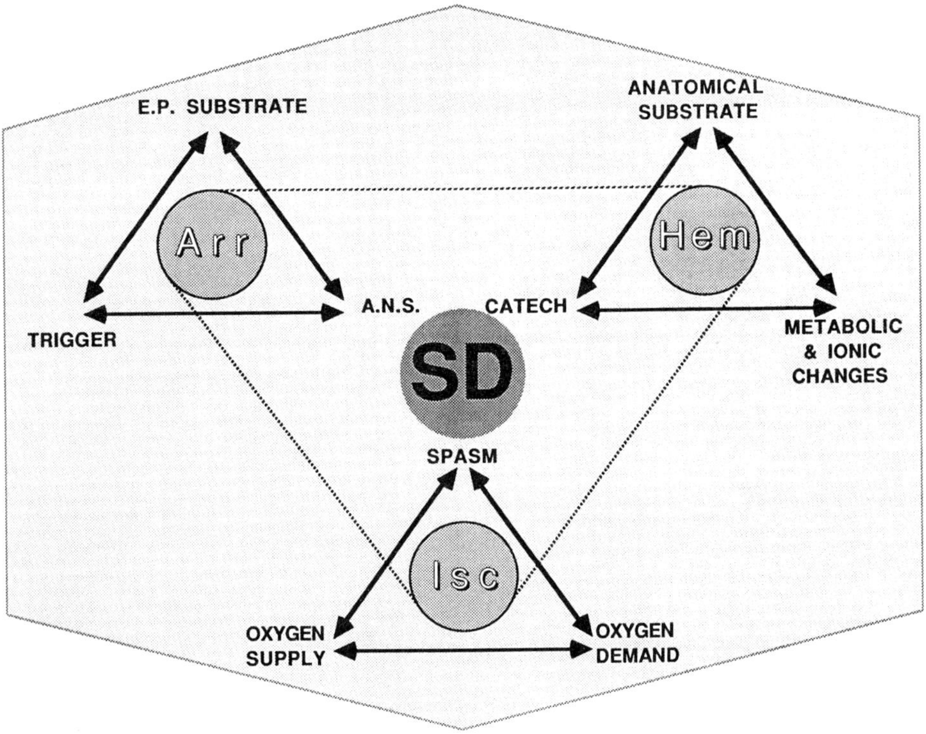

Figure 5 The "sudden death" polygon. One can draw any polygon including the various determinants of sudden death. However, all the factors may be interactive in the setting of arrhythmic, hemodynamic, and ischemic primary component. Overall, one can note that the various functions of the autonomic nervous system are always more or less involved in some form. This may explain why treatments dedicated only to arrhythmic, ischemic, or hemodynamic symptoms are insufficient to prevent sudden death, and can even be detrimental by modifying delicate balances. Beta-blockade addresses a common denominator of the various factors, and this mode of action may explain its better efficacy.

autonomic nervous system, interactions between arrhythmias and heart failure probably being the most important link. Not by chance but quite logically, beta-blockers are the drugs that can act on the common denominator of the various factors involved. One can conceive that they are particularly appropriate not to destabilize too rapidly critical balances, and to help break and revert vicious interactive mechanisms in complex pathophysiological situations.

REFERENCES

1. Vaughan-Williams EM. Beta-blockers in the control of arrhythmias. In: Zanchetti A, ed. Advances in beta-blocker therapy II. Amsterdam: Excerpta Medica, 1982:110-6.
2. Yussuf S, Peto R, Lewis J, Collins R, Sleight P. Beta-blockade during and after myocardial infarction. An overview of the randomized trials. Prog Cardiovasc Dis 1985; 77:335-71.
3. The Beta-Blocker Pooling Project Research Group. The beta-blocker pooling project (BBPP): subgroup findings from randomized trials in post infarction patients. Eur Heart J 1988; 9:8-16.
4. IMPACT Research Group. International mexiletine and placebo antiarrhythmic coronary trial. I. Report on arrhythmias and other findings. J Am Coll Cardiol 1984; 4:1148-58.
5. Gottlieb SH, Achuff SC, Mellits ED, Gerstenblith G, Baughmann KL, Becker L, Chandra NC, Henley S, Humphries JO, Heck C, Kennedy MM, Weisfeldt ML, Reid PR. Prophylactic antiarrhythmic therapy of high-risk survivors of myocardial infarction: lower mortality at 1 month but not at 1 year. Circulation 1987; 75:792-9.
6. The Cardiac Arrhythmia Suppression Trial (CAST) Investigators. Preliminary report: effect of encainide and flecainide on mortality in a randomized trial of arrhythmia suppression after myocardial infarction. New Engl J Med 1989; 321:406-12.
7. Bristow MR, Ginsburg R. $Beta_2$ receptors on myocardial cells in human ventricular myocardium. Am J Cardiol 1986; 57:3F-6F.
8. Cobbe SM, Hoffman E, Ritzenhoff A, Brachmann J, Kübler W, Senges J. Action of sotalol on potential reentrant pathways and ventricular tachyarrhythmias in concious dogs in the late postmyocardial infarction phase. Circulation 1983; 68:865-71.
9. Coumel P, Escoubet B, Attuel P. Beta-blocking therapy in atrial and ventricular tachyarrhythmias: experience with nadolol. Am Heart J 1984; 108: 1098-108.
10. Escoubet B, Leclercq JF, Maisonblanche P, Poirior JM, Gourmel B, Delhotal-Landes B, Coumel Ph. Comparison of four beta-blockers as assessed by 24-hour recordings. Clin Pharm Ther 1986; 39:361-8.

11. Hermida JS, De Jode P, Jarry G, Maison-Blanche P, Cauchemez B, Bernasconi P, Coumel P. Fréquence sinusale et écart-type des cycles cardiaques: influence de l'état myocardique et du traitement bêta-bloquant. Arch Mal Coeur 1989, in press.
12. Hamer A, Mandel WJ. Digitalis and beta-adrenergic blocking drugs for the treatment of tachycardias. In: Surawicz B, Reddy CP, Prystowsky EN, eds. Tachycardias. Boston: Martinus Nijhoff, 1984:431-59.
13. Kimura S, Bassett AL, Kohya T, Kozlovskis PL, Myerburg RJ. Automaticity, triggered activity, and responses to adrenergic stimulation in cat subendocardial Purkinje fibers after healing of myocardial infarction. Circulation 1987; 75:651-60.
14. Vincent HH, Man In't Veld AJ, Boomsma F, Schalekamp MADH. Prevention of epinephrine-induced hypokaliemia by nonselective beta-blockers. Am J Cardiol 1985; 56:10D-14D.
15. Williams ME, Gervino EV, Rosa RM, Landsberg L, Young JB, Silva P, Epstein FE. Catecholamine modulation of rapid potassium shifts during exercise. N Engl J Med 1985; 312:823-7.
16. Epstein FE, Rosa RM. Adrenergic control of serum potassium. N Engl J Med 1983; 309:1450-1.
17. Schwartz PJ, Vanoli E, Stramba-Badiale M, De Ferrari GM, Billman GE, Foreman RD. Autonomic mechanisms and sudden death. New insights from analysis of baroceptor reflexes in conscious dogs with and without a myocardial infarction. Circulation 1988; 78:969-79.
18. Schwartz PJ, Priori SG, Vanoli E, Zaza A, Zuanetti G. Efficacy of diltiazem in two experimental feline models of sudden cardiac death. J Am Coll Cardiol 1986; 8:661-8.
19. Coumel P. The management of clinical arrhythmias. An overview on invasive versus non-invasive electrophysiology. Eur Heart J 1987; 8:92-9.
20. Zimmermann M, Maisonblanche P, Cauchemez B, Leclercq JF, Coumel P. Determinants of the spontaneous ectopic activity in repetitive monomorphic idiopathic ventricular tachycardia. J Am Coll Cardiol 1986; 7:1219-27.
21. Nakagawa S, Yamamoto Y, Koiwaya Y. Ventricular tachycardia induced by clonidine withdrawal. Br Heart J 1985; 53:654-8.
22. Walden RJ, Hernandez J, Yu Y, Al-Khader A, Prichard BNC. Withdrawal of beta-blocking drugs. Am Heart J 1982; 104:515-20.
23. Coumel PH, Zimmermann M, Funck-Brentano C. Exercise test: arrhythmogenic or not? Eur Heart J 1987; 8D:7-15.
24. Lombardi F, Malfatto G, Belloni A, Garimoldi M. Effects of sympathetic activation on ventricular ectopic beats in subjects with and without evidence of organic heart disease. Eur Heart J 1987; 8:1065-74.
25. Zimmermann M, Maisonblanche P, Couchemez B, Leclercq JF, Coumel P. Déterminants de l'activité répétitive dans les tachycardies ventriculaires en salves. Arch Mal Coeur 1986; 79:1420-8.

26. Morady F, DiCarlo LA, Halter JB, de Buitleir M, Krol RB, Baerman JM. The plasma catecholamine response to ventricular tachycardia induction and external countershock during electrophysiologic testing. J Am Coll Cardiol 1986; 8:584-91.
27. Laclercq JF, Maison-Blanche P, Cauchemez B, Coumel P. Respective role of sympathetic tone and of cardiac pauses in the genesis of 62 cases of ventricular fibrillation recorded during Holter monitoring. Eur Heart J 1988; 9:1276-83.
28. Herre JM, Thames MD. Responses of sympathetic nerves to programmed ventricular stimulation. J Am Coll Cardiol 1987; 9:147-153.
29. Lombardi F, Ruscone TG, Malliani A. Premature ventricular contractions and reflex sympathetic activation in cats. Cardiovasc Res 1989; 23:205-12.
30. Welch WJ, Smith ML, Rea RF, Bauernfeind RA, Eckberg DL. Enhancement of sympathetic nerve activity by single premature ventricular beats in humans. J Am Coll Cardiol 1989; 13:69-75.
31. Coumel P, Rosengarten MD, Leclercq JF, Attuel P. Role of sympathetic nervous system in non-ischaemic ventricular arrhythmias. Br Heart J 1982; 47:137-143.
32. Anderson JL, Rodier HE, Green LS. Comparative effects of beta-adrenergic blocking drugs on experimental ventricular fibrillation threshold. Am J Cardiol 1983; 51:1196-202.
33. Gang ES, Bigger JT, Uhl EW. Effects of timolol and propranolol on inducible sustained ventricular tachyarrhythmias in dogs with subacute myocardial infarction. Am J Cardiol 1984; 53:275-81.
34. Patterson E, Scherlag BJ, Lazzara R. Mechanism of prevention of sudden death by nadolol: differential actions on arrhyhmia triggers and substrate after myocardial infarction in the dog. J Am Coll Cardiol 1986; 8:1365-72.
35. Duff HJ, Mitchell LB, Wyse DG. Antiarrhythmic efficacy of propranolol: comparison of low and high serum concentrations. J Am Coll Cardiol 1986; 8:959-65.
36. Woosley RL, Kornhauser DK, Smith RL. Suppression of chronic ventricular arrhythmias with propranolol. Circulation 1979; 60:819-27.
37. Heng MK, Zimmer I. Reduction of ventricular arrhythmias by atenolol. Am Heart J 1985; 109:1273-80.
38. Glasser SP, Clark PI, Laddu AR. Comparison of the antiarrhythmic effects of acebutolol and propranolol in the treatment of ventricular arrhythmias. Am J Cardiol 1983; 52:992-5.
39. Lui HK, Lee G, Dhurandhar R, Hungate EJ, Laddu A, Dietrich P, Mason DT. Reduction of ventricular ectopic beats with oral acebutolol: a double-blind, randomized crossover study. Am Heart J 1983; 105:722-6.
40. Podrid PJ, Lown B. Pindolol for ventricular arrhythmias. Am Heart J 1982; 104:491-6.
41. Morganroth J, Duchin KL. Effectiveness of low-dose nadolol for ventricular arrhythmias. Am J Cardiol 1986; 58:273-8.

42. Brodsky MA, Byron JA, Luckett CR, Capparelli EV, Wolff LJ, Henry WL. Antiarrhythmic efficacy of solitary beta-adrenergic blockade for patients with sustained ventricular tachyarrhythmias. Am Heart J 1989; 118:272-80.
43. Hermida JS, Coumel P, Leclercq JF, Cauchemez B, Maison-Blanche P, Leenhardt A, Slama R. Intérêt des bêta-bloquants dans le traitement des tachycardies ventriculaires récidivantes chez l'insuffisant cardiaque. Arch Mal Coeur 1987; 80:290-300.
44. Schwartz PJ. Idiopathic long QT syndrome. Progress and questions. Am Heart J 1985; 109:399-411.
45. Bayès de Luna A, Coumel P, Leclercq JF. Ambulatory sudden death: mechanisms of production of fatal arrhythmia on the basis of data from 157 cases. Am Heart J 1989; 117:151-9.
46. Olsson G, Odén A, Johansson L, Sjögren A, Rehnqvist N. Prognosis after withdrawal of chronic postinfarction metoprolol treatment: a 2-7 year follow-up. Eur Heart J 1988; 9:365-72.
47. Dollery CT. Beta-adrenoceptor blocking drugs in primary and secondary prevention of myocardial infarction. Eur Heart J 1987; 8M:131-4.
48. Chadda K, Goldstein S, Byington R, Curb JD. Effect of propranolol after acute myocardial infarction in patients with congestive heart failure. Circulation 1986; 73:503-10.
49. Olsson G, Rehnqvist N. Effect of metoprolol in postinfarction patients with increased heart size. Eur Heart J 1986; 7:468-74.
50. Malmberg K, Herlitz J, Hjalmarson A, Rydén L. Effects of metoprolol on mortality and late infarction in diabetics with suspected acute myocardial infarction. Retrospective data from two large studies. Eur Heart J 1989; 10: 423-8.
51. Australian and Swedish Pindolol Study group. The effect of pindolol on the two years mortality after complicated myocardial infarction. Eur Heart J 1983; 4:367-75.
52. Bethge KP, Andresen D, Boissel JP, von Leitner ER, Peyrieux JC, Schröder R, Tietze U. Effect of oxprenolol on ventricular arrhythmias: the european infarction study experience. J Am Coll Cardiol 1985; 6:963-72.
53. Kjekshus J. Heart rate reduction—a mechanism of benefit? Eur Heart J 1987; 8L:115-22.
54. Sheps DS, Heiss G. Sudden death and silent myocardial ischemia. Am Heart J 1989; 117:177-84.
55. Davies MJ, Thomas AC. Thrombosis and acute coronary artery lesions in sudden cardiac ischemic death. N Engl J Med 1984; 310:1137-40.
56. Quyyumi AA, Crake T, Wright C, Mockus L, Levy RD, Fox KM. The incidence and morphology of ischaemic ventricular tachycardia. Eur Heart J 1986; 7:1037-44.
57. The Multicenter DILTIAZEM Postinfarction Trial Research Group. The effect of diltiazem on mortality and reinfarction after myocardial infarction. New Engl J Med 1988; 319:385-92.

58. The Israeli Sprint Study Group. Secondary prevention reinfarction Israeli nifedipine trial (SPRINT). A randomized intervention trial of nifedipine in patients with acute myocardial infarction. Eur Heart J 1988; 9:354-64.
59. Wilcox RG, Hampton JR, Banks DC. Trial of early nifedipine in acute myocardial infarction: the Trent study. Br Med J 1986; 293:1204-8.
60. Danish Study Group on verapamil in myocardial infarction. The Danish studies on verapamil in myocardial infarction. Br J Pharmacol 1986; 21(suppl 2):197S-204S.
61. Raeder EA, Verrier RL, Lown B. Effects of sulfinpyrazone on ventricular vulnerability in the normal and the ischemic heart. Am J Cardiol 1982; 50: 271-5.
62. Rasmussen K, Lunde PI, Lie M. Coronary bypass surgery in exercise-induced ventricular tachycardia. Eur Heart J 1987; 8:444-8.
63. Codini MA, Sommerfeldt L, Eybel CE, DeLaria GA, Messer JV. Efficacy of coronary bypass grafting in exercise-induced ventricular tachycardia. J Thor Cardiovasc Surg 1981; 81:502-6.
64. CASS principal investigators and their associates. Myocardial infarction and mortality in the coronary artery surgery study (CASS) randomized trial. N Engl J Med 1984; 310:750-8.
65. Varnauskas E, European coronary surgery study group. Survival, myocardial infarction, and employment status in aprospective randomized study of coronary bypass surgery. Circulation 1985; 72(suppl V):90-101.
66. Chidsey CA, Braunwald E, Morrow AG, Mason JJ. Myocardial norepinephrine concentration in man. N Engl J Med 1963; 269:653-8.
67. Petch MC, Nayler WC. Uptake of catecholamines by human cardiac muscle in vitro. Br Heart J 1979; 41:336-9.
68. Baumann G, Riess G, Erhardt WD, Felix SB, Ludwig L, Blumel G, Blömer H. Impaired beta-adrenergic stimulation in the uninvolved ventricle post acute myocardial infarction: reversible defect due to excessive circulating catecholamine induced decline in number and affinity of beta-receptors. Am Heart J 1981; 101:569-81.
69. Mukherjee A, Bush LR, McCoy KE, Duke RJ, Hagler H, Buja LM, Willerson JT. Relationship between beta-adrenergic receptor numbers and physiological responses during experimental canine myocardial ischemia. Circ Res 1982; 50:735-41.
70. Bristow MR, Ginsburg R, Umans V. β_1 and β_2-Adrenergic-receptor subpopulations in non-failing and failing human ventricular myocardium: coupling of both receptor subtypes to muscle contraction and selective β_1-receptor down-regulation in heart failure. Circ Res 1986; 59:297-309.
71. Brodde OE, Zerkowski HR, Doetsch N, Motomura S, Khamssi M, Michel MC. Myocardial beta-adrenoceptor changes in heart failure: concomitant reduction in β_1 and β_2-adrenoceptor function related to the degree of heart failure in patients with mitral valve disease. J Am Coll Cardiol 1989; 14:323-31.

72. Pagani M, Lombardi F, Guzzetti F, Rimoldi O, Furlan R, Pizzinelli P, Sandrone G, Malfatto G, Dell'Orto S, Piccaluga E, Turiel M, Baselli G, Cerutti S, Malliani A. Power spectral analysis of heart rate and arterial pressure variables as a marker of sympatho-vagal interaction in man and conscious dog. Circulation Res 1986; 59:178-93.
73. Coumel P, Hermida JS, Leenhardt A, Maison-Blanche P, Cauchemez B, Leclercq JF, Wennerblöm B. Heart rate variability in myocardial hypertrophy and heart failure, and the effects of beta-blocking therapy. A non-spectral analysis of heart rate oscillations. Eur Heart J 1991; 12:412-22.
74. Lombardi F, Sandrone G, Pernpruner S, Sala R, Garimoldi M, Cerutti S, Baselli G, Pagani M, Malliani A. Heart rate variability as an index of sympathovagal interaction after acute myocardial infarction. Am J Cardiol 1987; 60:1239-45.
75. Kleiger RE, Miller JP, Bigger JT, Moss AJ, the Multicenter Post-Infarction Research Group. Decreased heart rate variability and its association with increased mortality after acute myocardial infarction. Am J Cardiol 1987; 59: 256-62.
76. Schwartz PJ, Zaza A, Pala M, Locati E, Beria G, Zanchetti A. Baroreflex sensitivity and its evolution during the first year after myocardial infarction. J Am Coll Cardiol 1988; 12:629-36.
77. Glover DR, Littler WA. Factors influencing survival and mode of death in severe chronic ischemic cardiac failure. Br Heart J 1987; 57:125-32.
78. Chakko CS, Gheorghiades M. Ventricular arrhythmias in severe heart failure: incidence, significance, and effectiveness of antiarrhythmic therapy. Am Hear J 1985; 109:497-504.
79. Packer M, Medina N, Yushak M. Hemodynamic and clinical limitations of long-term inotropic therapy with amrinone in patients with severe chronic heart failure. Circulation 1984; 70:1038-45.
80. Byington R, Goldstein S, and the BHAT research group. Association of digitalis therapy with mortality in survivors of acute myocardial infarction: observations in the beta-blocker heart attack trial. J Am Coll Cardiol 1985; 6:976-82.
81. Ferguson DW, Berg WJ, Sanders JS. Sympathoinhibitory responses to digitalis glycosides in heart failure patients. Direct evidence from sympathetic neural recordings. Circulation 1989; 80:65-77.
82. Swedberg K, Hjalmarson A, Waagstein F, Wallentin I. Beneficial effects of long-term beta-blockade in congestive cardiomyopathy. Br Heart J 1980; 44: 117-33.
83. Heilbrunn SM, Shah P, Bristow MR, Valantine HA, Ginsburg R, Fowler MB. Increased β-receptor density and improved hemodynamic response to catecholamine stimulation during long-term metoprolol therapy in heart failure from dilated cardiomyopathy. Circulation 1989; 79:483-90.
84. The Consensus Trial Study Group. Effects of enalapril on mortality in severe congestive heart failure. N Engl J Med 1987; 316:1429-35.

85. Webster MWI, Fitzpatrick MA, Nichols MG, Ikram H, Wells JE. Effect of enalapril on ventricular arrhythmias in congestive heart failure. Am J Cardiol 1985; 56:566-9.
86. Creager MA, Halperin JL, Bernard DB, Faxon DP, Melldossian CD, Gavras H, Ryan TJ. Acute regional circulatory and renal hemodynamic effects of converting-enzyme inhibition in patients with congestive heart failure. Circulation 1981; 64:483-9.
87. Wenting GJ, Man In'Tveld AJ, Woittiez AJ, Boomsma F, Laird-Meeter K, Simoons ML, Hugenholtz PG. Effects of captopril in acute and chronic heart failure: correlations with plasma levels of noradrenaline, renin, and aldosterone. Br Heart J 1983; 49:65-76.
88. Esler M. Assessment of sympathetic nervous function in humans from noradrenaline plasma kinetics. Clin Sci 1982; 62:247-54.
89. Cleland JGF, Dargie HJ, Hodsman GP, Ball SG, Robertson JIS, Morton JJ, East BW, Robertson I, Murray GD, Gillen G. Captopril in heart failure. A double blind controlled trial. Br Heart J 1984; 52:530-5.
90. Wilson JR, Schwartz JS, Sutton MS, Ferraro N, Horowitz LN, Reichek N, Josephson ME. Prognosis in severe heart failure: relation to hemodynamic measurements and ventricular ectopic activity. J Am Coll Cardiol 1983; 2: 403-10.
91. Franciosa JA, Wilen M, Ziesche S, Cohn JN. Survival in men with severe chronic left ventricular failure due to either coronary heart disease or idiopathic dilated cardiomyopathy. Am J Cardiol 1983; 51:831-6.
92. Packer M. Sudden unexpected death in patients with congestive heart failure: a second frontier. Circulation 1985; 72:681-5.
93. Furberg C, Yusuf R. Effects of vasodilators on survival in chronic congestive heart failure. Am J Cardiol 1985; 55:1110-3.
94. Maisel AS, Michel MC, Ziegy and late infarction in diabetics with suspected acute myocardial infarction. Retrospective data from two large studies. Eur Heart J 1989; 80:669-75.
95. Hugenholtz PG, Hagemeijer F, Lubsen J, Glazer B, VanDurme JP, Bogaert MG. One year follow-up in patients with persistent ventricular dysrhythmias after myocardial infarction treated with aprindine or placebo. In Sandoe E, Julian DG, Pell JW, eds. Management of ventricular tachycardia: role of mexiletine. Amsterdam: Excerpta Medica, 1978:572-8.
96. European Task Force. Cast and beyond. Circulation 1989; in press, and Eur Heart J 1989; in press.
97. Friedman LM, Byington RP, Capone RJ, Furburg CD, Goldstein S, Lichstein E. Effect of propranolol in patients with myocardial infarction and ventricular arrhythmia. J Am Coll Cardiol 1986; 7:1-8.
98. Lichstein E, Morganroth J, Harrist R, Hubble E, the BHAT study group. Effect of propranolol on ventricular arrhythmia. The Beta-Blocker Heart Attack Trial experience. Circulation 1983: 67(suppl I):5-10.

99. Olsson G, Rehnqvist N. Ventricular arrhythmias during the first year after acute myocardial infarction: influence of long-term treatment with metoprolol. Circulation 1984; 69:1129-34.
100. Rydén L, Ariniego R, Arman K. A double-blind trial on metoprolol in acute myocardial infarction. Effects on ventricular tachyarrhythmias. N Engl J Med 1983; 308:614-8.
101. Barber MJ, Mueller TM, Davies BG, Gill RM, Zipes DP. Interruption of sympathetic and vagal-mediated afferent responses by transmural myocardial infarction. Circulation 1985; 72:623-31.
102. Chilson DA, Peigh P, Mohamed Y, Zipes DP. Encircling endocardial incision interrupts efferent vagal-induced prolongation of endocardial and epicardial refractoriness in the dog. J Am Coll Cardiol 1985; 5:290-6.
103. Janse MJ, Schwartz PJ, Wilms-Schopman F, Peters RJG, Durrer D. Effects of unilateral stellate ganglion stimulation and ablation on electrophysiologic changes induced by acute myocardial ischemia in dogs. Circulation 1985; 72:585-95.
104. Schwartz PJ, Zaza A. The rational basis and the clinical value of selective cardiac sympathetic denervation in the prevention of malignant arrhythmias. Eur Heart J 1987; 7A:107-18.
105. Cinca J, Evangelista A, Montoyo J, Barutell C, Figueras J, Valle V, Rius J, Soler-Soler J. Electrophysiologic effects of unilateral right and left stellate ganglion block on the human heart. Am Heart J 1985; 109:46-54.
106. Wellens HJJ, Verneulen A, Durrer D. Ventricular fibrillation occuring on arousal from sleep by auditory stimuli. Circulation 1972; 46:661-5.
107. Coumel P, Leenhardt A. Mental activity, adrenergic modulation and cardiac arrhythmias in patients with heart disease. In: Mental stress as a trigger of cardiovascular events. Circulation 1991; 83:II 58-70.

4

Comparative Pharmacology of Beta-Adrenergic Blockers

William H. Frishman

The Albert Einstein College of Medicine and the Hospital of the Albert Einstein College of Medicine/Montefiore Medical Center, Bronx, New York

As a class of drugs, the beta-adrenoceptor blockers have been so successful that many of them have been synthesized and more than 15 are available on the world market (1). Selectivity for two subgroups of the beta-adrenoceptor population has also been taken advantage of: $beta_1$-receptors in the heart and $beta_2$-receptors in the peripheral circulation and bronchi (1,2). More controversial has been the introduction of beta-blocking drugs with alpha-adrenergic blocking actions, varying amounts of intrinsic sympathomimetic activity (ISA; partial agonist activity [PAA]), and nonspecific membrane-stabilizing effects (3). There also are pharmacokinetic differences among beta-blocking drugs that may be of clinical importance (2,4).

As of 1991, with the introduction of betaxolol, carteolol, and penbutolol, 12 beta-blockers are marketed for approved uses in the United States. These are propranolol for angina pectoris, arrhythmia, systemic hypertension, essential tremor, prevention of migraine headache, and reducing the risk of mortality of survivors of acute myocardial infarction; nadolol for angina pectoris and hypertension; timolol for hypertension, open angle glaucoma, and reducing the risk of mortality and reinfarction in survivors of acute myocardial infarction; atenolol and metoprolol for hypertension, angina pectoris, and reducing the risk of mortality in survivors of acute myocardial infarction; acebutolol for hypertension and ventricular arrhythmias; betaxolol, carteolol, penbutolol, and pincolol for hypertension; intravenous esmolol for supraventricular tachycardias; and labetalol for hypertension and hypertensive emergencies (2,3,5-8). Five beta-blockers (bisoprolol, bevantolol, carvedilol, celiprolol, d-sotalol) are now under consideration by the FDA for marketing approval or are being studied actively in clinical trials. Oxprenolol has been approved for use in hypertension but has not yet been marketed in the United States.

Despite the extensive experience with beta-blockers in clinical practice, there are no studies suggesting that one of these agents has major advantages or disadvantages over another for treatment of cardiovascular diseases. When any available beta-blocker is titrated properly, it can be effective in patients with arrhythmias, hypertension, or angina pectoris (2-9). However, one agent may be more effective in reducing adverse reactions in some patients and clinical situations.

POTENCY

Beta-adrenoceptor blocking drugs are competitive inhibitors of catecholamine binding at beta-adrenoceptor sites. In the presence of a beta-blocker, the dose-response curve of the catecholamine is shifted to the right; that is, a higher concentration of the catecholamine is required to provoke the response (2). The potency of a beta-blocker tells us how much of the drug must be administered in order to inhibit the effects of an adrenergic agonist. Potency can be assessed by noting the dose of the drug that is needed to inhibit tachycardia produced by an agonist or by exercise (10). Potency differs from drug to drug, with pindolol being the most potent and esmolol the least potent. While differences in potency explain the different dosages needed to achieve effective beta-adrenergic blockade, they have no therapeutic relevance, except when switching patients from one drug to another (2,11).

STRUCTURE-ACTIVITY RELATIONSHIPS

The chemical structure of most beta-adrenergic blockers have several features in common with the agonist isoproterenol (Fig. 1), which consists of an aromatic ring with a substituted ethanolamine side chain linked to it by an $-OCH_2$ group (2,3,12). Timolol has a catecholamine-mimicking side chain but a more complex ring.

Most beta-blockers exist as pairs of optical isomers and are marketed as racemic mixtures. Almost all of the beta-blocking activity is found in

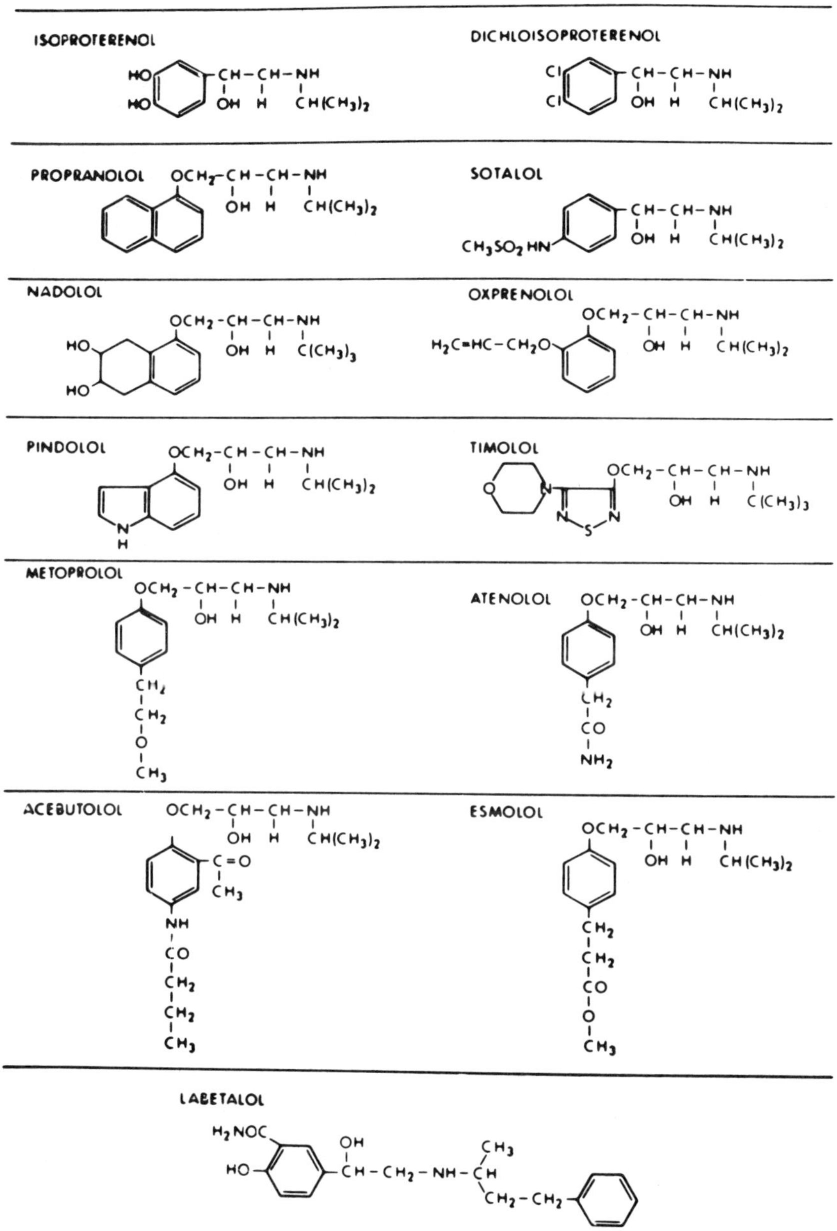

Figure 1 Molecular structure of the beta-adrenergic agonist isoproterenol and some beta-adrenergic blocking drugs. (From Ref. 10 with permission.)

the negative (−)levorotatory stereoisomer, which can be up to 100 times more active than the positive (+)dextrorotatory isomer. The two stereoisomers of beta-adrenergic blockers are useful to investigators seeking to differentiate between the pharmacologic effects of the beta-blockade and other unrelated effects. If the effect is produced when only a D-isomer is present, it can be assumed to be unrelated to catecholamine inhibitory actions. D-Isomers of beta-blocking drugs have, of themselves, no clinical value (2,11,12) except for D-sotalol, which has type III antiarrhythmic properties (13). Penbutolol and timolol are marketed only in the L-form.

MEMBRANE-STABILIZING ACTIVITY (MSA)

At very high concentrations, certain beta-blockers have a quinidine or local anesthetic effect on the cardiac action potential. This property is exhibited equally by the two stereoisomers of the drug, and is unrelated to beta-adrenergic blockade and major therapeutic antiarrhythmic actions. There is no evidence that MSA is responsible for any direct negative inotropic effect of the beta-blockers, since drugs with and without this property depress left ventricular function equally (2,14). Only during massive beta-blocker intoxication is the activity manifested (10,15,16).

BETA$_1$-SELECTIVITY

The beta-adrenoceptor blockers can be classified as selective or nonselective, according to their relative abilities to antagonize the actions of sympathomimetic amines in some tissues at lower doses than those required in other tissues (2,5). When used in low doses, beta$_1$-selective blocking agents, such as acebutolol, esmolol, atenolol, and metoprolol inhibit cardiac beta$_1$-receptors but have less influence on bronchial and vascular beta-adrenoceptors (beta$_2$). In higher doses, however, beta$_1$-selective blocking agents also block beta$_2$ receptors. Accordingly, beta$_1$-selective agents may be safer than nonselective ones in patients with obstructive pulmonary disease since beta$_2$-receptors remain available to mediate adrenergic bronchodilatation. However, even selective beta-blockers may aggravate bronchospasm in certain patients, and so these drugs should generally not be used in patients with bronchospastic disease.

A second theoretical advantage is that, unlike nonselective beta-blockers, selective beta$_1$k-blockers also have a less inhibitory effect on the beta$_2$-receptors that mediate dilation of arterioles, and are thus less likely to impair peripheral blood flow. In the presence of epinephrine, nonselective beta-blockers can cause a pressor response by blocking $beta_2$-receptor mediated vasodilation (since alpha-adrenergic vasoconstriction receptors remain operative). Selective $beta_1$-blockers may not induce this effect in the presence of epinephrine and may lessen the impairment of peripheral blood flow. It is possible that leaving the $beta_2$-receptors unblocked and responsive to epinephrine may be functionally important in some patients with asthma, hypoglycemia, hypertension, or peripheral vascular disease treated with beta-adrenergic blocking drugs (2,3,5).

ISA (PARTIAL AGONIST ACTIVITY [PAA])

Certain beta-adrenoceptor blockers possess ISA (PAA) at $beta_1$-adrenoceptor receptor sites, $beta_2$-adrenoceptor receptor sites, or both. In a beta-blocker, this property is identified as a slight cardiac stimulation, which can be blocked by propranolol (2,3,8,9). The beta-blocking drugs with this property slightly activate the beta-receptor in addition to preventing the access of natural or synthetic catecholamines to the receptor (Fig. 2).

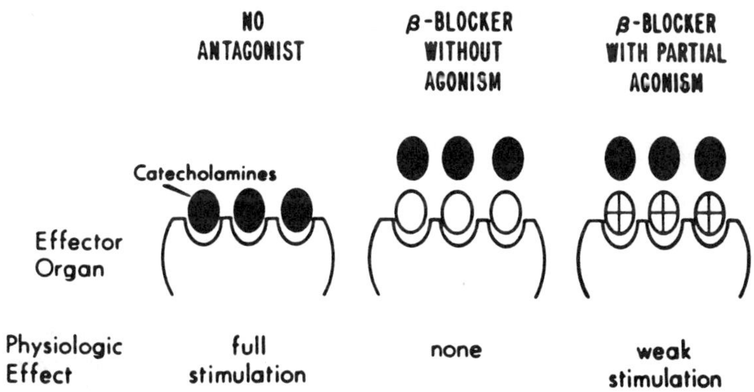

Figure 2 Physiologic effects of beta-adrenergic blocking drugs with and without partial agonist activity in the presence of circulating catecholamines. When circulating catecholamines (●) combine with beta-adrenergic receptors, they produce a full physiologic response. When these receptors are occupied by a beta-blocker lacking partial agonist activity (○), no physiologic effects from catecholamine stimulation can occur. A beta-blocking drug with partial agonist activity (⊕) also blocks the binding of catecholamines to beta-adrenergic receptors, but the drug also causes a relatively weak stimulation of the receptor. (From Ref. 8 with permission.)

Dichloroisoprenaline, the first beta-adrenoceptor blocking drug synthesized, exerted such marked PAA that it was unsuitable for clinical use (9). However, compounds with less PAA are effective beta-blocking drugs. The PA effects of beta-adrenoceptor blocking drugs such as a pindolol and oxprenolol differ from those of the agonist epinephrine and isoproterenol in that the maximum pharmacological response that can be obtained is low, although the affinity for the receptor is high. In the treatment of patients with arrhythmia, angina of effort, and hypertension, drugs with mild to moderate PAA appear to be as efficacious as are beta-blockers lacking this property. It is still debated whether the presence of PAA in a beta-blocker constitutes an overall advantage or disadvantage in cardiac therapy (8). Drugs with PAA cause less slowing of the heart rate at rest than do propranolol and metoprolol, although the increments in heart rate with exercise are similarly blunted. Beta-blocking agents with nonselective PAA (pindolol) and selective $beta_2$-agonism (celiprolol) reduce peripheral vascular resistance and may also cause less depression of atrioventricular conduction than drugs lacking these properties (8). Some investigators claim that PAA in a beta-blocker protects against myocardial depression, lipid abnormalities, bronchial asthma, and peripheral vascular complications, as caused by propranolol (8,17). The evidence supporting all these claims is not definite, and more definitive clinical trials will be necessary to resolve these questions.

ALPHA-ADRENERGIC ACTIVITY

Labetalol is a beta-blocker with antagonistic properties at both alpha- and beta-adrenoceptors, and it has direct vasodilator activity (3,10,18). Labetalol has been shown to be 6-10 times less potent than phentolamine at alpha-adrenoceptors and 1.5-4 times less potent than propranolol at beta-adrenoceptors, and is itself 4-16 times less potent at alpha- than at beta-adrenoceptors (3,10,18). Like other beta-blockers, it is useful in the treatment of hypertension and angina pectoris (10,19,20). However, unlike most beta-blocking drugs, the additional alpha-adrenergic blocking action does result in a reduction of peripheral vascular resistance, which may maintain cardiac output (10,18). Whether concomitant alpha-adrenergic blocking activity is actually advantageous in a beta-blocker remains to be determined.

PHARMACOKINETIC PROPERTIES

Although the beta-adrenergic blocking drugs have similar therapeutic effects, their pharmacokinetic properties differ significantly (see Tables

2,3) (3,11,14,21,22). Among individual drugs, there are differences in completeness of GI absorption, amount of first-pass hepatic metabolism, lipid solubility, protein binding, extent of distribution in the body, penetration into the brain, concentration in the heart, rate of hepatic biotransformation, pharmacological activity of metabolites, and renal clearance of the drug and its metabolites, which may influence the clinical usefulness of these drugs in some patients (2,3,11,14). The desirable pharmacokinetic characteristics in this group of compounds are a lack of major individual differences in bioavailability and in metabolic clearance of the drug and a rate of removal from active tissue sites that is slow enough to allow longer dosing intervals (2,3).

On the basis of their pharmacokinetic properties, the beta-blockers can be classified into two broad categories: those eliminated by the hepatic metabolism (with relatively short half-lives) and those eliminated unchanged by the kidney (which tend to have longer half-lives) (2). Drugs in the first group, for example, propranolol and metoprolol, are lipid soluble, are almost completely absorbed by the small intestine, and are largely metabolized by the liver. They tend to have highly variable bioavailability and relatively short plasma half-lives (3,5,11). A lack of correlation between the duration of clinical pharmacological effect and plasma half-life may allow these drugs to be administered once or twice daily (2). In contrast, drugs in the second category are more water soluble, are incompletely absorbed through the gut, and are eliminated unchanged by the kidney (6,7). They show less variable bioavailability in patients with normal renal function, in addition to longer half-lives, allowing one dose a day (6,7). The longer half-lives may be useful in patients who find compliance with frequent beta-blocker dosing a problem (6).

A long-acting, sustained-release preparation of propranolol has been approved for marketing (see Tables 2,3) (23). The propranolol is part of a soluble matrix inside tiny spheroids made of an insoluble membrane. GI fluid enters the spheroids, and propranolol exits via a concentration gradient into the gut lumen and then the bloodstream (23). The absorption of long-acting propranolol is not dependent on gastric acidity or enzymatic action. Studies have shown that this compound provides a much smoother curve of daily plasma levels than comparable divided doses of conventional propranolol and that it has fewer side effects (24,25). A similar sustained-release preparation of metaprolol has just become available for marketing in the United States.

Ultra-short-acting beta-blockers, with a half-life of no more than 10 minutes, also offer advantages to the clinician, for example, in patients with questionable congestive heart failure where beta-blockers may be harmful. One of these compounds, esmolol, a beta$_1$-selective drug (Tables 1,2,3) has been shown to be useful in the treatment of perioperative hypertension and supraventricular tachyarrhythmias (26). Another drug, flestolol, is under evaluation in clinical trials (27). The short half-life (approximately 15 minutes) relates to the rapid metabolism of the drug by blood

Table 1 Pharmacodynamic Properties of Beta-Adrenoceptor Blocking Drugs

Drug	Beta$_1$-blockade potency ratio (propranolol = 1.0)	Relative Beta$_1$-selectivity	Intrinsic sympathomimetic activity	Membrane-stabilizing activity
Acebutolol	0.3	+	+	+
Atenolol	1.0	+ +	0	0
Bevantolol	0.3	+ +	0	0
Bisoprolol	10.3	+ +	0	0
Bucindolol[a]		0	+	0
Carteolol	10.0	0	+	0
Carvedilol[b]	10.0	0	0	+ +
Celiprolol[c]	9.4	+	+	0
Dilevalol[d]	1.0	0	+	0
Esmolol	0.02	+ +	0	0
Labetalol[a]	0.3	0	+	0
Metoprolol	1.0	+ +	0	0
Nadolol	1.0	0	0	0
Oxprenolol	0.5-1.0	0	+	+
Penbutolol	1.0	0	+	0
Pindolol	6.0	0	+ +	+
Propranolol	1.0	0	0	+ +
Sotalol[e]	0.3	0	0	0
Tertatolol		0	0	0
Timolol	6.0	0	0	0
Isomer: D-propranolol				+ +

[a]Bucindolol and labetalol have additional alpha$_1$-adrenergic blocking activity and direct vasodilatory actions (beta$_2$-agonism).
[b]Carvedilol has additional alpha$_1$-adrenergic blocking activity without peripheral beta$_2$-agonism.
[c]Celiprolol may have additional peripheral alpha$_2$-adrenergic blocking activity at high doses.
[d]Dilevalol is an isomer of labetalol adrenergic with peripheral beta$_2$-agonism but no alpha$_1$-blocking activity.
[e]Sotalol has additional type of antiarrhythmic activity.
Source: Ref. 10.

Table 2 Pharmacokinetic Properties of Various Beta-Adrenoceptor Blocking Drugs

Drug	Extent of absorption (% of dose)	Extent of bioavailability (% of dose)	Dose-dependent bioavailability (major first-pass hepatic metabolism)	Interpatient variations in plasma levels	Beta-blocking plasma concentrations	Protein binding (%)	Lipid solubility[a]
Acebutolol	≃70	≃40	No	7-fold	0.2-2.0 μg/ml	25	Moderate
Atenolol	≃50	≃40	No	4-fold	0.2-5.0 μg/ml	>15	Weak
Bevantolol	≃90	≃55	No	4-fold	0.13-3.0 μg/ml	95	Moderate
Carteolol	≃90	≃90	No	2-fold	40-160ng/ml	20-30	Weak
Celiprolol	≃30	≃30	No	3-fold		≃30	Weak
Esmolol[b]	NA	NA	NA	5-fold	0.15-1.0 μg/ml	55	Weak
Labetalol	>90	≃33	Yes	10-fold	0.7-3.0 μg/ml	≃50	Weak
Metoprolol	>90	≃50	No	7-fold	50-100ng/ml	12	Moderate
Nadolol	≃30	≃30	No	7-fold	50-100ng/ml	≃30	Weak
Oxprenolol	≃90	≃40	No	5-fold	80-100ng/ml	80	Moderate
Penbutolol	>90	≃90	No	4-fold		98	High
Pindolol	>90	≃90	No	4-fold	5-15 ng/ml	57	Moderate
Propranolol	>90	≃30	Yes	20-fold	50-100ng/ml	93	High
Long-acting propranolol	>90	≃20	Yes	10- to 20-fold	20-100ng/ml	93	High
Sotalol	≃70	≃60	No	4-fold	0.5-4.0 μg/ml	0	Weak
Timolol	>90	≃75	No	7-fold	5-10 ng/ml	≃10	Weak

[a]Determined by the distribution ratio between octanol and water.
[b]Ultrashort-acting beta-blocker only available in intravenous form. NA indicates not applicable.
Source: Ref. 10.

Table 3 Elimination Characteristics of Beta-Adrenoceptor Blocking Drugs

Drug	Elimination half-life (II)	Total body clearance (ML IIIVMIN)	Urinary Recovery of unchanged drug (% of dose)	Total urinary recovery (% of dose)	Predominant route of elimination[a]	Active metabolites	Drug accumulation in renal disease
Acebutolol	3-1[b]	6-15	≃40	>90	RE (≃40% unchanged and HM)	Yes	Yes
Atenolol	6-9	130	≃40	>95	RE	No	Yes
Bevantolol	2-4	960	1	74	HM	No	No
Carteolol	5-6	497	40-68	90	RE	Yes	Yes
Celiprolol	5	500	≃90	≃30	RE (≃50% unchanged and HM)	Yes	No
Esmolol[c]	9 min	27,000	<2	70-90	BE[d]	No	No
Labetalol	3-4	2,700	<1	>90	HM	No	No
Metoprolol	3-4	1,100	≃3	>95	HM	No	No
Nadolol	14-24	200	70	70	RE	No	Yes
Oxprenolol	2-3	380	2-5	70-95	HM	No	No
Penbutolol	27	350	50-70	>90	RE	No	No
Pindolol	3-4	400	≃40	>90	RE (≃40% unchanged and HM)	No	No
Propranolol	3-4	1,000	<1	>90	HM	Yes	No
Long-acting propranolol	10	1,000	<1	>90	HM	Yes	No
Sotalol	9-10	150	≃60	>90	RE	No	Yes
Timolol	4-5	660	≃20	65	RE U (≃20% unchanged and HM)	No	No

[a]RE denotes renal excretion; HM, hepatic metabolism.
[b]Acebutolol has an active metabolite with elimination half-life of 8-13 hours.
[c]Ultrashort-acting beta-blocker only available in intravenous form.
[d]Metabolized by blood esterases.
Source: Ref. 10.

and hepatic esterases. Metabolism does not seem to be altered by disease states (28).

In medical practice, the pharmacokinetic properties of the different beta-adrenergic blockers become important (1,3). The dose of the drug, for example, depends on its first-pass metabolism; if the first-pass effect is extensive, not much of an orally administered drug will reach the systemic circulation (2,3,11,21), and so dosage will have to be larger than the intravenous dose would be (5,11,21). Knowing if the drug is transformed into active metabolites as opposed to inactive metabolites is important in gauging the total pharmacological effect (29). The total pharmacological effect therefore depends on the amount of the drug administered and its active metabolites (2,22). Characteristics of lipid solubility have been associated with the entry of these drugs into the brain (2,3), resulting in side effects that are probably unrelated to beta-blockade, such as lethargy, mental depression, and even hallucinations (2,7). Whether drugs that are less lipid soluble cause fewer of these adverse reactions remains to be determined (6,7,32-34).

RELATIONSHIP BETWEEN DOSE, PLASMA LEVEL, AND EFFICACY

Attempts have been made to establish a relationship between the oral dose, the plasma level measured by gas chromatography, and the pharmacological effect of each beta-blocking drug. After administration of a certain oral dose, beta-blocking drugs that are largely metabolized in the liver show large interindividual variation in circulating plasma levels (2,3). Many explanations have been proposed to explain wide individual differences in the relation between plasma concentrations of beta-blockers and any associated therapeutic effect. First, patients may have different levels of "sympathetic tone" (circulating catecholamines and active beta-adrenoceptor binding sites) and may thus require different drug concentrations to achieve adequate beta-blockade (11). Second, many beta-blockers have flat plasma drug-level response curves (22). Third, active drug isomers and active metabolites are not specifically measured in many plasma assays. Fourth, the clinical effect of a drug may last longer than the period suggested by the drug's half-life in plasma (11), since recycling of the beta-blocker between receptor site and neuronal nerve endings may occur. Despite the lack of correlation between plasma levels and therapeutic effect, there is some evidence that a relationship does exist between the logarithm of the plasma level and the beta-blocking effect (blockade of exercise- or isoproterenol-induced tachycardia) (5,11,22). Plasma levels have

Table 4 Pharmacodynamic Properties and Cardiac Effects of Beta-Adrenoceptor Blockers

Drug	Relative $beta_1$ selectivity[a]	Partial agonist activity	Membrane-stabilizing activity	Resting heart rate	Exercise heart rate	Resting myocardial contractility	Resting blood pressure	Exercise blood pressure	Resting atrioventricular conduction	Antiarrhythmic effect
Acebutolol	+	+	+	↓↔	↓	↓↔	↓	↓	↓↔	+
Atenolol	++	0	0	↓	↓	↓	↓	↓	↓	+
Betaxolol	++	0	+	↓	↓	↓	↓	↓	↓	+
Bevantolol	++	0	0	↓	↓	↓	↓	↓	↓	+
Carteolol	0	+	0	↓↔	↓	↓↔	↓	↓	↓	+
Carvedilol[b]	0	+	0	↓↔	↓	↓↔	↓	↓	↓↔	+
Celiprolol[c]	+	+	0	↓↔	↓	↓↔	↓	↓	↓↔	+
Dilevalol[d]	0	+	0	↓↔	↓	↓↔	↓	↓	↓↔	+
Esmolol	++	0	0	↓	↓	↓	↓	↓	↓	+
Labetalol[e]	0	+	0	↔	↓	↓↔	↓	↓↓	↓↔	+
Metoprolol	++	0	0	↓	↓	↓	↓	↓	↓	+
Nadolol	0	0	0	↓	↓	↓	↓	↓	↓	+
Oxprenolol	0	+	+	↓↔	↓	↓↔	↓	↓	↓↔	+
Penbutolol	0	+	0	↓↔	↓	↓↔	↓	↓	↓↔	+
Pindolol	0	++	0	↓↔	↓	↓↔	↓	↓	↓↔	+
Propranolol	0	0	++	↓	↓	↓	↓	↓	↓	+
Sotalol	0	0	0	↓	↓	↓	↓	↓	↓	+
Timolol	0	0	0	↓	↓	↓	↓	↓	↓	+
Isomer: D-propranolol	0	0	++	↔	↔	↔↓[f]	↔	↔	↔↓[f]	+[f]

[a]$Beta_1$ selectivity is seen only with low therapeutic drug concentrations. With higher concentrations, $beta_1$ selectivity is not seen.
[b]Carvedilol has additional $alpha_1$-adrenergic blocking activity without $beta_2$-agonism.
[c]Celiprolol has peripheral $beta_2$ agonism and may have additional $alpha_2$-adrenergic blocking activity at high doses.
[d]Dilevalol is an isomer of labetalol with peripheral $beta_2$ agonism but no $alpha_1$-blocking activity.
[e]Labetalol has additional $alpha_1$-adrenergic blocking properties and direct $beta_2$-adrenergic vasodilator activity.
[f]Effects of D-propranolol with doses in human beings well above the therapeutic level. The isomer also lacks beta-blocking activity.

Two pluses indicate a strong effect; one plus, modest effect; zero, absent effect; upward-pointing arrow = elevation; downward-pointing arrow = reduction; double-headed horizontal arrow = no change.

Source: Ref. 10.

little to offer as therapeutic guides, except for ensuring compliance and for diagnosis of overdose. Pharmacodynamic characteristics and clinical response should be used as guides in determining efficacy.

CLINICAL EFFECTS AND THERAPEUTIC APPLICATIONS

The therapeutic efficacy and safety of beta-adrenoceptor blocking drugs has been well established in patients with angina pectoris, cardiac arrhythmias, and hypertension, and for reducing the risk of mortality and possibly nonfatal reinfarction in survivors of acute myocardial infarction (Table 4) (2,3,10,33). These drugs may be useful as a primary protection against cardiovascular morbidity and mortality in hypertensive patients (34). The drugs are also used for a multitude of other cardiac and noncardiac conditions.

ANTIARRHYTHMIC EFFECTS: ELECTROPHYSIOLOGICAL EFFECTS

Beta-adrenoceptor blocking drugs have two main effects on the electrophysiological properties of specialized cardiac tissue (Table 5) (35). The first results from the specific blockade of adrenergic stimulation of cardiac pacemaker potentials. In concentrations causing significant inhibition of adrenergic receptors, the beta-blockers produce little change in the transmembrane potentials of cardiac muscle. However, by competitively inhibiting adrenergic stimulation, beta-blockers decrease the slope of phase 4 depolarization and the spontaneous firing rate of sinus or ectopic pace-

Table 5 Antiarrhythmic Mechanisms of Beta-Blockers

Beta-Blockade:
Electrophysiology—depress excitability; depress conduction
Prevention of ischemia—decrease automaticity; inhibit reentrant mechanisms
Membrane-Stabilizing Effects:
Local anesthetic "quinidinelike" properties—depress excitability; prolong refractory period; delay conduction
Clinically—probably not significant
Special Pharmacological Properties:
$Beta_1$-selectivity and intrinsic sympathomimetic activity do not appear to contribute to antiarrhythmic effectiveness

makers, therefore decreasing automaticity. Arrhythmias occurring in the setting of enhanced automaticity, as seen in myocardial infarction, digitalis toxicity, hyperthyroidism, and pheochromocytoma, would therefore be expected to respond well to beta-blockade (10,35).

The second electrophysiological effect of beta-blockers involves MSA, also known as "quinidine-like" or "local anesthetic" action, which is observed only at very high-dose levels. This property is unrelated to inhibition of catecholamine action and is possessed equally by both the D- and L-isomers of the drugs (D-isomers have almost no beta-blocking activity) (35). Characteristic of this effect is a reduction in the rate of rise of the intracardial action potential without an effect on the spike duration of the resting potential (35). This effect and its attendant changes have been explained by inhibition of the depolarizing inward sodium current (35).

Sotalol is unique among the beta-blockers in that it possesses Class III antiarrhythmic properties, causing prolongation of the action potential period, and thus delaying repolarization (13). Clinical studies have verified the efficacy of sotalol in control of arrhythmias (13), but additional

Table 6 Effects of Beta-Blockers in Various Arrhythmias

SUPRAVENTRICULAR:
Sinus Tachycardia—treat underlying disorder; excellent response to beta-blocker, if needed to control rate (e.g., ischemia)
Atrial Fibrillation—beta-blockers reduce rate, rarely restore sinus rhythm, may be useful in combination with digoxin
Atrial Flutter—beta-blockers reduce rate, sometimes restore sinus rhythm
Atrial Tachycardia—effective in slowing ventricular rate, may restore sinus rhythm; useful in prophylaxis
VENTRICULAR:
Premature Ventricular Contractions—good response to beta-blockers, especially digitalis-induced, exercise (ischemia)-induced, mitral valve prolapse, or hypertrophic cardiomyopathy
Ventricular Tachycardia—effective as quinidine, most effective in digitalis toxicity or exercise (ischemia)-induced
Ventricular Fibrillation—electrical defibrillation is treatment of choice. Beta-blockers can be used to prevent recurrence in cases of excess digitalis or sympathomimetic amines; appear to be effective in reducing the incidence of ventricular fibrillation and sudden death postmyocardial infarction)

Source: Ref. 10.

investigation will be required to determine whether its Class III antiarrhythmic properties contribute significantly to its efficacy as an antiarrhythmic agent.

The most important mechanism underlying the antiarrhythmic effect of beta-blockers, with the possible exclusion of sotalol, is thought to be beta-blockade with resultant inhibition of pacemaker potentials. The contribution of MSA does not appear to be clinically significant. In vitro experiments with human ventricular muscle have shown that the concentration of propranolol required for MSA is 50-100 times the concentration usually associated with inhibition of exercise-induced tachycardia and at which only beta-blocking effects occur (35). Moreover, D-propranolol, which possesses MSA but no beta-blocking action, is a weak antiarrhythmic even in high doses, while beta-blockers devoid of MSA (atenolol, esmolol, metoprolol, nadolol, pindolol) have been shown to be effective antiarrhythmic drugs (3,10,26). Differences in overall clinical usefulness are related to their other associated pharmacological properties (3,10).

THERAPEUTIC USES IN CARDIAC ARRHYTHMIAS

Beta-adrenergic blocking drugs have become an important treatment modality for various cardiac arrhythmias (Table 6) (3,10,35). It has long been thought that beta-blockers are more effective in treating supraventricular than ventricular arrhythmias, and only recently has it been appre-

Table 7 Possible Mechanisms by Which Beta-Blockers Protect the Ischemic Myocardium

Reduction in myocardial oxygen consumption, heart rate, blood pressure, and myocardial contractility
Augmentation of coronary blood flow—increase in diastolic perfusion time by reducing heart rate; augmentation of collateral blood flow—redistribution of blood flow to ischemic areas
Alterations in myocardial substrate utilization
Decrease in microvascular damage
Stabilization of cell and lysosomal membranes
Shift to oxyhemoglobin dissociation curve to the right
Inhibition of platelet aggregation
Prevention of atherosclerotic plaque rupture in vulnerable coronary lesions by decreasing blood pressure, heart rate, and myocardial contractility

Source: Refs. 10, 39.

ciated that this may not be the case. These agents can be quite useful in the treatment of ventricular tachyarrhythmias in the setting of myocardial ischemia (Table 7), mitral valve prolapse, and other cardiovascular conditions (35-39).

REFERENCES

1. Cruickshank JM, Prichard BNC. Beta-blockers in clinical practice. Edinburgh: Churchill Livingstone, 1987.
2. Frishman WH. Beta-adrenoceptor antagonists: new drugs and new indications. N Engl J Med 1981; 305:500-6.
3. Frishman WH. Beta-adrenergic blockers. Med Clin N Amer 1988; 72:37-81.
4. Frishman WH. The beta-adrenoceptor blocking drugs. Intl J Cardiol 1982; 2:165-78.
5. Koch Weser J. Metoprolol. N Engl J Med 1979; 301:698-703.
6. Frishman WH. Atenolol and timolol, two new systemic adrenoceptor antagonists. N Engl J Med 1982; 306:1456-62.
7. Frishman WH. Nadolol: a new beta-adrenoceptor antagonist. N Engl J Med 1981; 305:678-82.
8. Frishman WH. Pindolol: a new beta-adrenoceptor antagonist with partial agonist activity. N Engl J Med 1983; 308:940-4.
9. Frishman W, Silverman R. Clinical pharmacology of the new beta-adrenergic blocking drugs. Part III: Comparative clinical experience and new therapeutic applications. Am Heart J 1979; 98:119-31.
10. Frishman WH. Clinical pharmacology of the beta-adrenoceptor blocking drugs, 2nd ed. Norwalk, CT: Appleton-Century-Crofts, 1984.
11. Frishman W. Clinical pharmacology of the new beta-adrenergic blocking drugs. Part 1: Pharmacokinetic and pharmacodynamic properties. Am Heart J 1979; 97(5):663-70.
12. Conolly ME, Kerstting F, Dollery CT. The clinical pharmacology of beta-adrenoceptor blocking drugs. Prog Cardiovasc Dis 1976; 19:203-34.
13. Singh BN, Deedwania P, Nademanee K, Ward A, Sorkin EM. Sotalol: a review of its pharmacodynamic and pharmacokinetic properties and therapeutic use. Drugs 1987; 34:311-49.
14. Opie LH. Drugs and the heart: I. Beta-blocking agents. Lancet 1980; 1: 693-8.
15. Frishman W, Jacob H, Eisenberg E, Ribner H. Clinical pharmacology of the new beta-adrenergic blocking drugs. Part VIII: Self-poisoning with beta-adrenoceptor blocking drugs: recognition and management. Am Heart J 1979; 98:798-811.
16. Henry JA, Cassidy SL. Membrane stabilizing activity: A major cause of fatal poisoning. Lancet 1986; 1:1414-17.

17. Taylor SH, Silke B, Lee PS. Intravenous beta-blockade in coronary heart disease: is cardioselectivity or intrinsic sympathomimetic activity hemodynamically useful? N Engl J Med 1982; 306:631-5.
18. Frishman W, Halprin S. Clinical pharmacology of the new beta-adrenergic blocking drugs. Part VII: New horizons in beta-adrenoceptor blocking therapy: labetalol. Am Heart J 1979; 98:660-5.
19. Frishman WH, Strom J, Kirschner M, Poland M, Klein N, Halprin S, LeJemtel T, Kram M, Sonnenblick EH. Labetalol therapy in patients with systemic hypertension and angina pectoris: Effects of combined alpha- and beta-adrenergic blockade. Am J Cardiol 1981; 48:917-28.
20. Frishman WH. Properties of labetalol, a combined beta- and alpha-adrenergic blocking agent relevant to the treatment of myocardial ischemia. Cardiovasc Drug Ther 1988; 2:343-53.
21. Waal-Manning HJ. Hypertension: which beta-blocker? Drugs 1976; 12:412-41.
22. Johnsson G, Regardh CG. Clinical pharmacokinetics of beta-adrenoceptor blocking drugs. Clin Pharmacokinet 1976; 1:233-63.
23. Frishman WH, Teicher M. Long-acting propranolol. Cardiovasc Rev Rep 1983; 4:1100-2.
24. Halkin H, Vered I, Saginer A, Rabinowitz B. Once-daily administration of sustained release propranolol capsules in the treatment of angina pectoris. Eur J Clin Pharmacol 1979; 16:387-91.
25. Parker JO, Porter A, Parker JD. Propranolol in angina pectoris: comparison of long-acting and standard formulation propranolol. Circulation 1982; 65:1351-5.
26. Frishman WH, Murthy VS, Strom JA. Ultra-short acting beta-adrenergic blockers. Med Clin N Amer 1988; 72:359-72.
27. Strom J, Josephson M, Frishman WH. Hemodynamics of flestolol—a titratable short-acting intravenous beta-adrenergic receptor blocker. J Clin Pharmacol 1988; 28:276-82.
28. Murthy VS, Frishman WH. Controlled beta-receptor blockade with esmolol and flestolol. Pharmacotherapy 1988; 8:168-82.
29. Frishman WH. Acebutolol. Cardiovasc Rev & Rep 1985; 6:979-82.
30. Wurzelmann J, Frishman W, Aronson M, Masur D, Ooi WL. Neuropsychological effects of antihypertensive drugs in the old old. Cardiol Clinics 1987; 5:689-99.
31. Carney RM, Rich MW, te Velde A, Saini J, Clark K, Freedland KE. Prevalence of major depressive disorders in patients receiving beta-blocker therapy versus other medications. Am J Med 1987; 83:223-6.
32. Drayer DE. Lipophilicity, hydrophilicity, and the central nervous system side effects of beta-blockers. Pharmacother 1987; 7:87-91.
33. Frishman WH, Furberg CD, Friedewald WT. Beta-adrenergic blockade for survivors of acute myocardial infarction. N Engl J Med 1984; 310:830-7.
34. Wikstrand J, Warnold I, Olsson G, Tuomilehto J, Elmfeldt D. Primary prevention with metoprolol in patients with hypertension. JAMA 1988; 259:1976-82.

35. Frishman WH, Laifer LI. Beta-adrenergic blockade in the therapy of arrhythmias. In Horowitz L, ed. A.N. Richards Symposium of the Philadelphia Physiological Society. Baltimore: Urban & Schwarzenberg, 1984:207-48.
36. Pratt C, Lichstein E. Ventricular anti-arrhythmic effects of beta-adrenergic blocking drugs: a review of mechanism and clinical studies. J Clin Pharmacol 1982; 22:335-47.
37. Ryden L, Ariniego R, Arnman K, Herlitz J, Hjalmarson A, Holmberg S, Reyes C, Smedgard P, Svedberg K, Vedin A, Waagstein F, Walendstrom A, Wilhelmsson C, Wedel H, Yamamoto M. A double-blind trial of metoprolol in acute myocardial infarction: effects on ventricular tachyarrhythmias. N Engl J Med 1983; 308:614-18.
38. Lichstein E, Morganroth J, Harrist R, Hubble E. Effect of propranolol on ventricular arrhythmias—the beta-blockers: Preliminary data from the heart attack trial experience. Circulation 1983; 67(6: Part 2):I5-I10.
39. Frishman WH, Lazar EJ. Reduction in mortality, sudden death, and nonfatal reinfarction with beta-adrenergic blockers in survivors of acute myocardial infarction: A new hypothesis regarding the cardioprotective action of beta-adrenergic blockade. Am J Cardiol 1990; 66:66G-70G.

II

Beta-Blockers in Survivors of Acute Myocardial Infarction

5

Mechanisms and Rationale for the Use of Beta-Blockers in Survivors of Acute Myocardial Infarction

Bramah N. Singh
Veterans Affairs Medical Center of West Los Angeles and University of California at Los Angeles School of Medicine, Los Angeles, California

Since the introduction of beta-adrenergic blockers into cardiovascular therapeutics in the early 1960s, the role of this unique class of pharmacological agent has undergone considerable redefinition and expansion (1). In the earliest phases of their clinical application, the major focus was on the symptomatic control of myocardial ischemia; this was followed by a phase of rapid growth for their use in the treatment of hypertension, certain forms of ventricular and supraventricular tachyarrhythmias, and in hypertrophic cardiomyopathy. Subsequently, an increasing body of clinical and experimental evidence clearly demonstrated that the dominant action of beta-blockers, as was the original intent in synthesizing them, was to inhibit the deleterious effects of excessive or inappropriate stimulation of the sympathetic nervous system. In recent years this issue has assumed particular importance in terms of the effects of cardioactive agents on mortality in the survivors of acute myocardial infarction. This subset of patients, comprising those with clinically identifiable correlates of infarction as well as those experiencing essentially silent myocardial necrosis (2), probably form the largest group susceptible to a high risk for sudden cardiac death (3). Three major factors have been considered to be the critical determinants of risk: Reduced ventricular function reflecting the overall size of infarct or infarcts, latent or manifest persisting myocardial ischemia, and the presence of the so-called potentially malignant ventricular arrhythmias resulting from electrical instability appear to provide the milieu for the development of sudden death in these patients. A plethora of antiarrhythmic drugs and antiischemic agents has been tested to determine whether the mortality figures might be reduced by pharmacological therapy in the survivors of myocardial infarction.

As discussed elsewhere in this monograph, an area of beta-blocker therapy that has drawn a great deal of interest in the last decade or so is the use of prophylactic treatment in the survivors of acute myocardial infarction. It has been shown that when these drugs are commenced between 4 and 28 days following acute infarction and continued for 90 days or longer, there is a consistent and highly significant reduction (18 to 39%) in sudden cardiac death and a fall in the reinfarction rate between 35 and 40% (3-6) in the first year following infarction. The reduction in mortality occurred regardless of age, sex, race, site of infarction, or the comparative risk profile of the patients, although, as might be expected, the beneficial effect was more readily demonstrable in those at the highest risk for a coronary event. This was particularly striking in the case of postinfarct patients with markedly reduced ventricular function. It should also be stressed that the beneficial effect could not be related systematically to the associated properties of different beta-blockers such as cardioselectivity or the local anesthetic effects. As it will be emphasized later in this chapter, the beneficial effect was somewhat linearly correlated with the degree of heart rate reduction indicating that the fundamental mechanism stemmed from the blocking of beta-receptors.

While the impact of beta blockade on the mortality figures is beyond dispute, the precise mechanism(s) mediating the observed salutary effect is in doubt. From pooled data from 18,000 postinfarct patients, the average reduction in mortality from randomized trials was about 20% (3). The exact details of individual trials are presented elsewhere in this monograph. The reduction in sudden death by beta-blockers was even more striking than in the reduction of total mortality. It was about 30% with 95% confidence limits of 20 to 40% (3).

Since pharmacological therapy is unlikely to substantively alter the level of ventricular function resulting from blighted myocardium, the roles of the other two factors need to be considered as the basis for the salutary effects. The first relates to the effects of beta-blockers on myocardial ischemia and its hemodynamic and metabolic determinants. The other stems from the actions of these agents on the electrical instability occurring independently of ischemia. The purpose of this chapter is to critically examine experimental and clinical studies to see whether data from specific pharmacological probes might provide insights into these two potential mechanisms. The emerging data indicate the critical role of heart rate reduction as the key to the efficacy of pharmacological agents in reducing sudden death in patients surviving acute myocardial infarction.

POTENTIAL ROLE OF EFFECTS ON ISCHEMIA IN MEDIATING THE REDUCTION OF SUDDEN DEATH BY BETA BLOCKADE

Both calcium channel blockers and beta-blockers have been tested for their cardioprotective effects in the survivors of acute myocardial infarction. There is limited data on the effects of nitrates and they will not be discussed here. There is convincing in vitro and in vivo experimental data that beta-blockers and calcium channel blockers exert a significant cardioprotective effect in the ischemic myocardium (7,8-27). They exert a beneficial effect on ischemic ventricular arrhythmias (12,21,22), reduce myocardial infarct size (16,26,27), improve segmental ventricular wall motion abnormalities (28), and elevate ventricular fibrillation threshold (18,25). In the open-chest as well as closed-chest canine model of experimental myocardial ischemia, calcium channel blockers have been shown to significantly increase endocardial perfusion (17,28); such an effect appeared less striking in the case of beta-blockers although clearly significant (28). Numerous experimental studies indicate a marked beneficial effect of calcium channel blockers in ventricular reperfusion arrhythmias (29) as well as in the model of "stunned" myocardium (30). Consistent with these experimental data are the findings from extensive clinical studies with subjective and objective end points indicating that both calcium channel blockers and beta-blockers exert equipotent or close to equipotent anti-ischemic effects in patients with coronary artery disease. However, there are differences between the two classes of drugs that need emphasis. Calcium channel blockers do not adversely affect the lipid profile of patients; in experimental animals they have been shown to exert an antiatherogenic action (31), and, at least in one recent study (32), they have been shown to prevent the development of new atherosclerotic lesions during serial coronary angiography. Such data have not been reported for beta-blockers, which have the propensity to increase plasma lipids.

CALCIUM CHANNEL BLOCKERS AND CARDIOPROTECTION: SIGNIFICANCE OF THEIR VARIABLE EFFECTS ON HEART RATE

There is, therefore, a compelling reason for calcium channel blockers to exert a favorable effect on sudden death by ameliorating ischemia in the survivors of acute myocardial infarction in the event the data obtained to date have been either negative, inconclusive, or demonstrating a possibly deleterious effect (33). For example, in the case of verapamil, the first calcium antagonist which has been investigated with the aim to reduce mortality and reinfarction rate in infarct survivors, the results are inconclusive (34-37). In this 1436-patient study, 717 were treated with verapamil and 719 with placebo. At the end of 6 months, the mortality in the treated group was 12.8% and 13.9% in the placebo series. At 12 months the corresponding figures were 15.2% versus 16.4%. Although a trend in mortality reduction was evident in this study, it is clear that the drug, given early, did not significantly influence early mortality from acute myocardial infarction.

Yusuf and Furberg (33) have recently reviewed most of the randomized trials of calcium antagonists following acute myocardial infarction. They combined all the mortality data by the Mantel-Haenszel method (33) for each of the calcium antagonists for which data were available from short-term and long-term trials and for all the trials in total. They calculated a pooled odds ratio and its 98% confidence limits aimed at providing a typical estimate of the effects of the individual agents on mortality.

The data summarized in Table 1 indicate that 13,139 patients were studied in nine randomized controlled trials (33). It is noteworthy that eight of the nine trials showed *a small excess of mortality* in the treated group, although the difference from the effects of placebo did not reach a statistical significance. There were 574 deaths among the 6567 patients randomized to the active treatment group (8.7%); in the control group there were 545 deaths in a population of 6572 (8.3%). This gave an odds ratio of 1.06 with 95% confidence interval of 0.94-1.20. The results were similar when the data were split according to whether the trials evaluated early treatment or when treatment was delayed 1-2 weeks following myocardial infarction. It was of interest that an excess but nonsignificant mortality was consistently observed with all of the above agents (38-42). However, while the data on verapamil (one trial with 3464 patients), lidoflazine (one trial with 1792 patients), and nifedipine (5 trials with 7309 patients) were

Table 1 An Overview of Mortality in Trials Evaluating Calcium Channel Blockers Following Myocardial Infarction

Agent (no. studies)	Deaths/Patients Calcium blockers	Deaths/Patients Controls	Observed expected	Variance
Acute, short-term studies				
Verapamil (1)	0/8	2/9	−0.9	0.5
Nifedipine (4)	171/2509	157/2521	+7.5	76.7
Diltiazem (1)	11/287	9/289	+1.0	4.8
Subtotal (6)	182/2802	168/2819	+7.6	82.0
Long-term studies				
Nifedipine (1)	66/1140	64/1139	+1.0	30.7
Lidoflazine (1)	177/896	168/896	+4.5	69.7
Subtotal (2)	243/2036	232/2035	+5.5	100.4
Acute and long-term studies				
Verapamil (1)	149/1729	145/1718	+1.5	67.2
Total (9)	574/6567	545/6572	+14.6	249.6

Typical odds ratio of 1.06; 95% confidence interval (CI) of 0.94 to 1.2, N.S. See text for further details.
Source: Ref. 33.

from reasonably large population samples, the data on diltiazem are limited (only 576 in one trial). Thus, the potential beneficial effect of diltiazem on mortality in patients with myocardial infarction cannot be excluded. This possibility is of particular interest as diltiazem is the calcium antagonist that perhaps has the highest potency for reducing heart rate. The issue of heart rate reduction is of particular importance in this context, especially in the case of diltiazem, in light of more recent trials involving the compound. It so happens that reduction in heart rate appears to be the common denominator in the case of beta-blockers having a salutary effect on sudden death and reinfarction rate in patients surviving infarction (43). Kjekshus (43) carried out an analysis of the most significant beta-blocker trials in the survivors of acute infarction; he found that a linear correlation existed between the degree of heart reduction effected by a beta-blocker and the percentage reduction in sudden death that resulted during chronic prophylaxis with the compound (Fig. 1). It was of interest that those beta-blockers that reduced the heart rate significantly were the only ones that were effective. In contrast, those (e.g., oxprenolol

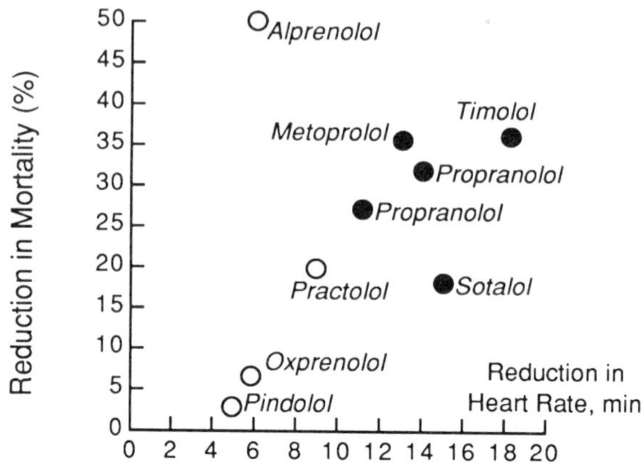

Figure 1 Relationship between heart rate reduction and reduction in mortality induced by beta-blockers in survivors of acute infarction. Note that beta-blockers that have a significant intrinsic sympathomimetic activity with little or no bradycardia effects exert little or no effect on mortality. (From Ref. 43 with the permission of the author and of the Editor of the American Journal of Cardiology.)

or pindolol) that had a marked intrinsic sympathomimetic action and little or no bradycardic response at rest either had no effect on sudden death or tended to *increase* its incidence.

Calcium channel blockers exert variable effects on the 24-hour profile of heart rate. The dihydropyridines either have no effect or tend to increase heart rate over 24 hours while preserving its circadian periodicity. In contrast, both verapamil and diltiazem tend to produce a modest decrease (Figs. 2 and 3), but their effects do not approach those of beta-blockers without intrinsic sympathomimetic actions (Fig. 3). A rate-lowering beta-blocker consistently decreases heart rate markedly and attenuates its circadian periodicity (Fig. 3). Thus, as stressed by Yusuf and Furberg (33), the variable effect of calcium channel blockers on heart rate in men may account for the unexpectedly disappointing results on mortality following calcium antagonists consistent with the failure of this class of drugs to exhibit unequivocally beneficial effect on infarct size, development of myocardial infarction, or reinfarction in trials of myocardial infarction or unstable angina (45). However, the positive data from the recent trial of diltiazem in patients with non-Q wave infarction merits consideration (40). This multicenter randomized double-blind trial (40) involved 576

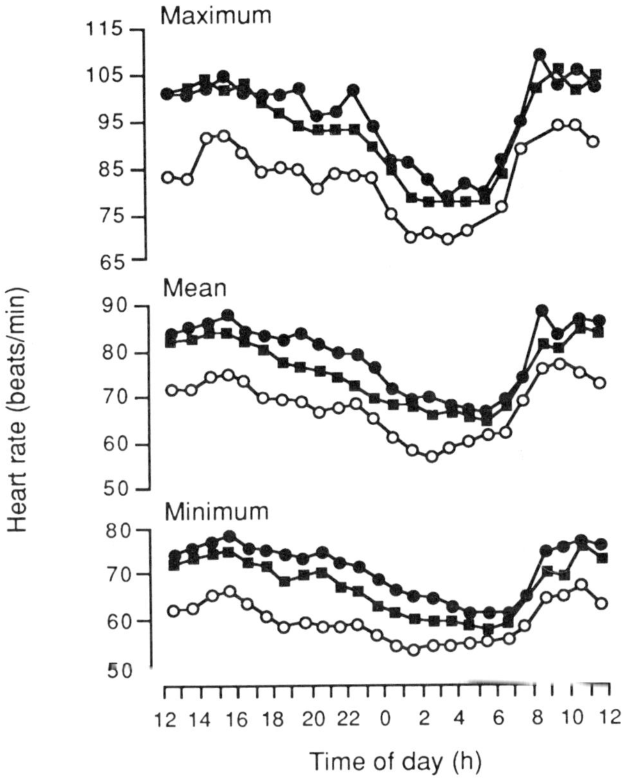

Figure 2 The hourly maximum, mean, and minimum heart rate during double-blind trial comparing verapamil 120 mg three times a day (○) with nifedipine, 20 mg three times a day (●), and placebo in 28 patients (■). Note that the circadian rhythmicity in heart rate is maintained; nifedipine tends to *increase* the heart rate and verapamil to slow it but the mean and maximum heart rates are still high and do not reach the levels induced by beta-blockade. (From Ref. 44 with the permission of the author and of the Editor of the American Journal of Cardiology.)

patients recovering from non-Q wave infarction. Diltiazem (360 mg/day) was given to 278 patients, placebo to 289, for 14 days after acute myocardial infarction. The two groups were identical. The 14-day mortality was similar in both groups, but reinfarction occurred in 26 patients on placebo and 11 in the diltiazem group. The difference of 42% was significant ($p < 0.04$). It is striking that there was a very low incidence of mortality (3%)

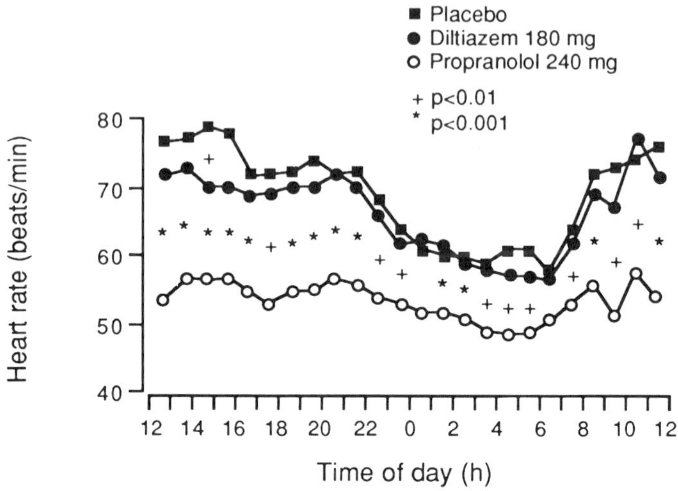

Figure 3 The 24-hour ambulatory minimum heart rate on placebo, diltiazem, 180 mg/day, in 14 patients with stable angina. Note that diltiazem hardly affects the minimum heart rate during the 24-hour monitoring while propranolol (240 mg/day) consistently and significantly reduces it. (From Ref. 44 with the permission of the author and of the Editor of American Journal of Cardiology.)

in both the treated as well as the placebo groups, but one important feature of the patients entering the study was that 61% of them were treated concurrently with beta-blockers. It may well be that the demonstrated salutary effect of diltiazem on reinfarction may be greatest in the presence of beta blockade, a finding also noted in trials involving patients with unstable angina (45) in which a calcium antagonist was combined with a beta-blocker. A major reduction in heart rate is likely during a combination regimen of diltiazem and a beta-blocker. An analysis of changes in heart rate in patients taking both beta-blockers and diltiazem versus diltiazem alone relative to the beneficial effect might have been of much interest.

An intriguing observation was made in another larger trial (46) in which 2466 patients surviving Q and non-Q wave acute infarction and being treated with or without beta-blockers were randomized in a double-blind fashion into one group given diltiazem and one given placebo. The data showed that the cumulative mortality and reinfarction rates were similar in diltiazem-treated and placebo-treated patients who were followed for a mean period of 25 ± 8 months. There was no significant effect of dilti-

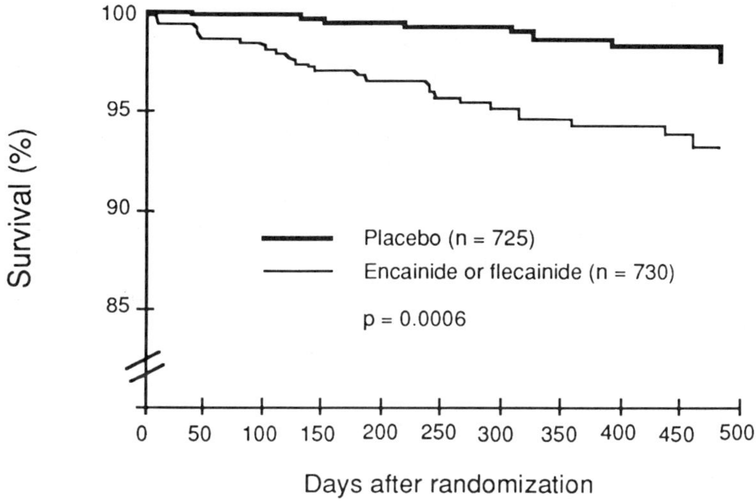

Figure 4 Effects of flecainide, encainide, and placebo on sudden arrhythmic deaths in the survivors of acute myocardial infarction with high-density premature ventricular contractions (PVCs). At the end of about ten months of follow-up, there was about threefold *increase* in mortality on flecainide/encainide despite a substantial degree of suppression of PVCs. It is assured that the excess in mortality in the drug-treated limbs compared to placebo is due to the pro arrhythmic actions of Class 1c agents (see text for more details). (From Ref. 58.)

azem on mortality for the entire group. However, when a subset analysis was performed, it was clear that for patients who had history of pulmonary congestion reflecting a lower ejection fraction, mortality over the follow-up period was *increased*; in the group without pulmonary congestion, there was a significant reduction in mortality. The reason for the difference is not clear. However, the data is in marked contrast to those with beta-blockers in which benefit was evident at all levels of function and appeared to be greater in those with cardiomegaly and pulmonary congestion (47).

BETA-BLOCKADE, HEART RATE, AND MYOCARDIAL ISCHEMIA INTERRELATIONSHIPS

The fact that calcium channel blockers for the most part, do not exert a significant effect in reducing sudden death in the survivors of acute infarction does not negate the possibility that the efficacy of beta-blockers in this regard is mediated at least in part through an action on myocardial ischemia. there are experimental and theoretical reasons for thinking that slowing of heart rate by whatever means might be beneficial in ischemia. As emphasized by Clusin (48), perhaps the most potent means of modulating the severity of ischemia is through the regulation of heart rate (49). The major effect of heart rate on ischemia is generally attributed to alterations in myocardial oxygen demand. However, recent experimental data indicate that changes in oxygen consumption may be less critical (50) than theretofore believed. The major effect of heart rate may stem from the modulation of calcium influx and retention by the ischemic myocardium (48). It is known that myocardial calcium channels open and inactivate during each action potential. Therefore, the number of action potentials per unit time will exert a marked influence on calcium ingress. Since Ca^{2+}-Na^{+} exchange over the plateau range of potentials is voltage-dependent, an increase in time at the plateau voltages will have a significant effect on overall cell calcium load (48). An increase in subendocardial blood flow per minute and per beat in the ischemic zone may also relate, in part, to a reduced number of systolic contractions with a longer period for diastolic perfusion (51). This may be a mechanism to account for increased subendocardial flow per beat after beta-blockade; the longer diastolic period may also allow for recovery of metabolism per beat and over successive beats may contribute to the increased regional contraction in the ischemic zone (28).

The crucial significance of lower rate as an integral component of the action of beta-blockade on regional ischemia during exercise is suggested by studies on exercise after beta-blockade in which the lowered heart rate was returned to the predrug value by atrial pacing (52). The beneficial effects on blood flow as well as on regional contractile function in the ischemic zone evident at lower heart rate were completely abolished at the higher rate produced by pacing (52). These observations are consistent with a recent report that the beneficial effect of propranolol in a model of stunned myocardium was negated by atrial pacing at a rate that was identical to the control heart rate (53). These findings on the importance of lowering heart in ischemia is further emphasized by the use of a specific bradycardic agent (UL FS-49, Thomae Pharmaceutical, Biberach, FRG) in studies in a canine model of chronic coronary artery stenosis (54). As in the case of beta-blockade, a marked improvement in the regional function occurred when changes before and after drug administration were compared during exercise; the change was accompanied by a twofold increase in subendocardial blood flow (54). These experimental data on the effects of specific bradycardic agents is of crucial practical importance. These agents constitute pharmacological probes that may be used to determine the relative importance of the negative chronotropic and inotropic effects in mediating the observed salutary effects of beta-blockers in the survivors of acute myocardial infarction and other ischemic myocardial syndromes. If it can be demonstrated that the beneficial effect in terms of electrical stability and amelioration of ischemia stems largely from heart rate reduction, the data will have important therapeutic implications for the treatment of coronary artery disease, hypertensive heart disease, and other conditions with ventricular hypertrophy such as hypertrophic cardiomyopathy.

REDUCTION IN SUDDEN DEATH BY BETA BLOCKADE BY CONTROLLING VENTRICULAR ARRHYTHMIAS

That adrenergic transmitters play a significant role in the genesis of ventricular arrhythmias has been recognized for many decades (21). For example, it was shown that reserpinization of experimental animals prevented the development of ventricular fibrillation due to cardiac glycoside intoxication in experimental animals (21,22). It has also been found that regional cardiac sympathectomy (23) and left stellate ganglionectomy (24) led to a control of recalcitrant ventricular arrhythmias in man. It is, therefore, assumed that antiarrhythmic actions of beta-blockers stem directly from their ability to reverse the deleterious electrophysiological effects of catecholamines. In recent years, beta-blockers as antiarrhythmic agents have gained prominence, especially in reducing the incidence of sudden cardiac death in the survivors of acute myocardial infarction (4-6), and in the control of recurrent ventricular fibrillation or torsades des pointes in patients with the long QT_c interval syndrome (55). It is, however, far from clear whether the reduction in sudden death by beta-blockers in the survivors of acute myocardial infarction results simply from suppression of asymptomatic ventricular arrhythmias. There are, nevertheless, numerous studies which indicate that most beta-blockers have a significant suppressant effect on PVCs in patients with as well as without cardiac disease (56). The effect is characterized by (1) a significant effect in about 50% of the patients in various series, (2) a higher degree of suppression with respect to the higher grades of PVCs, especially runs of ventricular tachycardia, and (3) abolition or a marked attenuation of the circardian pattern of PVC distribution when present.

There are a number of reasons why it is unlikely that the beneficial effect of beta-blockers on sudden death in survivors of infarction is mediated via the suppression of PVCs. It is known that only about 12-30% of the patients in the postinfarct period have complex ectopic activity, especially runs of ventricular tachycardia (57). Thus, in the various beta-blocker trials a relatively small number of patients with the so-called potentially life-threatening ventricular arrhythmias would have been included. The observed benefit must have occurred independently of effects on PVCs. It has been reported that PVCs tend to increase from the early hospital phase to about 6 weeks after infarction in patients on placebo. On beta-blockers, the tendency was blunted somewhat but not dramatically reduced. A formal analysis of the influence of arrhythmia suppression in the Beta-Blocker Heart Attack Trial (BHAT) showed that patients without the arrhythmia derived as much benefit from the beta-blocker as those who had the arrhythmia on the Holter recordings. Thus, it appears unlikely that such a modest effect on PVCs might lead to a significant effect on sudden death, although this possibility cannot be excluded in certain subsets of patients.

Even with more powerful suppressant agents, a reduction in sudden death in this subset of patients has not been reported. The recent results (58) of the so-called Cardiac Arrhythmia Suppression Trial (CAST) are of particular interest in this regard. CAST was designed to test the effect of flecainide, encainide, and ethmozine versus placebo in the survivors of myocardial infarction with complex PVCs and at high risk for sudden death. After 2 years into the study, it was clear that rather than reducing the incidence of death in the group with encainide or flecainide, there was an *increase* in mortality compared to placebo despite over 80% suppression of PVCs and elimination of ventricular tachycardia beats. The preliminary results of CAST involving 1500 patients revealed that of the 730 patients assigned to encainide or flecaindie and treated an average of 10 months, 56 died or suffered cardiac arrest, while among the 725 given a placebo 23 had died or suffered cardiac arrest. In fact, over a mean treatment duration of 10 months, patients receiving encainide and flecainide sustained a 3.64-fold increase in arrhythmic death/cardiac arrest compared to their respective placebo (Fig. 4). The difference is disturbing and cannot be ignored; rightfully the two drugs were withdrawn from the trial, which is continuing with ethmozine and placebo. The data raise an additional and broader and perhaps a more fundamental issue, suspected for some time, that the reduction of PVCs (it being doubtful whether it is indeed possible to eliminate every PVC that is generated in the heart), however

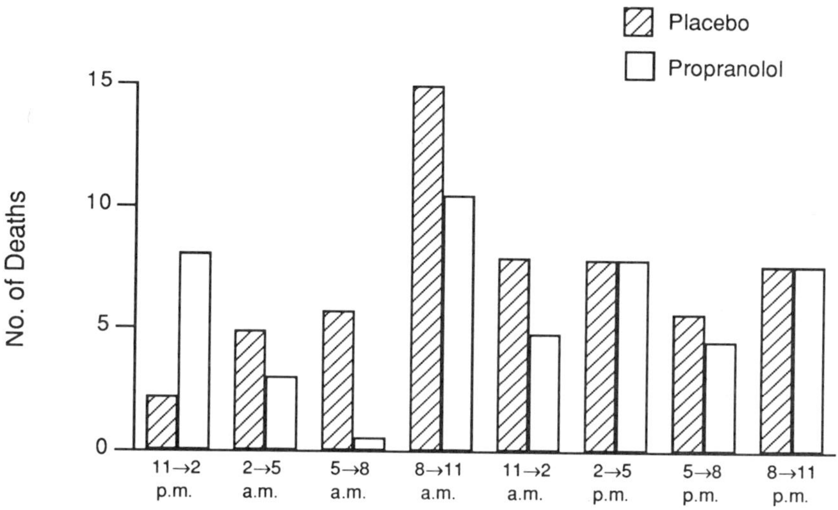

Figure 5 Circadian rhythmicity in the occurrence of sudden death in the Beta-Blocker Heart Attack Trial (BHAT). Note that the effects of propranolol is greatest at a time when the heart rate is lowest (see text for discussion). (From Ref. 66 with the permission of the authors and of the Editor of the American Journal of Cardiology.)

achieved, may not lead directly to a reduction in sudden death. In any event, never has it been established clearly what percentage PVC reduction is needed to effect a meaningful clinical outcome. The CAST results support this premise, at least with respect to the drugs that have a marked propensity to slow conduction. An analysis of the available data on the effects of various antiarrhythmic agents (exclusive of beta-blockers) performed by Furberg (59) indicates either an unfavorable trend with slight increase in mortality or no effect in survivors of acute infarction (Table 2). His analysis of the data taken in conjunction with the CAST results does not appear to support the use of the clinical end point of PVC suppression or of treating asymptomatic arrhythmias as realistic or desirable approaches to a reduction of arrhythmic deaths. As indicated in Table 3, there appears to be no systematic relationship between PVC suppression induced by different antiarrhythmic drugs and their property or preventing VT/VF induction by programmed electrical stimulation of the heart. A lack of concordance in this regard might indicate that the density and

Table 2 Antiarrhythmic Agents and Their Effects on Inducibility of Ventricular Tachycardia and Fibrillation and on PVCs

Test drug by class		Prevention of inducibility of VT/VF by PES [% of patients]	Suppression of PVCs (by >75%) [% of patients]	Suppression of VT beats (by >90%) [% of patients]
Class IA	Quinidine	15-20	60	? 70
	Procainamide	15-25	60	? 70
	Disopyramide	10-20	60	? 70
Class IB	Mexiletine	15	60	>70
	Tocainide	10-15	60	? >70
	Ethmozine	15-20	60	? >70
Class IC	Encainide	10-15	80	90-100
	Flecainide	10-15	80	90-100
	Propafenone	10-20	70	90-100
	Indecainide	10-15	70	90-100
Class II	Beta-blockers (without ISA)	?1-2	50	?70-80
Class III	Amiodarone	8-40	90	90-100
	Sotalol	40-45	50-60	80
Class IV	Verapamil	1-2	≤10	≤10
	Diltiazem	?	≤10	≤10

Data included herein are crude estimates from controlled and uncontrolled studies reported in the literature. However, they provide a reasonable approximation of the overall effects of various antiarrhythmic agents in affecting two major end points used in determining the efficacy of pharmacological therapy of (life-threatening) ventricular arrhythmias. Note the lack of concordance between PVC suppression and the suppression of inducible VT/VF.

Table 3 Retrospective Evaluation of Randomized Antiarrhythmic Trials

Class		Randomized (Pts) active/placebo	Death (Pts) active/placebo
Type IA		1642/1563	122/112
Type IB		6177/6076	196/150
Type IC		1278/1117	97/65
Total		9097/8756	415/327 (+22%)
Type II	Short-term	13,815/13,721	513/586 (−14%)
	Long-term	12,140/11,551	917/1090 (−22%)
Type III		204/193	22/20 (+4%)
Type IV		8870/8887	673/825 (+6%)

Source: Ref. 59.

complexity of PVCs do not provide reliable information about the electrical instability of the substrate for lethal arrhythmias. On the other hand, the possibility is not excluded that reduction or elimination in repetitive beats by agents which have different electrophysiological profiles with no effect on conduction (e.g., beta-blockers) or those with modest depressant effect on conduction (e.g., amiodarone) might be effective in altering mortality in patients with potentially life-threatening ventricular arrhythmias. However, the so-called PVC hypothesis can not be tested with such drugs as they have a complex electrophysiological profile. PVC suppression produced by them may only be a component, perhaps not the most important one, in their overall pharmacological effects that contribute to mortality reduction. Thus, in the case of beta-blockers it remains speculative whether PVC suppression by these agents contributes to their observed salutary effect on mortality in the survivors of acute infarction.

ADRENERGIC BLOCKADE, HEART RATE, AND VENTRICULAR FIBRILLATION THRESHOLD INTERRELATIONSHIPS

One must stress that the beta-blocker trials unlike CAST were *not* suppression trials and the effects on arrhythmias were not evaluated. The reduction in mortality in these trials occurred regardless of age, sex, race, site of infarction, or the comparative risk profile of the patients, although, as might be expected, the beneficial effect was more readily demonstrable in those at the highest risk for a coronary event. When the drugs were given intravenously early during the course of infarction, the frequency of occurrence of ventricular fibrillation was significantly reduced (60, 61). Norris et al. (61) showed that when propranolol was administered about the time of presumed coronary occlusion and continued subsequently, it significantly reduced the incidence of ventricular fibrillation in hospital when its effects were compared to those of a matching placebo. The metoprolol study (60) showed no effects of the beta-blocker on PVCs but had a significant effect on the occurrence of VF. There were 17 cases of VF in the placebo group (out of 697 patients) but only 6 episodes of VF in the beta-blocker treated group from 698 patients ($p < 0.05$). Clearly, the antiectopic effects of beta-blockers are dissociated from their antifibrillatory actions. It is known that ischemia and catecholamines reduce ventricular fibrillation threshold; beta-blockers might abort sudden death by elevating it (25). The benefit of beta-blockers could not be correlated with the associated properties of beta-blockers, namely, cardioselectivity or local anesthetic actions. As indicated above, the observed benefit was, however, correlated negatively with their sympathomimetic actions. For example, drugs such as pindolol or oxprenolol with significant sympathomimetic activity either had no effect or were deleterious. The effects of beta-blockers that have a marked sympathomimetic effect (e.g., pindolol) on ventricular fibrillation threshold is not known. As already indicated, the reduction in mortality from sudden death could be correlated linearly with the decrease in heart rate (see Fig. 1) emphasizing the significance of antiadrenergic effect. It is of interest that other causes of bradycardia might also exert antifibrillatory effects. For example, recently it was shown that in rabbits made hypothyroid, the ventricular fibrillation threshold was significantly elevated compared to euthyroid controls and markedly reduced in rabbits made thyrotoxic by thyroid hormone injection (62). In these studies, the changes in ventricular fibrillation threshold was correlated inversely but significantly with heart rate. It is also known that reduction of heart rate to levels below control by vagal stimulation has antifibrillatory effects (48). Scherlag et al. (63) found that vagal stimulation abolished arrhythmias during coronary occlusion in an open-chest canine model of experimental infarction. These observations indicating an inverse correlation between the occurrence of ventricular fibrillation and heart rate are likely to have important clinical implications. They emphasize the importance of slow heart rate in maintaining electrical stability in the ischemic myocardium.

What might be the "ideal" heart rate for patients with various ischemic myocardial syndromes, nonetheless, remains essentially a matter for conjecture. However, before the days of routine beta-blocker therapy Norris et al. (64) showed that in postinfarct survivors the average heart rate at the time of hospital discharge was an important determinant of prognosis. Those with lower heart rates had better survival during follow-up. It is also known that the circadian rhythmicity in sudden death closely parallels that of heart rate and catecholamine surges (65). The fewest deaths occurred between midnight and 8 a.m. In the BHAT data, the effects of propranolol on circadian rhythmicity was examined by Peters et al. (66). Propranolol had a variable effect on the incidence of sudden death between 8 a.m. and 11 p.m. In contrast, the beta-blocker produced a most striking decrease on the incidence of sudden death between the hours of 2 and 8 a.m. (see Fig. 5), undoubtedly coincident with the most pronounced bradycardic response, emphasizing again the significance of lowering heart rate in the postinfarct patient. It should be emphasized that the exaggerated reduction in heart rate on a beta-blocker in the early hours of the morning might be due in part to a vagal dominance resulting from the block of sympathetic impulse traffic to the sinus node. This suggests that the slowing of heart rate by interventions that reduce the action of sympathetic transmitters to the heart might be beneficial in the setting of acutely or chronically ischemic myocardium in part by augmenting vagal activity, which has been demonstrated to be associated with an antifibrillatory activity in the ventricle (63).

BRADYCARDIA, PROLONGED REPOLARIZATION, AND VENTRICULAR FIBRILLATION THRESHOLD: INSIGHTS FROM STUDIES ON AMIODARONE

In a series of studies, an interesting observation has been reported by Raine and Vaughan Williams (67) on the changes in the cardiac action potentials in the rabbit myocardium from animals chronically treated with a variety of beta-blockers. They found that agents such as propranolol and acebutolol produced a modest but significant lengthening of the action potential duration (67) but without effect on the upstroke velocity of phase 0. It was postulated that such a change represented a physiological adaptation to chronic sympathetic blockade. The observed prolongation of the action potential duration was therefore considered a mechanism for the reduction of sudden death by beta-blockade. The clinical counterparts of these studies have been conflicting. There have been studies with the monophasic action potential measurements using suction electrodes which have both confirmed as well as denied the prolongation of repolarization (68,69). Measurements of the QT_c intervals in man following chronic beta-blockade have shown that repolarization may shorten, prolong, or not change at all (69,70). However, to date the circadian rhythmicity of QT/QT_c changes induced by chronic beta-blockade has not been determined. Such a rhythmicity for QT_c in normal subjects is known to be out of phase with the heart rate being longest when the sinus frequency is the lowest (71). Therefore, it is possible that beta-blockers do prolong the QT_c but only during the sleep cycle. The effect of homogeneously prolonging repolarization with a corresponding increase in the ventricular effective refractory period might be antifibrillatory and contribute to sudden death reduction in the early hours of the morning. Whether the ventricular effective refractory period does increase as a function of chronic beta-blockade has not been determined, but, in light of these considerations, it clearly is a relevant issue for verification.

A clinical context which on many counts resembles the long-term administration of beta-blockers is the chronic administration of amiodarone. The drug is a complex iodinated molecule that slows the heart rate in a stepwise fashion as a function of time, exhibits significant antiischemic properties, antagonizes sympathetic excitation, and elevates ventricular fibrillation threshold (72). It has a significant effect in suppressing PVCs and in both experimental models as well as in man it prevents the occurrence of sudden death (72) being effective in over two thirds of patients with life-threatening ventricular arrhythmias when other agents fail. For this reason, the effects of amiodarone, *a complex agent that consistently and markedly reduces heart rate* (74), on mortality in the survivors of acute infarction is of interest. Preliminary data from a recent study (73) in which 312 patients following myocardial infarction with complex PVCs were randomized into three treatments are of importance. The first group ($n = 114$) were not given antiarrhythmic treatment; the second group ($n = 100$) was given conventional antiarrhythmic treatment with agents and doses adjusted to produce a define degree of PVC suppression; and a third group ($n = 98$) was treated with amiodarone with an initial loading dose followed by a low maintenance dose. The follow-up period was 12 months. At the end of this period there were 15 cases of sudden deaths in the untreated group, 12 in the group with individualized antiarrhythmic therapy, and 5 in the amiodarone group ($p < 0.05$ compared to the first group). The data indicated that amiodarone had the potential to reduce sudden death in the survivors of myocardial infarction, but the numbers of patients in each of the groups were too small to permit an analysis of the link between sudden death and the degree of suppression of complex PVCs. It is likely that, as in the case of beta-blockers, the beneficial effect is related to the antifibrillatory actions of the drug rather than its antiectopic property. A number of larger and placebo-controlled trials are being initiated to determine whether the results of this pilot study will be confirmed. In the meantime, the use of amiodarone in patients surviving myocardial infarction and having complex ventricular ectopy cannot be recommended in a routine fashion; its use in this context should take cognizance of its complex and potentially deleterious side effects relative to the expected beneficial effect on mortality. Nevertheless, the properties of the drug and those of beta-blockers clearly provide important pharmacological probes to define the critical determinants of efficacy of a compound for mortality reduction in high risk survivors of myocardial infarction.

COMMENTS AND CONCLUSIONS

There is now little doubt that beta-blockers reduce the incidence of sudden death and reinfarction in the survivors of acute myocardial infarction. However, the precise mechanism mediating the salutary effect is not known. It is likely to be complex and multifactorial, perhaps resulting largely from the competitive attenuation of the ischemic and arrhythmogenic influences of sympathetic stimulation. From the available techniques, it appears difficult to precisely quantify the relative importance of effects on collateral blood flow, myocardial substrate utilization, myocardial oxygen demand, platelet aggregability or even triggers of sustained electrical disturbances in the ischemic myocardium. What has emerged somewhat compellingly from a growing experimental and clinical database is the key role of heart rate in modulating not only the severity of ischemia but also the vulnerability to ventricular fibrillation in the ischemic myocardium. The evidence stems not only from the acute and chronic effects of beta-blockade on indices of ischemia and electrical stability but also from other bradycardic situations such as sustained vagal stimulation, chronic amiodarone administration, and hypothyroidism. Preliminary experimental and clinical data with a novel class of specific bradycardic agents are also consistent. The importance of these agents as pharmacological probes to elucidate the significance of selective reduction in heart rate in ameliorating ischemia and electrical instability in the survivors of infarction and in other subsets of patients with coronary artery disease should be emphasized. In this context, the preliminary data of Beere et al. (77) indicating a retarding effect of lowered heart rate on coronary atherosclerosis is of importance. They produced bradycardia in six cynamolgus monkeys by sinoatrial nodel ablation by surgery; eight animals undergoing a sham operation served as controls. Both series of monkeys were fed on an atherogenic high cholesterol diet for 6 months. Heart rates were monitored for 24-hour test periods repeatedly.

At the end of 6 months, the extent of coronary atherosclerosis in animals with postoperative heart rates lower than the preoperative mean for all of the animals that underwent surgery was less than half that of the animals with heart rates above the mean or of diet-fed control animals not subjected to surgery. These data indicate that heart rate per se may contribute to mechanisms responsible for the development of coronary artery disease since the two groups did not differ in blood pressure, serum lipids, or body weight. In a similar recent study (78) involving 26 months' duration, propranolol given chronically was found to inhibit coronary atherosclerosis in behaviorally predisposed monkeys fed an atherogenic diet. Thus, in determining mechanisms that mediate the cardioprotective effects of pharmacological agents in ischemic heart disease not only the short-term effects on ischemia and electrical instability merit consideration but also their antiatherogenic potential. It is likely that the heart rate lowering effect of beta-adrenergic blockade plays an integral role both during short-term as well as long-term drug administration in the survivors of acute infarction.

ACKNOWLEDGMENTS

I am much indebted to Francesca Frederick and Lawrence Kimble for help in preparing this chapter. The work was supported by grants from the Medical Research Service of the Veterans Administration and the American Heart Association, the Greater Los Angeles Affiliate, Los Angeles, California.

REFERENCES

1. Cruickshank JM, Prichard BNC. Beta-blockers in Clinical Practice. Edinburgh: Churchill Livingstone, 1987:1-1003.
2. Kannel WB, Abbott RD. Incidence and prognosis of unrecognized myocardial infarction. N Engl J Med 1984; 311:1144-50.
3. Yusuf S, Peto R, Lewis J, Collins R, Sleight P. Beta-blockade during and after myocardial infarction: an overview of the randomized trials. Prog Cardiovasc Dis 1985; 27:235-371.
4. Norwegian Multicenter Study Group. Timolol induced reduction in mortality and reinfarction in patients surviving acute myocardial infarction. New Engl J Med 1981; 304:801-6.
5. Beta-Blocker Heart Attack Trial Research Group. A randomized trial of propranolol in patients with acute myocardial infarction. I. Mortality results. JAMA 1982; 247:1707-15.
6. ISIS-1 Collaborative Group. Randomized trial of intravenous atenolol among 16,027 cases of suspected acute myocardial infarction. Lancet 1986; 2:57-66.
7. Singh BN, Nayler WG. The role of calcium antagonists in acute myocardial infarction. In: E. Rapaport, ed. Early interventions in acute myocardial infarction. Boston: Kluwer Academic Publications, 1989:123-42.
8. Nayler WG, Ferrari R, Williams A. Protective effect of pretreatment with verapamil, nifedipine and propranolol on mitochondrial function in the ischemic and reperfused myocardium. Am J Cardiol 1980; 46:242-8.
9. Bourdillon PD, Poole-Wilson PA. The effects of verapamil, quiescence and cardioplegia on calcium exchange and mechanical function in ischemic rabbit myocardium. Circ Res 1982; 50:360-8.

10. Reimer KA, Lowe JE, Jennings RB. Effect of the calcium antagonist verapamil on necrosis following temporary coronary artery occlusion in dogs. Circ 1977; 55:581-7.
11. Nayler WG. The pharmacological protection of the ischemic heart: The use of calcium antagonists and beta-adrenoceptor antagonists. Europ Heart J 1980; 1:5-13.
12. Kaumann AJ, Aramendia P. Prevention of ventricular fibrillation induced by coronary ligation. J Pharm Exp Ther 1968; 166:326-40.
13. Henry PD, Shuchleib R, Davis J, Weiss ES, Sobel BE. Myocardial contracture and accumulation of mitochondrial calcium in ischemic rabbit heart. Am J Physiol 1977; 233:H677-H684.
14. Nayler WG. Protection of the myocardium against post-ischemic reperfusion damage. J Thorac Cardiovasc Surg 1982; 84:897-905.
15. Hamm CW, Opie LH. Protection of infarcting myocardium by slow-channel inhibitors. Circ Res (Suppl 1) 1983; 52:129-38.
16. Smith HJ, Singh BN, Nisbet HD, Norris RM. Effects of verapamil on infarct size following experimental coronary occlusion. Cardiovasc Res 1975; 9:569-78.
17. Henry PD, Shuchleib R, Borda LJ, Roberts R, Williams JR, Sobel BE. Effects of nifedipine on myocardial perfusion and ischemic injury in dogs. Circ Res 1978; 43:372-80.
18. Thandroyen FT. Protective action of calcium channel antagonist agents against ventricular fibrillation in the isolated perfused rat heart. J Mol Cell Cardiol 1982; 14:21-32.
19. Opie LH, Coetzee WA, Dennis SC, Thandroyen FT. A potential role of calcium ions in early ischemic and reperfusion arrhythmias. Ann NY Acad Sci 1988; 522:464-77.
20. Blake K, Clusin WT. Reduction of ischemic myocardial depolarization and extracellular potassium accumulation by diltiazem. Europ J Pharmacol 1988; 127:261-5.
21. Singh BN, Jewitt DE. β-Adrenoceptor blocking drugs in cardiac arrhythmias. Drugs 1974; 7:426-43.
22. Jewitt DE, Singh BN. The use of adrenergic blockade in myocardial infarction. Prog Cardiovasc Dis 1976; 16:421.
23. Ebert PA, Allgood RJ, Sabiston DC. The anti-arrhythmic effects of cardiac denervation. Ann Surg 1968; 168:728.
24. Cox WV, Robertson HF. The effect of stellate ganglionectomy on the cardiac function of intact dogs and its effect on extent of myocardial infarction and on cardiac function following coronary artery occlusion. Am Heart J 1936; 12:285.
25. Anderson JL, Rodier HE, Green LA. Comparative effects of β-adrenergic drugs on experimental ventricular fibrillation threshold. Am J Cardiol 1983; 51:1096-102.
26. Maroko PR, Braunwald E. Modification of myocardial infarct size after coronary occlusion. Ann Int Med 1973; 79:720-9.

27. Peter CT, Norris R, Clarke ED, Heng M, Singh BN. Propranolol in the treatment of acute myocardial infarction. Circ 1974; 57:1091-5.
28. Ross J. Mechanisms of regional ischemia and anti-anginal drug action during exercise. Prog Cardiovasc Dis 1989; 21:455-66.
29. Opie LH, Coetzee NA. Role of calcium ions in reperfusion arrhythmias: relevance to pharmacologic intervention. Cardiovasc Drugs and Ther 1988; 2:623-636.
30. Bush LR, Buja LM, Tilton G, Wathan M, Appril P, Ashton J, Willerson JT. Effects of propranolol and diltiazem alone or in combination on the recovery of left ventricular segmental function after temporary coronary occlusion and long-term reperfusion in porcine hearts. J Amer Coll Cardiol 1987; 10:906-16.
31. Rouleau J-L, Parmley WW, Stevens J, Wikman-Coffelt J, Sievers R, Mahley RM, Hovel RJ. Verapamil suppresses atherosclerosis in cholesterol-fed rabbits. J Amer Coll Cardiol 1:1453-60.
32. Lichtlen PR, Hugenholtz P, Rofflenbeul W, Jost S, Hecker H, and the INTACT Study Group for Retardation of the Progression of Coronary Artery Disease with Nifedipine. Results of INTACT. Circ 1989; 80:II-382.
33. Yusuf S, Furberg CD. Effects of calcium-channel blockers on survival after acute myocardial infarction. Cardiovasc Drugs and Thera 1987; 1:343-4.
34. Hansen JF, Sigurd B, Mellemgaard K, Lynby I. Verapamil in acute myocardial infarction. Dan Med Bull 1980; 27:105-9.
35. Danish Multicenter Study Group. Verapamil in myocardial infarction. Clin Pharmacol Exp Physiol 1982; 6:89-96.
36. Danish Multicenter Study Group. Verapamil in myocardial infarction. Europ Heart J 1984; 4:516-28.
37. Danish Multicenter Study Group. Verapamil in myocardial infarction. Am J Cardiol 1984; 54:24E-28E.
38. Crea F, Deanfield J, Crean P, Sharom M, Davies G, Maseri A. Effects of verapamil in preventing early post infarction angina and reinfarction. Am J Cardiol 1985; 55:900-4.
39. Norwegian Nifedipine Group. Nifedipine in acute myocardial infarction. No influence on enzymatic infarct size. Acta Med Scan 1983; 68:22 (abstr).
40. Gibson RS, Boden WE, Theroux P, Strauss HD, Pratt CM, Gheorghiade M, Capone RJ, Crawford MH, Schlant RC, Kleiger RE, Young PM, Schechtman K, Perryman MB, Roberts R. Diltiazem and reinfarction in patients with non-Q wave MI. NEJM 1986; 315:423-9.
41. de Geest R, Kesteloot H, Piessens J. Secondary prevention ischemic heart disease: a long-term controlled lidoflazine study. Acta Cardiol 1979; 24:7-26.
42. The Israeli SPRINT Study Group. Secondary prevention reinfarction Israeli nifedipine trial (SPRINT): a randomized intervention trial of nidedipine in patients with acute myocardial infarction. Eur Heart J 1988; 9:354-64.
43. Kjekshus JK. Importance of heart rate in determining beta-blocking efficacy in acute and long-term myocardial infarction trials. Amer J Cardiol 1986; 57:43F-49F.

44. Balasubramanian BV. Clinical and research applications of ambulatory Holter ST-segment and heart rate monitoring. Amer J Cardiol 1986; 58:11B-20B.
45. Holland Interuniversity Nifedipine/Metoprolol Trial (HINT) Research Group. Early treatment of unstable angina in the coronary care unit: a randomized, double-blind placebo controlled comparison of recurrent ischemia in patients treated with nifedipine or metoprolol or both. Br Heart J 1986; 56:400-13.
46. The Multicenter Diltiazem Post Infarction Trial Research Group. The effect of diltiazem on mortality and reinfarction after myocardial infarction. N Engl J Med 1988; 319:385-92.
47. Chadda K, Goldstein S, Byington R, Curb JD. Effect of propranolol after acute myocardial infarction in patients with heart failure. Circ 1986; 73:503-10.
48. Clusin WT. What is the solution to sudden cardiac death: calcium modulation or arrhythmia clinics? Cardiovasc Drugs and Therapy 1987; 1:335-42.
49. Blake K, Smith NA, Clusin WT. Rate-dependence of ischemic myocardial depolarization-evidence for a novel membrane current. Cardiovasc Res 1986; 20:557-62.
50. Clusin WT, Opie LH, Thandroyen F. Drastic reduction of cardiac work fails to mimic the antifibrillatory effect of low calcium. Circulation 1984; 70: II-346.
51. Bache RJ, Cobb FR. Effect of maximal coronary vasodilation on transmural perfusion during tachycardia in the awake drug. Circ Res 1977; 41:648-53.
52. Guth BD, Heusch G, Seiteberger R, Ross J Jr. Mechanism of beneficial effect of beta-adrenergic blockade on exercise-induced-ischemia in conscious dogs. Circ Res 1987; 738-46.
53. Al-Wathiqui MH, Farber N, Pele L, Gross GJ, Brooks HL, Warltier DC. Improvement in functional recovery of stunned canine myocardium by long-term pretreatment with oral propranolol. Amer Heart J 1987; 117:791-8.
54. Guth BD, Heusch G, Ross J Jr. Elimination of exercise-induced regional myocardial dysfunction by a bradycardia agent in dogs with chronic coronary stenosis. Circ 1987; 75:661-9.
55. Schwartz PH. Idiopathic long QT syndrome: progress and questions. Am Heart 1985; 109:399-410.
56. Singh BN, Nademanee K. Antihypertensive compounds as anti-arrhythmic agents: focus on beta-blocking drugs in ventricular arrhythmias. Am Heart J 1987; 114:1040-50.
57. Bigger JT. Definition of benign versus malignant ventricular arrhythmias: target for treatment. Am J Cardiol 1983; 52:47c-53c.
58. The Cardiac Arrhythmia Suppression Trial (CAST) Investigators Preliminary Report. Effect of encainide and flecainide on mortality in a randomized trial of arrhythmia suppression after myocardial infarction. New Engl J Med 1989; 321:406-12.
59. Furberg CD. Effects of antiarrhythmic drugs on mortality after myocardial infarction. Am J Cardiol 1983; 53:32c-36c.

60. Ryden L, Arciniego R, Arnonan K. A double-blind trial of metoprolol in acute myocardial infarction: Effects on ventricular tachyarrhythmias. N Engl J Med 1983; 308:614-18.
61. Norris RM, Brown MA, Clarke ED, Barney PF, Geary GG, Logan RI. Prevention of ventricular fibrillation during acute myocardial infarction by intravenous propranolol. Lancet 1984; 2:883-6.
62. Venkatesh N, Kuhle WE, Feld GK, Singh BN. Hypothyroidism elevates ventricular fibrillation threshold in rabbits. J Amer Coll Cardiol 1988; 11:41A.
63. Scherlag BJ, El-Sherif N, Hope R, Lazzara R. Characterization and localization of ventricular arrhythmias resulting from myocardial ischemia and infarction. Circ Res 1974; 35:372-77.
64. Norris RM, Mercer CJ, Yeates BE. Sinus rate in acute myocardial infarction. Brit Heart J 1972; 9:901-4.
65. Willich SN, Levy D, Rocco MB, Tofler GH, Stone PH, Muller JE. Circadian variation in the incidence of sudden cardiac death in the Framingham Heart Study Population. Am J Cardiol 1987; 60:801-6.
66. Peters RW, Muller JE, Goldstein G, Byington R, Friedman LM. Effect of beta-blockers on circadian variation of sudden cardiac death in survivors of myocardial infarction. Am J Cardiol 1987; 63:1518-20.
67. Raine AEG, Vaughan Williams EM. Adaptation to prolonged beta-blockade on rabbit atrial, Purkinje and ventricular potentials and papillary muscle contractions. Circ Res 1981; 48:804.
68. Edvaardson N, Olsson B. Effects of acute and chronic beta-blockade on ventricular repolarization in man. Brit Heart J 1981; 45:626-32.
69. Duff H, Roden DM, Brorson L, Wood AJJ, Dawson AK, Primm K, Oates JA, Smith RF, Woosley RL. Electrophysiologic actions of high plasma concentrations of propranolol in human subjects. J Amer Coll Cardiol 1983; 2:1134-40.
70. Stern S, Eisenberg S. The effect of propranolol on the electrocardiogram of normal subjects. Brit Heart J 1969; 77:192-6.
71. Sarma JSM, Venkataraman K, Nicod P, Polikar R, Smith J, Schoenbaum MP, Singh BN. Circadian rhythmicity of rate-corrected QT interval in hypothyroidism: significance for the development of Class III antiarrhythmic agents. Amer J Cardiol 1990.
72. Singh BN. Amiodarone: historical development and pharmacologic profile. Am Heart J 1983; 106:788-96.
73. Nademanee K, Stevenson WG, Weiss J, Singh BN. The role of amiodarone in the survivors of sudden arrhythmic deaths. In: Singh BN, ed. Control of Cardiac Arrhythmias by Lengthening Repolarization. Mt. Kisco, NY: Futura Publishing Co., 1988:489-508.
74. Pritchard DA, Singh BN, Hurley PJ. Effects of amiodarone on thyroid function in patients with ischemic heart disease. Brit Heart J 1975; 37:856-61.
75. Burkart F, Pfisterer M, Kiowski W, Burckhardt D, Follath F. Improved survival of patients with sympatomatic ventricular arrhythmias after myocardial infarction with amiodarone: a randomized controlled trial. Circ 1989; 80:II-119.

76. Indolfi C, Guth BD, Miura T, Miyazaki S, Schulz R, Ross J. Mechanisms of improved ischemic regional dysfunction by bradycardia: studies on UL-FS49 in swine. Circ 1989; 80:983-93.
77. Beere PA, Glagov S, Zarins CK. Retarding effect of lowered heart rate on coronary atherosclerosis. Science 1985; 226:180-2.
78. Kaplan JR, Manuck SB, Adams MR, Weingard KW, Clarkson TB. Propranolol inhibits coronary atherosclerosis in behaviorally predisposed monkeys fed on atherogenic diet. Circ 1987; 76:1364-72.

6

Effects of Beta-Blockers on Cardiac Arrhythmia in Acute Myocardial Infarction: The BHAT Experience

Edgar Lichstein
Maimonides Medical Center and State University of New York—Health Science Center at Brooklyn, Brooklyn, New York

PROPRANOLOL DECREASES MORTALITY AFTER MYOCARDIAL INFARCTION

Beta-blockers decrease mortality after myocardial infarction. This statement is no longer controversial since the publication of several large well-controlled studies (1-4). Yusuf (5), in an extensive review, concluded that all available data support the conclusion that beta-adrenergic blocking agents decrease mortality, the incidence of nonfatal reinfarction, and sudden death after infarction.

The only questions that remain are whether or not this is a class action of all beta-blockers and what is the mechanism of action. The European Infarction Study (6) studied the effects of oxprenolol and was one of the few studies with negative results. The study had to be stopped prematurely because of an increase in mortality noted in the study group. It is thought that the negative results may have been due to the intrinsic agonist activity of oxprenolol (7).

POSSIBLE EXPLANATIONS FOR DECREASED MORTALITY

Mortality following myocardial infarction may be due to recurrent ischemia, arrhythmia, or left ventricular dysfunction (8). Possible mechanisms by which beta-blockers protect ischemic myocardium include (9): (1) blockade of beta-receptors resulting in a decrease in myocardial oxygen consumption, (2) blockade of beta-receptors and of sympathetic nervous activity, (3) alteration of substrate utilization, (4) increase in collateral blood flow, (5) decrease of microvascular damage, and (6) stabilization of cell membranes (11). It may be difficult to separate the effects of ischemia from arrhythmia in the postinfarction patient. Catecholamines increase myocardial oxygen consumption and may, therefore, increase ischemia (10). Beta-blocking drugs reduce the effects of these catecholamines by decreasing blood pressure, heart rate, and myocardial contractility. Cyclic adenosine monophosphate (AMP), which accumulates in ischemic zones of animals with myocardial infarction, is arrhythmogenic, and its occurrence may be prevented by beta-blockers (11).

Ventricular arrhythmia after myocardial infarction is a marker for increased mortality. Although it is difficult to separate ventricular arrhythmia from ventricular function, it does appear that complex forms of ventricular arrhythmia are independent markers of mortality (12).

BETA-BLOCKERS DECREASE VPB FREQUENCY AFTER MYOCARDIAL INFARCTION

Beta-blockers have been used for many years in treating ventricular arrhythmias. Woosley et al (13) evaluated the antiarrhythmic efficacy of propranolol in 32 patients with chronic high frequency VPBs and various forms of cardiac disease. They attempted to relate propranolol level to VPB suppression and found that the antiarrhythmic effect of propranolol in many patients required plasma concentrations higher than usually associated with beta blockade. They postulated that suppression of renin release also occurs at these dose levels and might play a role in arrhythmia suppression.

Koppes et al. (14) evaluated the use of propranolol in treating VPBs in 32 patients within 2 months of myocardial infarction. All patients had more than 30 VPBs per hour with bigeminy, couplets, multifocal complexes, or ventricular tachycardia. With an average dose of propranolol of 160 mg per day, a significant decrease in complexity and frequency of VPBs was noted.

In the Swedish Metoprolol trial (4), there were 23 patients with recorded episodes of ventricular fibrillation: 17 of 697 patients taking placebo and 6 of 698 taking metoprolol. This was a highly significant difference. Arrhythmia data is also available on 107 patients in the British Sotalol trial (15); patients taking sotalol had fewer episodes of ventricular tachycardia and fewer ventricular couplets than those on placebo. It was concluded that the drug reduces VPBs. In addition, sotalol, like propranolol, appears to blunt the increase in VPB rate from baseline to 1 month after myocardial infarction.

Sloman and Stannard (16) reported on a randomized study of 49 patients who received propranolol after acute myocardial infarction. The drug was given intravenously at the time of hospital admission and was followed by a dose of 60 mg daily for 3 weeks. Significant ventricular arrhythmia occurred in 3 of 26 patients treated with propranolol and in 5 of 23 of the placebo patients. This difference was not statistically significant. This lack of treatment effect with propranolol is thought to be due to the low dose of drug used in the study. More recent studies, including the beta-blocker heart attack trial (BHAT), used much higher doses of propranolol.

Although these and other studies report the prevalence of ventricular arrhythmia after myocardial infarction, they are difficult to compare with BHAT data. This difficulty is due to the fact that there were differences in length of time of recording, time after myocardial infarction, and differences in method of classifying VPBs.

RELATIONSHIP BETWEEN VPBs AND INCREASED MORTALITY

The interest in suppressing VPBs has increased because of a number of epidemiological and clinical studies, which have focused attention on VPBs as a marker of patients at increased risk for subsequent sudden death. A great deal of information is available from studies involving survivors of acute myocardial infarction.

Two hundred and thirty-five out of 2035 men (12%) in the placebo group of the coronary drug project had one or more VPBs on the standard 12 lead electrocardiogram at entry into the trial (17). During a 3-year follow-up period, there were twice the number of deaths in those men having any VPBs compared to those with no VPBs on the baseline electrocardiogram. A further access risk of death was noted if frequent VPBs, pairs, or runs of ventricular tachycardia were present on the entry electrocardiogram.

Kotler et al. (18) reported on the follow-up of 160 male survivors of myocardial infarction. Serial 12-hour EKG recordings were performed, and the follow-up period ranged from 30-54 months. Of the patients with significant VPBs (frequent multifocal paired or ventricular tachycardia), 13.8% experienced sudden death as opposed to 3% of those not manifesting these ventricular arrhythmias.

Studies by Vismara et al. (19) have shown that ventricular arrhythmias noted late in the hospitalization period are more likely predictive of subsequent sudden death than early ventricular arrhythmias.

A large study by Ruberman et al. (20) confirmed the importance of VPBs in the setting of coronary artery disease. Ruberman performed 1-hour EKG recordings on 1739 men with recent myocardial infarction. These men were then followed for a mean of 24.4 months of the sudden deaths in the follow-up period. Those patients manifesting complex VPBs on the initial 1-hour EKG recording had a risk of sudden death three times that of men free of complex VPBs during the hour of EKG recording.

Moss et al. (12) evaluated the role of VPBs in identifying patients who died of cardiac causes in 940 patients who survived acute myocardial infarction. Six-hour Holter recordings were obtained before hospital discharge, and VPBs were classified as complex (bigeminal, multiform, repetitive, or R on T), simple (one or more VPBs that did not have complex patterns), or not present. Patients were followed for an average of 36 months, and cardiac mortality was characterized as sudden (≤1 hour) or nonsudden. They found that complex VPBs were associated with a significantly increased cardiac death rate, but the VPB frequency did not discriminate between sudden and nonsudden cardiac death. Simple VPBs were associated with a cardiac mortality rate in between those with complex and those with no VPBs. This relationship between complex VPB's and cardiac mortality was independent of 10 relevant clinical variables including left ventricular dysfunction.

Bigger et al. (21) examined the relationship between ventricular arrhythmia, left ventricular dysfunction, and mortality after myocardial infarction in 766 patients enrolled in a multicenter trial. Left ventricular ejection fraction was determined by radionuclide ventriculography and dichotomized at 30%. VPB frequency was divided into three categories: (1) less than one per hour, (2) 1-2.9 per hour, and (3) 3 or more per hour. Repetitiveness of VPBs was also divided into three categories: (1) no repetitive VPBs, (2) paired VPBs, and (3) VPB runs. There were no significant interactions among the variables with respect to the effects of risk of mortality. There was a suggestion of an interaction between each risk variable and time after infarction. Low ejection fraction was a better predictor of early mortality (less than 6 months), while the presence of ventricular arrhythmia was a better predictor of late mortality (after 6 months). These investigators concluded that ventricular arrhythmia and left ventricular dysfunction were independently related to mortality risk.

BHAT STUDY

The Beta Blocker Heart Attack Trial (BHAT) was a placebo controlled, randomized, double-blind, clinical trial of the long-term administration of propranolol in patients with at least one documented myocardial infarction. The primary objective of the study was to determine whether the daily administration of propranolol to these patients would result in a significant reduction in mortality from all causes during a 2- to 4-year follow-up period. Secondary objectives of the trial were to study the effect of chronic administration of propranolol on coronary heart disease mortality and specifically sudden death. A total of 3837 patients at 31 centers were divided into two groups: 1916 patients received propranolol in a dose of 180 to 240 mg/day, and 1921 patients received a matching placebo. All patients were followed for an average of 25 months. Baseline comparability between the two groups was excellent. The patients were similar with regard to cardiovascular risk factors, use of medications, past medical history, and laboratory data. The average time from the infarction to randomization was 13.8 days.

All patients initially received 40 mg of propranolol or a matching placebo three times a day. A serum propranolol level was measured several days after enrollment and was used to further adjust the dose of study medication. A maintenance dose of 60 mg three times a day or 80 mg three times a day was prescribed at the 1-month follow-up visit depending on these serum levels. Patients were seen every 3 months for evaluation. Intervention was originally scheduled to end in June 1982.

The trial was stopped 9 months earlier than scheduled with a publication of a preliminary report (22), which reported a mortality of 9.5% in the placebo group (183 deaths) and 7% in the propranolol group (135 deaths). This represented a reduction of 26%. All patients were analyzed according to treatment assignment regardless of subsequent compliance. The analysis of mortality indicated that both sudden and nonsudden coronary heart disease mortality was decreased in the propranolol group (1). Propranolol appeared to benefit patients with either anterior or inferior myocardial infarction. Patients with nontransmural myocardial infarction did not show any benefit. The majority of observed deaths were from cardiovascular disease. Most of the deaths were due to coronary heart disease, and about half of these deaths were sudden. Sudden cardiac death was seen in 3.3% of the propranolol patients and 4.6% among the placebo patients. A subsequent report (2) reported on coronary event incidents (coronary heart disease mortality + nonfatal myocardial infarction) and nonfatal events. Coronary event incidents were 23% lower in the propranolol-treated group, and nonfatal reinfarction was 16% lower.

The results of BHAT are consistent with those of the Norwegian Timolol Trial (3) and the Metoprolol Trial (4). The percent reduction in mortality at 1 year seen in the Timolol Trial was approximately 33% and similar to the 39% reduction seen in 1 year in BHAT. The dose of propranolol used in the BHAT study was thought to have a beta-blocking effect comparable to the doses used in the timolol and metoprolol studies. Eighty-two percent of the BHAT patients received 180 mg of propranolol per day while 18% received 240 mg of study medication per day.

HOLTER MONITORING

Twenty-four-hour Holter monitoring was performed at baseline in the majority of patients. At the 6-week visit, a second 24-hour ambulatory recording was performed on 840 randomly selected patients, which represented approximately 25% of the total population. The initial 24-hour recording was successfully performed in 85.8% of those randomly assigned to propranolol (1644 of 1916) and 85.1% of those randomly assigned to placebo (1635 of 1921).

The 24-hour two-channel reel-to-reel Holter magnetic tapes were generated on Avionic recorders (Model 445) and processed by Cardio Data System, which is digital software-based (Worchester Polytechnic Institute) and capable of differentiating up to 25 different EKG variables involving rate and rhythm change. Electrocardiogram complexes are noted by the computer and an operator verifies the decision, thus providing human interaction with the computer. The Cardio Data System analysis method has been validated both for accuracy and precision for ventricular beat detection.

DEFINITION OF ARRHYTHMIA

Since ventricular arrhythmias are categorized by different criteria in the literature, the BHAT data were evaluated using seven definitions, which will allow comparison to data from other studies (23).

1. Average VPBs per hour greater than 0.
2. Average VPBs per hour equal to or greater than 10.
3. Average VPBs per hour equal to or greater than 10 and at least one run of ventricular tachycardia or VPB pairs.
4. Average VPBs per hour equal to or greater than 10 and at least one run of ventricular tachycardia or VPB pairs and multiform beats.
5. Average VPBs per hour equal to or greater than 30.
6. Average VPBs per hour equal to or greater than 30 and at least one run of ventricular tachycardia or VPB pairs.
7. At least one run of ventricular tachycadia or VPB pairs.

A total of 419 propranolol and 407 placebo patients had successful monitoring at both baseline and 6 weeks. The paired data provided an opportunity to compare the change in arrhythmia status at these two points in time. Since there is a considerable normal variation in VPB frequency, the following definitions were developed to determine if a significant change had occurred. A decrease in arrhythmia was defined as a 75% reduction in average VPB frequency between baseline and 6 weeks with no ventricular tachycardia, couplets, or multiform beats present at 6 weeks. For participants with some VPBs at baseline an increase in arrhythmia was defined as a 10-fold or greater increase in the hourly VPB frequency couplets or ventricular tachycardia beats.

The group of major interest were those with complex ventricular premature beats as defined in the protocol. Complex ventricular premature beats were defined as the presence of one or more of the following features on the 24-hour recording: multiform VPBs, an average of at least 10 VPBs per hour, and at least 1 VPB pair or run of ventricular tachycardia. Multiform ventricular premature beats were defined as beats with varying configuration in either channel noted visually by the scanning technician and confirmed by the supervising cardiologist.

Because ventricular ectopic activity is characterized by different criteria in other reports, three different patients subgroups were also considered. These were (1) patients with at least one VPB during the 24-hour period, (2) patients with an average of at least 10 VPBs per hour, and (3) patients with an average of at least 10 VPBs per hour plus at least one pair or run of ventricular premature beats plus multiform ventricular premature beats.

EFFECT OF PROPRANOLOL ON VENTRICULAR ARRHYTHMIA

Analysis of the baseline Holter recordings in the BHAT study revealed that slightly more than 80% of the patients had VPBs during the 24-hour monitoring period (23). Thirteen percent of the patients had an average of at least 10 VPBs per hour, and 7% had an average of at least 30 VPBs per hour. Twenty percent had ventricular tachycardia or ventricular couplets. This data is summarized in Table 1.

The group of patients with at least 10 VPBs per hour and at least one run of ventricular tachycardia or ventricular couplet were examined in detail. Although the prevalence of ventricular arrhythmia varied according to the criteria used, the same trends were noted for all definitions of ventricular arrhythmia. Ventricular arrhythmia appears to increase with age, past history of myocardial infarction, and use of diuretics. Other factors, including sex, CPK ratio, history of smoking, diabetes, hypertension, and infarct location seemed less clearly associated with the prevalence of ventricular arrhythmia.

The change in prevalence of ventricular arrhythmia was noted by examining paired data from patients having Holter recordings both at baseline and at 6 weeks. Again, the category of patients having at least 10 VPBs per hour and at least one run of ventricular tachycardia or ventricular couplet is used for illustration. Thirty-three of 407 placebo patients (8.1%) and 30 of 419 propranolol patients (7.2%) had this ventricular arrhythmia at baseline ($Z = 0.51$). By the sixth week, this increased to 104 patients (25.6%) in the placebo group and to only 61 patients (14.6%) in the propranolol group. This difference was statistically significant ($Z = 3.95$). Examination of the entire placebo group revealed that 72.7% continued to have ventricular arrhythmia at 6 weeks compared with 53.3% in the propranolol group ($Z = 1.60$). Of those in the placebo group who

Table 1 Ventricular Arrhythmia on Baseline 24-Hour Holter

Arrhythmia	No. patients	%
VPB>0	2735	83.6
VPB≥10	434	13.2
VPB≥10 &	251	7.7
VT or Couplets	233	7.1
VPB≥10 &		
VT or Couplets & Multiform		
VPB≥30	225	6.9
VPB≥30 & VT or Couplets	159	4.8
VT or Couplets	667	20.3

Source: Ref. 23.

showed no ventricular arrhythmia at baseline, 21.4% did have ventricular arrhythmia at 6 weeks, compared to only 11.6% in the propranolol group, who developed arrhythmia at 6 weeks (Z = 3.67).

Examination of the patients with ventricular arrhythmia at baseline revealed that 11.6% in the placebo group showed a decrease at 6 weeks compared with 15.4% showing a decrease in the propranolol group (Z = 1.49). In the placebo group, 41.6% of the patients had an increase in ventricular arrhythmia, while only 30.3% in the propranolol group showed an increase (Z = 3.12). Among those with no VPBs at baseline, 29.5%

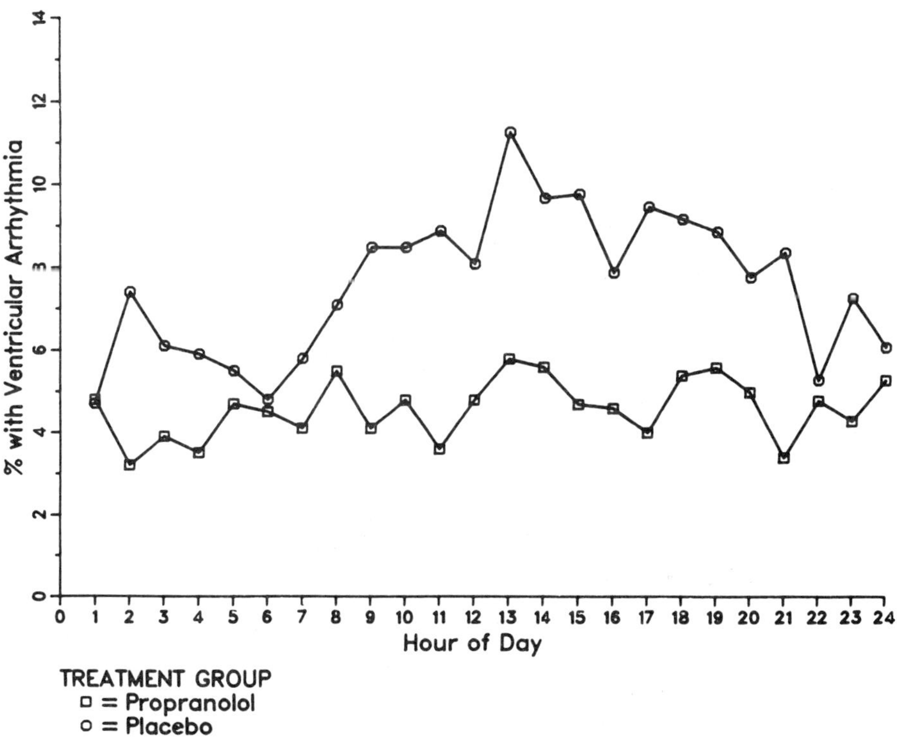

Figure 1 Proportion of patients having ventricular arrhythmia (10 or more ventricular premature beats and at least one run of ventricular tachycardia or a pair of ventricular premature beats). Data are shown for the placebo (○) and the propranolol (□) groups for 24 hours, starting at midnight.

of the placebo group and 36.2% of the propranolol group showed an increase in ventricular arrhythmia (Z = 0.81).

Figure 1 shows the percentage of patients at 6 weeks having at least 10 VPBs per hour and at least one run of ventricular tachycardia or ventricular couplet for both placebo and propranolol patients by the hour of the day. It is noted that a greater proportion of placebo patients had ventricular arrhythmia during waking hours than during sleep. This increase during waking hours was not seen for the propranolol patients and is described as a blunting effect.

Peters et al. (24) noted an increase in the frequency of sudden cardiac death during the morning in patients enrolled in the BHAT study. His analysis showed that there were six deaths in the placebo group during the hours of 5 to 8 a.m. compared with none in the propranolol group. Of 56 deaths occurring in the placebo group, 25 (38%) occurred in a 6-hour period (5 to 11:00 a.m.) compared with 11 of 45 (24%) in the propranolol group. At other times during the day, there was nearly an equal number of sudden cardiac deaths in both the propranolol and placebo groups. Of interest, however, is the fact that ventricular arrhythmias did not show a midmorning peak in this study population. This dissociation between frequency of ventricular arrhythmia and sudden cardiac death, noted by Peters, suggests that sudden cardiac death may not be triggered by the arrhythmias that we are monitoring.

The BHAT experience has shown that shortly after myocardial infarction, frequent and complex ventricular arrhythmia is associated with age, previous myocardial infarction, and diuretic usage. Ventricular arrhythmia increases after hospital discharge, and this increase was blunted by propranolol therapy.

EFFECT OF PROPRANOLOL IN PATIENTS WITH MYOCARDIAL INFARCTION AND COMPLEX VENTRICULAR ARRHYTHMIA

Analysis of BHAT data shows that patients on propranolol had decreased mortality and a lower incidence of sudden death. The data also shows that propranolol has an effect on ventricular arrhythmia. This raises the question of whether or not the improved mortality was specifically due to the decrease in ventricular arrhythmia. One of the specific subgroup hypotheses of the Beta Blocker Heart Attack Trial was that propranolol would be particularly effective in reducing sudden death in patients with complex ventricular arrhythmia. Table 2 shows the percentage of coronary

Table 2 Outcome by Classification of Arrhythmia According to Treatment Group

Arrhythmia, VPB ⩾ 10/hr or VT or multiform	*n*	CHD mortality (%)	R.R.	Sudden death (%)	R.R.
Present					
Propranolol	672	10.4	0.69	5.5	0.72
Placebo	666	15.2		7.7	
Absent					
Propranolol	978	4.8	0.75	2.1	0.84
Placebo	974	6.4		2.6	

R.R. = relative risk.
Source: Ref. 25.

heart disease mortality and percentage of sudden death for patients with complex ventricular arrhythmia, which is defined as VPBs ⩾10/hr or ventricular tachycardia runs or multiform VPBs. The amount of risk of having one of these outcome events is shown for those on propranolol compared with those in the placebo group. The amount of risk of sudden death for this subgroup was 0.72 vs. 0.84 for the subgroup without complex ventricular arrhythmia. This difference is not statistically significant and does not support the subgroup hypothesis that sudden death would be preferentially reduced in patients with complex ventricular arrhythmia. The presence of complex ventricular arrhythmia did identify a group of patients with almost twice the risk of death as those without this arrhythmia, although similar relative benefit from propranolol was seen. If the same number of patients were treated, those in the high-risk group would have a greater absolute benefit from the drug with more lives being saved per number treated (23).

Table 3 shows that very little benefit is obtained from propranolol in patients with the arrhythmia classification of VPBs ⩾10/hr + runs + multiform ventricular beats. This is in contrast to the benefit obtained by propranolol in the patients without this arrhythmia. This could be explained by the fact that these patients are not only at high risk of sudden death, but also at higher risk of being harmed by beta-blockers (25). It was also noted that compliance in taking study medication was not as good in this subgroup possibly limiting the ability to detect benefit, if any, from propranolol.

Table 3 Outcome by Classification of Arrhythmia According to Treatment Group

Arrhythmia, VPB > 10/hr + VT + multiform	*n*	CHD mortality (%)	R.R.	Sudden death (%)	R.R.
Present					
Propranolol	122	15.6	0.87	10.7	0.99
Placebo	112	17.9		10.7	
Absent					
Propranolol	1528	5.4	0.67	2.9	0.70
Placebo	1528	8.0		0.70	

R.R. = relative risk.
Source: Ref. 25.

A finding that patients without arrhythmia benefit relatively as much from propranolol as those with the arrhythmia implies that propranolol has other mechanisms of action other than reducing ventricular arrhythmia. Propranolol has been demonstrated to increase ventricular fibrilation threshold (26). This effect on ventricular fibrillation threshold appears to be completely different from an effect on suppressing ventricular ectopic beats. It has also been postulated that the benefit of propranolol might be due to its antiischemic effect (27). Propranolol, which is a nonselective beta-blocker, may also function by blocking $beta_2$ receptors. This action will serve to decrease arrhythmia mediated through catecholamine-induced hypokalemia (28).

The hypothesis that propranolol would be of special benefit to patients who had ventricular arrhythmia was not supported. This was true regardless of a classification of ventricular arrhythmia that was used for analysis. The finding of ventricular arrhythmia on a Holter recording still identifies high-risk patients. Since mortality is higher in these patients with ventricular arrhythmia, even the same relative benefit would lead to a greater absolute benefit in those receiving propranolol since more lives would be saved per number treated.

POSSIBLE MECHANISMS OF PROPRANOLOL'S BENEFICIAL EFFECT

A retrospective trial was done in which the patients from the BHAT were divided into four subgroups (29). This included those with electrical prob-

Table 4 All-Cause Mortality (%) by Risk Group

	Propranolol		Placebo		
Risk group	No. pts	Mortality	No. pts	Mortality	Relative risk
None	1047	6.2	1079	6.6	0.94
Electrical	443	5.2	423	10.9	0.48
Mechanical	201	10.4	202	16.8	0.62
Electrical and mechanical	225	12.9	217	17.1	0.76

Source: Ref. 29.

lems, those with mechanical or pump problems, those with both, and those with neither. The subgroup of patients with electrical problems (including ventricular fibrillation immediately prior to enrollment) seemed to benefit most from propranolol. In the large subgroup of patients with no reported complications, the 25-month mortality was low and the observed benefit of propranolol was small. The patients with electrical complications only had intermittent mortality and a pronounced effect of treatment. Those with mechanical complications had the highest mortality and experienced an intermittent relative benefit of beta-blocker therapy; this data is summarized in Table 4. A more detailed analysis of the individual electrical and mechanical complications is shown in Table 5. The patients who had an episode of ventricular tachycardia made up the largest subgroup. Among these patients, mortality was 44% lower in the

Table 5 All-Cause Mortality (%) by Complications

	Propranolol		Placebo		
Complication	No. pts	Mortality	No. pts	Mortality	Relative risk
Ventricular fibrillation	104	6.7	99	18.2	0.37
Ventricular tachycardia	441	6.8	446	12.1	0.56
Pulmonary edema	52	19.2	51	19.6	0.98
Rales	58	13.8	57	22.8	0.60

Source: Ref. 29.

propranolol group than in the controls. The lowest relative risk that suggests that patients receive special benefit from propranolol therapy was observed in the subgroup of patients experiencing ventricular fibrillation before randomization. There were 104 patients in the propranolol group who had ventricular fibrillation and experienced a 6.7% mortality. This is contrasted to the 99 patients in the placebo group who had ventricular fibrillation and experienced an 18.2% mortality rate. The effect of beta-blockers on ventricular fibrillation has been noted previously. Anderson et al. (26) demonstrated an increase in VF threshold with five different beta-blockers using the anesthetized chest dog model. In the five agents tested, all had different beta-blocking characteristics, but each was effective in changing ventricular fibrillation threshold. The relationship between ventricular fibrillation threshold and cardiac sympathetic stimulation is suggested by noting that ventricular fibrillation threshold increases after bilateral stellate ganglionectomy (26). These studies suggest that the effect of the beta-blockage itself and not any of the accessory properties explain the drug's beneficial effect on VF threshold. This conclusion is reached since Anderson found no significant difference between drugs that had membrane-stabilizing properties or cardioselectivity. Anderson concludes that the data is consistent with a general class effect of beta-blocking drugs on ventricular fibrillation threshold. He feels that this effect presumably relates primarily to blocking the $beta_1$ receptor since this is an action that all the drugs that he tested held in common.

The metopolol study (30) showed no effect on ventricular premature beats but a significant effect on preventing ventricular fibrillation. In this study, they noted 17 cases of ventricular fibrillation in the placebo group (697 patients) and only 6 episodes of ventricular fibrillation in the metopolol group (698 patients $p < 0.05$). During the hospital stay, significantly fewer patients receiving metopolol (16 versus 38) ($p < 0.01$) required lidocaine. These authors point out the fact that the mechanisms behind ventricular premature contractions and ventricular fibrillation are not the same. This is consistent with the observation in the BHAT study where propranolol was more effective in patients with ventricular fibrillation and was not as effective in suppression of ventricular premature beats. It has been suggested that a rise in cyclic AMP may induce a electrophysiological substrate for ventricular fibrillation (31). Beta-blockers may be effective by blocking the rise in cyclic AMP and thereby diminish the risk of ventricular fibrillation.

These studies indicate that an antifibrillatory effect may be seen when an antiectopic effect is not. It is possible that micro reentry, which is necessary for ventricular fibrillation, may be prevented in situations in which macro reentry, which is necessary for ventricular premature beats, is not prevented (32).

REFERENCES

1. Beta Blocker Heart Attack Trial Research Group. A randomized trial of Propranolol in patients with acute myocardial infarction. JAMA 1982; 247: 1707-14.
2. Beta Blocker Heart Attack Trial Research Group. A randomized trial of Propranolol in patients with acute myocardial infarction. JAMA 1983; 250: 2814-9.
3. The Norwegian Multicenter Study Group. Timolol induced reduction in mortality and reinfarction in patients surviving acute myocardial infarction. N Engl J Med 1981; 304:801-7.
4. Hjalmarson A, Elmfeldt D, Herlitz J, Holberg S, Malek I, Nyberg G, Ryden L, Swedberg K, Vedin A, Waagstein F, Waldenstrom A, Waldenstrom J, Wedel H, Wilhelmensen L, Wilhelmsson C. Effect on mortality of metoprolol in acute myocardial infarction. Lancet 1981; 2:823-6.
5. Yusuf S, Peto R, Lewis J, Collins R, Sleight P. Beta blockade during and after myocardial infarction: an overview of the randomized trials. Prog Cardiovasc Dis 1985; 27:335-71.
6. The European Infarction Study Group. European Infarction Study (Eis). A secondary prevention study with slow release oxprenolol after myocardial infarction: morbidity and mortality. Eur Heart J 1984; 5:189-202.
7. Lichstein E. Why do beta-receptor blockers decrease mortality after myocardial infarction? JACC 1985; 6:973-5.
8. Bigger JT, Coromilas J. How do beta blockers protect after myocardial infarction. Ann Intern Med 1984; 101:256-8.
9. Braunwald E, Mueller JE, Kloner RA, Maroko PR. Role of beta adrenergic blockade in the therapy of patients with myocardial infarction. Am J Med 1983; 74:113-23.
10. Koch-Weser J, Frishman WH, Furberg CD, Friedenwald WT. Beta adrenergic blockade for survivors of acute myocardial infarction. N Engl J Med 1984; 310:830-7.
11. Pratt C, Lichstein E. Ventricular antiarrhythmic effects of beta adrenergic blocking drugs: a review of mechanism and clinical studies. J Clin Pharmacol 1982; 22:335-47.
12. Moss AJ, Davis HT, DeCamilla J, Bayer LW. Ventricular ectopic beats and their relation to sudden and nonsudden cardiac death after myocardial infarction. Circulation 1979; 60:998-1003.
13. Woosley RL, Kornhauser D, Smith R, Reele S, Higgins SB, Nies AS, Shand DG, Oates JA. Suppression of chronic ventricular arrhythmias with propranolol. Circulation 1979; 60:819-23.

14. Koppes GM, Beckmann CH, Jones FG. Propranolol therapy for ventricular arrhythmias two months after acute myocardial infarction. Am J Cardiol 1980; 46:322-9.
15. Julian DJ, Prescott RJ, Jackson FS, Szekely P. A controlled trial of Sotalol for one year after myocardial infarction. Lancet 1982; 1:114-18.
16. Sloman G, Stannard M. Beta adrenergic blockade and cardiac dysrhythmias. Br Med J 1967; 4:508-12.
17. Coronary Drug Project. Prognostic importance of premature beats following myocardial infarction. JAMA 1973; 223:1116-24.
18. Kotler M, Tabatznik M, Mawer M, Tominaga S. Prognostic significance of ventricular ectopic beats with respect to sudden death in late post infarction period. Circulation 1973; 33:959-67.
19. Vismara M, Amsterdam E, Mason D. Relation of arrhythmias in the late hospital phase of acute myocardial infarction to sudden death after a hospital discharge. Am J Med 1975; 59:6-12.
20. Ruberman W, Wernblatt E, Goldberg J, Frank C. Shapiro S. Ventricular premature beats and mortality after myocardial infarction. N Engl J Med 1977; 297:750-7.
21. Bigger TJ, Fleiss JL, Kleiger R, Miller PJ, Rolnitzky LM. The relationships among ventricular arrhythmias, left ventricular dysfunction and mortality in the 2 years after myocardial infarction. Circulation 1984; 69:250-8.
22. The Beta Blocker Heart Attack Trial Preliminary Report. JAMA 1981; 256: 2073-4.
23. Lichstein E, Morganroth J, Harrist R, Hubble E. Effect of propranolol on ventricular arrhythmia—the beta-blocker heart attack trial experience. Circulation 1983; 6(suppl I):5-10.
24. Peters RW, Muller JE, Goldstein S, Byington R, Friedman LM. Propranolol and the morning increase in the frequency of sudden cardiac death (BHAT study). Am J Cardiol 1989; 63:1518-20.
25. Friedman LM, Byington RP, Capone RJ, Furberg CD, Goldstein S, Lichstein E. Effect of propranolol in patients with myocardial infarction and ventricular arrhythmia. JAMA 1986; 7:1-8.
26. Anderson JL, Rodier HE, Green LS. Comparative effects of beta adenergic blocking drugs on experiment ventricular fibrillation threshold. Am J Cardiol 1983; 51:1196-202.
27. Frishman WH, Furberg CD, Friedewald WT. Beta adrenergic blockade for survivors of acute myocardial infarction. N Engl J Med 1984; 310:830-7.
28. Vincent HH, Manin T, Veld AJ, Boomsma F, Derkx FHM, Wenting GJ, Schalekamp MA. Cardio protection by blockade of beta 2 adrenergic receptors. Eur Heart J 1983; 4:109-15.
29. Furberg CD, Hawkins M, Lichstein E. Effect of propranolol in post infarction patients with a mechanical or electrical complications. Circulation 1984; 69:761-5.
30. Ryden L, Ariniego R, Arnman K. A double blind trial of metoprolol in acute myocardial infarction. Effects on ventricular tachyarrhythmias. N Engl J Med 1983; 308:614-18.

31. Opie LH, Lubbe WF. Catecholamine mediated arrhythmias in acute myocardial infarction. Experimental evidence and role of beta adrenergic blockade. South Afri Med J 1979; 56:871-80.
32. Cardinal R, Janse MJ, VanEeden I, Werner G. The effect of lidocaine on intracellular and extracellular potentials, activation and ventricular arrhythmias during acute regional ischemia in the isolated porcine heart. Circulation Res 1981; 49:792-806.

7

Effect of Beta-Blockers on Circadian Variation of Sudden Cardiac Death in Survivors of Myocardial Infarction

Robert W. Peters
Veterans Affairs Medical Center and the University of Maryland School of Medicine, Baltimore, Maryland

INTRODUCTION

There are almost half a million sudden cardiac deaths in the United States every year, many of them occurring in patients who were previously healthy and might otherwise have been expected to live for many more years. In the hope of implementing effective preventive measures, several investigators have sought to identify specific predisposing factors for sudden cardiac death which might be used to identify high-risk populations suitable for possible intervention. Whether or not there are premonitory symptoms, the vast majority of these deaths in the United States and Western Europe occur in the setting of atherosclerotic coronary artery disease. In particular, the 6-week period immediately following acute myocardial infarction is associated with high risk of sudden cardiac death. This increased likelihood of sudden cardiac death gradually diminishes until 6-12 months after the acute infarct, when it becomes comparable to that of the population with stable coronary artery disease. Presumably this period of increased susceptibility to malignant arrhythmias is due to a vulnerable substrate (myocardial cells in varying degrees of necrosis, ischemia, and healing, creating the ideal milieu for reentrant arrhythmias) in the setting of enhanced ventricular irritability. Efforts to reduce the incidence of sudden cardiac death through control of arrhythmias have been disappointing, in part, perhaps because of the relative inefficacy and toxicity of presently available antiarrhythmic drugs. As a consequence, efforts to diminish the incidence of sudden cardiac death have focused on a variety of different fields. In this chapter, the potential role of circadian rhythms in the causation of pathological events will be discussed. It is an area that has gained increasing recognition as a clinically relevant issue in the evolution of ischemic heart disease and the occurrence of sudden cardiac death. Several studies in the past few years have noted morning peaks or morning and evening peaks in sudden cardiac death and the onset of symptoms of acute myocardial infarction (1-3). This chapter will address in detail the circadian variation in sudden cardiac death and the effects of beta-blockers with specific reference to the large multicenter NHLBI-sponsored Beta Blocker Heart Attack Trial (BHAT) (4).

CIRCADIAN RHYTHMS

Circadian rhythm can be defined as the regular or repetitive occurrence of a biological process on a daily or 24-hour basis (Table 1). For example, plasma and urinary catecholamines, steroids, the renin-angiotensin aldosterone system, and insulin as well as platelet aggregate ability, fibrinolytic

Table 1 Normal Circadian Rhythms (Biological Processes That Display Circadian Periodicity)

1. Hormonal Factors
   A. Urinary (17) keto-steroids
   B. Plasma cortisol
   C. Urinary and plasma catecholamines
   D. Immunoreactive insulin
   E. Antidiabetic hormone
   F. ACTH
   G. Plasma renin and aldosterone
2. Other Factors
   A. Heart rate
   B. Blood pressure
   C. Arterial oxygen saturation
   D. Renal function
   E. Platelet aggregability
   F. Fibrinolytic activity

activity, and vascular tone all display regular peaks and valleys that recur every 24 hours. Related to these hormonal cycles, at least in part, are daily fluctuations in body temperature, heart rate, and blood pressure (5-13). Although the mechanisms underlining circadian rhythms are poorly understood, these cycles are apparently affected by the waking-sleeping-activity sequence, especially the time of arising, exposure to light, and the timing of meals, as well as a variety of other apparently less important factors. In light of the complexity of these biorhythms, it is not surprising that the body's response to pharmacological agents (bioavailability, pharmacokinetics, metabolism, excretion, and pharmacodynamics) as well as to noxious stimuli, such as allergens or infectious agents, also displays circadian periodicity. For example, allergic rhinitis tends to produce its most troubling symptoms in the early and mid-morning hours, while fevers tend to peak in the late afternoon and early evening.

CIRCADIAN RHYTHMS AND ACUTE CARDIAC EVENTS

Circadian rhythms appear to assume major clinical importance in studies of acute cardiovascular events. Circadian periodicity has been demonstrated with respect to the time of onset of acute myocardial infarction, transient myocardial ischemia, cerebrovascular accidents, and sudden cardiac death (1-3,14-16) (Table 2). Our ability to collect information in these areas has been greatly helped by the development of sophisticated monitoring techniques. With current monitoring systems, it is readily feasible to detect changes in heart rate and rhythm, blood pressure, and even identify periods of myocardial ischemia on a 24- or even a 48-hour basis. Such information permits confirmation of circadian rhythms as key factors in these pathological events. When serum sampling is combined with analysis of recordings, the relation between circadian rhythms

Table 2 Cardiovascular Events and Abnormalities That Display Circadian Periodicity

A. Myocardial infarction
B. Sudden cardiac death
C. Cerebrovascular accidents
D. Transient myocardial ischemia
E. Ventricular arrhythmias

and the hormonal fluctuations mentioned earlier may be more completely explored. Preliminary observations suggest that further research into these interactions will help to elucidate the mechanisms involved.

Based upon newer information, circadian rhythms are recognized to fit into the framework of the pathogenesis of acute myocardial infarction and sudden cardiac death. These events appear to occur as a direct consequence of the development of fresh thrombus which either partly or completely occludes a major epicardial coronary artery, usually at the site of preexisting disease. Davies and Thomas performed postmortem examinations in 100 patients who experienced sudden ischemic cardiac death and found that 95 had recent luminal or intimal thrombi, presumably precipitated by fissuring of a lipid-laden endothelial plaque (17). In contrast, no intraluminal and only eight intraintimal thrombi were found in a group of age-matched controls, only three of whom revealed plaque fissuring of any type. Similar findings have been described for acute myocardial infarction and unstable angina pectoris (18-21). Ordinarily, the coronary artery endothelium, directly and through chemical mediators, has both antiplatelet aggregating and vasodilatory effects which help to preserve vascular integrity. However, damaged endothelium loses these properties and becomes susceptible to a variety of noxious stimuli which mediate adverse changes in vascular tone, platelet aggregation, and perhaps hormonal factors. It is likely that the role for circadian rhythms as a trigger to acute cardiac events operates by influencing this sequence of local vascular events. The etiology of endothelial damage has not been conclusively established in all cases, but there is considerable evidence to implicate atherosclerotic plaque disruption with extrusion of thrombogenic material into the vessel lumen or intima (19,22). Of particular note is a recent report by Little and coworkers, who reviewed coronary arteriograms in a group of consecutive patients who had undergone angiography before and up to 1 month after acute myocardial infarction (23). The infarct-producing occlusion was always found at a site of preexisting disease, but in 66% of patients, the artery that subsequently occluded displayed less than 50% stenosis on the first angiogram, while more highly stenosed segments remained stable. Thus, factors that promote plaque instability, rather than high grade stenosis alone, seem to play a crucial role in the genesis of acute cardiac events. It is likely that these factors display circadian periodicity.

BETA-BLOCKERS AND CIRCADIAN RHYTHMS

Several large, randomized, double-blind trials completed in the past decade have demonstrated that beta-blockers reduce overall mortality and the incidence of sudden cardiac death and recurrent infarction in survivors of acute myocardial infarction (4,24-26). The exact mechanism underlying these beneficial effects remains to be elucidated; it is likely that multiple factors are involved (27,28). These reports helped to stimulate several groups to investigate the effect of beta-blockers upon the circadian periodicity of acute cardiac events in the hope of gaining further insight into the pathophysiology. Muller and associates examined the large MILIS (Multicenter Investigation of Limitation of Infarct Size) database to study the timing of acute myocardial infarction (1). They found the onset of infarction to be significantly more frequent in the time period between 6 a.m. and noon but that this apparent peak was not evident in individuals receiving beta-blockers (Fig. 1). Similar data were reported from the Intravenous Streptokinase in Myocardial Infarction (ISAM) study (29). In

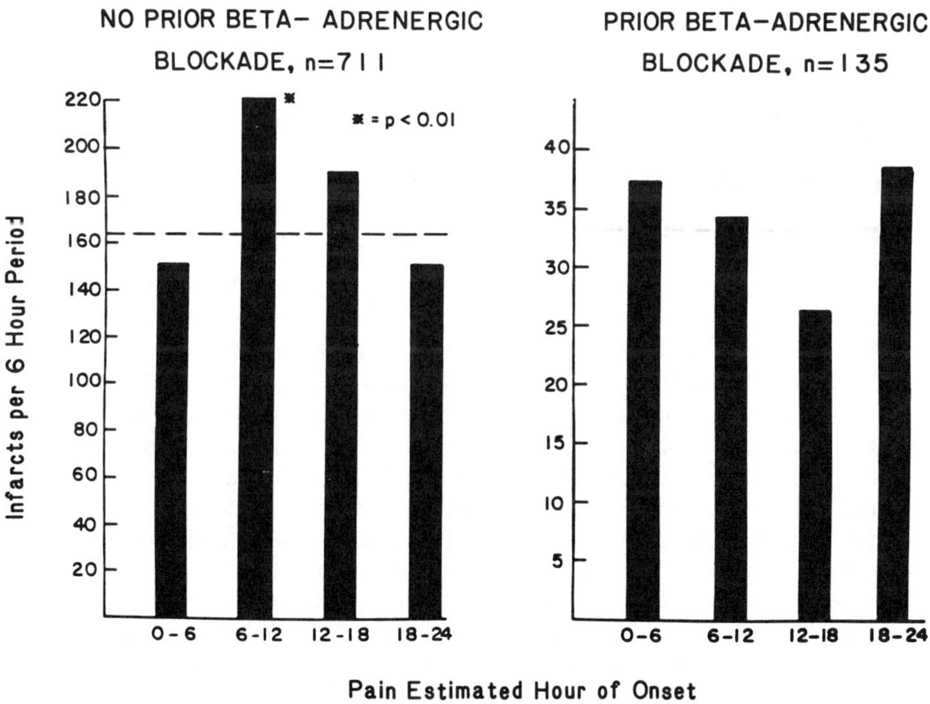

Figure 1 The time of onset of myocardial infarction in the Multicenter Investigation of Limitation of Infarct Size (MILIS) in patients not receiving (left) and receiving (right) beta-blockers. (From Ref. 1.)

contrast, Hjalmarson et al., in a large multicenter study supported by the Specialized Center of Research (SCOR) on ischemic heart disease at the University of California in San Diego, found that the onset of acute myocardial infarction occurred in two nearly equal peaks (morning and evening) and that this pattern was not affected by beta-blockers (30). The dose of beta-blockers is not specified in any of these three studies, so it is difficult to directly compare them. Mulcahy and coworkers performed ambulatory electrocardiographic monitoring (Holters) in 15 patients with documented atherosclerotic coronary artery disease who had been withdrawn from antianginal therapy and found a major peak in ischemic-appearing ST segments changes in the morning and a lesser peak in the evening (14). Subgroups were then randomized to receive either atenolol or nifedipine, and the ambulatory monitoring was repeated. It was found that the morning peak was abolished in the atenolol-treated patients but not in the group receiving nifedipine. This suggests that the effect of beta-blockers in transient myocardial ischemia may be similar to their action in acute myocardial infarction.

CIRCADIAN RHYTHM AND SUDDEN CARDIAC DEATH IN THE BETA-BLOCKER HEART ATTACK TRIAL (BHAT)

Description of Study

With the background information provided by the MILIS study, the ISAM study and others, the extensive database from the very large and carefully followed BHAT population was analyzed to determine whether the previously reported circadian variation in sudden cardiac death could be confirmed and to ascertain whether this pattern would be affected by the use of beta-blockers. BHAT is the subject of many previous reports (4,31,33) and is described in detail in another chapter of this book, so this brief overview of study design concentrates on areas relevant to analysis of circadian rhythms. The primary objective of BHAT was to determine whether long-term oral therapeutic doses of propranolol would prolong life in a large cohort of patients, aged 35 to 69, who had survived a documented acute myocardial infarction. Specifically excluded were patients with either an indication (for example, postinfarction angina) or a contraindication (for example, decompensated congestive heart failure or marked sinus bradycardia) to the use of beta-blockers. Following the recording of a 24-hour ambulatory electrocardiogram (Holter), patients were randomized to receive either propranolol 180 or 240 mg daily in three divided doses, or matching placebo (in a double-blind manner), 5-21 days after acute myocardial infarction.

Follow-up visits were scheduled at 6 weeks, 3 months, and at 3-month intervals thereafter. Standard data obtained included information about cardiac signs and symptoms, quality of life, and medication compliance. All deaths were investigated in detail, first by the individual clinical centers and later by a central Mortality Classification Committee. Mortality investigation included interviews with friends, relatives, and bystanders at the scene of the death. Copies of the death certificate and postmortem examination report were forwarded to the Mortality Classification Committee along with a detailed mortality form, which included a narrative summary prepared by the principal investigator. In the mortality investigation, particular attention was devoted to the presence of acute or prodromal signs and symptoms and the patient's activities in the 24-hour period preceding death. Completed mortality forms for each death were reviewed separately by two committee members who coded the deaths (disagreement between coders were adjudicated by a vote of the entire committee) based upon the predetermined described below.

Definition of Terms

Cardiovascular death—death from any cardiac or vascular cause.

Sudden cardiac death—a cardiovascular death (or death of unknown cause) occurring either instantaneously or within one hour of the onset of symptoms. The timing of deaths were decided to the nearest hour based upon the available clinical information (for example, a wife reported that she last saw her husband alive at 6:30 a.m. when he arose to go to the bathroom. Subsequently, she found him dead in the bathroom at 6:45 a.m. when she was awakened by the alarm clock. This death was coded as a sudden cardiac death occurring between 6:00 and 7:00 a.m.). All individuals involved in patient care, data collection and tabulation, and coding of deaths were blinded as to treatment group. The decision that a death was sudden was not necessarily based upon autopsy data or definitive evidence of an arrhythmia since these data were frequently nonexistent. The analysis described in the present chapter was limited to events that were initiated outside of either a hospital or medical emergency room. Specifically excluded were deaths that could not be coded to the nearest hour (for example, an individual who lived alone and was found dead in bed 2 days after last being seen).

Clinical death—point of spontaneous cessation of respiration and circulation accompanied by permanent loss of consciousness. Thus, if a patient suffered a cardiac arrest but was kept "alive" without regaining consciousness by means of a respirator for another 2 weeks, clinical death would be considered to have occurred at the time of the initial collapse. Clinical death, rather than official death, was used in the present analysis.

Official death—the official time of death stated on the death certificate.

Results (BHAT Mortality Data Analysis)

Some of the more important demographics of the BHAT population are shown in Table 3. The population is predominantly male and middle-aged with a moderately high incidence of coronary risk factors. Over a 25-month (mean) follow-up period, overall mortality was reduced by 26% in the propranolol-treated group with slightly lesser reductions in sudden cardiac death and nonfatal reinfarction (Table 4). Approximately one third of the out-of-hospital sudden cardiac deaths in both treatment groups had to be excluded from the time-of-death analysis because the time of clinical death (to the nearest hour) could not be determined.

The frequency distribution of out-of-hospital sudden cardiac deaths is detailed in Figure 2. The majority of deaths occurred at home; few were associated with heavy or even moderate exertion. As can be seen, excluding the 6-hour period between 5 and 11 a.m., there were a nearly equal number of deaths in the propranolol and placebo groups. Of particular note is the 3-hour period between 5 and 8 a.m. when there were six deaths in the placebo group compared with none in the patients receiving propranolol.

Table 3 Baseline Demographics of Propranolol and Placebo Group in the Beta Blocker Heart Attack Trial (BHAT)

	Propranolol (n = 1916)	Placebo (n = 1921)
Mean age (hr)	57.4	54.9
Male (%)	83.6	85.0
Current smoker (%)	57.4	57.0
Prior myocardial infarction (%)	13.9	13.2
Hypertension (%)	41.4	40.1
Angina (%)	35.8	36.5
Diabetes (%)	11.7	11.3
Race (% Caucasian)	89.3	88.4
Anterior myocardial infarction (%)	27.8	25.7
History of congestive heart failure (%)	9.0	9.4

Table 4 Acute Cardiac Events in the Beta-Blocker Heart Attack Trial

	Propranolol	Placebo	Total
Total deaths	127	171	298
Nonfatal reinfarction	85	101	186
Coronary incidence	192	249	441
Cardiovascular deaths	127	171	298
All sudden cardiac deaths[a]	64	89	153
Sudden cardiac deaths analyzed in this chapter[b]	45	56	101

[a]Instantaneous death or death within one hour of onset of symptoms.
[b]Out of hospital sudden cardiac deaths in whom the timing of collapse (in instantaneous death) or the onset of symptoms could be determined to the nearest hour.

Detailed analysis of the circumstances surrounding death failed to reveal any difference between groups which might explain the dissimilar frequency distribution.

Comments

Our findings from retrospective analysis of prospectively obtained BHAT data confirm those of previous studies, which report a mid-morning peak

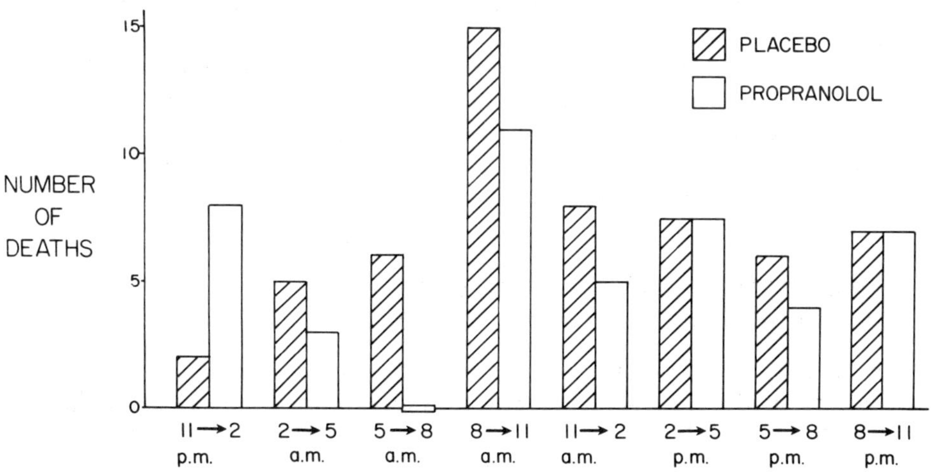

Figure 2 The time of onset of sudden cardiac death in the Beta-Blocker Heart Attack Trial (BHAT) in patients receiving placebo or propranolol. (From Ref. 16.)

in the incidence of sudden cardiac death. In addition, these data provide the first evidence that beta-blockers blunt or abolish this peak. Not surprisingly, these findings do not provide insight into the mechanisms by which beta-blockers exert their beneficial effects but suggest that circadian rhythms must be included as factors to be studied in future attempts to elucidate the reduction in mortality and reinfarction following myocardial infarction.

An intriguing aspect of the BHAT data is the apparent lack of correlation between the frequency distribution of ventricular arrhythmias and that of sudden cardiac death. As reported by the Lichstein et al., ventricular arrhythmias in BHAT, as determined by 24-hour Holter, were elevated throughout waking hours and did not display circadian periodicity (34, 35). This dissociation between the temporal distribution of arrhythmias and sudden cardiac death adds further clinical evidence supporting the hypothesis that the mechanism of sudden cardiac death is not solely arrhythmic. Other factors, particularly thrombosis and ischemia, appear to play an important, if not central, role. Whether the mediating event in the pathogenesis of sudden cardiac death is thrombosis, ischemia, a primary arrhythmia, or a combination of factors, beta-blockers are likely to be of benefit because of their multiplicity of actions. Thus, Willich and associates studied the effect of metoprolol on silent myocardial ischemia and platelet agreeability in a randomized, double-blind, placebo-controlled crossover trial in 10 patients with documented coronary artery disease (29). They found that although metoprolol did not affect the basal level or morning increase in platelet aggregability, it markedly diminished the duration and number of silent ischemic episodes. This antiischemic effect was accompanied by a reduction in heart rate and blood pressure, suggesting a decrease in myocardial oxygen demand. Interestingly, the four episodes of silent ischemia that were not prevented by metoprolol occurred in the same mid-morning and late afternoon distribution apparent in the placebo-treated patients.

Limitations of BHAT Data on Circadian Variation of Sudden Cardiac Death

Although derived from a prospective study, the data analysis regarding time of sudden cardiac death was performed retrospectively and could be subject to the bias inherent in all retrospective analysis. However, careful blinding as to treatment group of all individuals involved should have minimized the bias. It is unfortunate that comparable data are not available from other large postinfarction trials of beta-blockers to either confirm or contradict our findings. Ironically, it is the very success of beta-blockers in reducing mortality in these studies that will make it difficult to study beta-blockers in placebo-controlled trials in the future.

Another potential limitation of these data is that the findings apply only to an outpatient population. Hospitalized patients were excluded because they are subject to a variety of interventions which may artificially alter the sleeping-waking-activity cycle (for example, being admitted to critical care unit where there is little fluctuation in artificial light for the entire 24-hour period, being awakened to take medication during the middle of the night, etc.) or which may actually prevent sudden cardiac death (for example, a monitored bed with a defibrillator in the room, etc.) and thus might tend to mask circadian rhythms.

Determining the time of death required a great deal of effort on the part of the Mortality Classification Committee, and it can be argued that the morning peak in sudden cardiac death may be an artifact secondary to a spouse awakening and discovering the death when, in fact, the patient died at some time during the night. However, it was felt that death could be accurately timed to the nearest hour in the majority of cases, especially when the death was preceded by symptoms. Nonetheless, approximately one third of the sudden cardiac deaths in each treatment group had to be excluded from analysis, because of inability to determine the time of death.

Unfortunately, there is no information in the BHAT database regarding the usual sleeping-waking-activity cycle and very incomplete information about the timing of the last several doses of the study medication (in some cases it was uncertain whether or not the study medication was taken at all in the 24 hours preceding death). Since TID dosing was encouraged (rather than every 8 hours), it is likely that the serum concentration was lowest when it was needed most (at the time of arising). In addition, the degree of beta blockade was not routinely verified, a factor that may be important given the marked interindividual variation in response to oral propranolol. Thus, the study results may underestimate the potential beneficial effects of beta-blockers so that larger doses or longer-acting medication might have been even more effective and further attenuated the early morning peak in sudden cardiac death.

SUMMARY AND CONCLUSION

This chapter has focused on some of the processes that display circadian rhythms, particularly those factors thought to be relevant to acute cardiac events. Changing concepts regarding the pathogenesis of sudden cardiac death and their relation to circadian periodicity are emphasized, and clinical data are presented suggesting that beta-blockers abolish or blunt circadian rhythms. Although precise mechanisms remain obscure, the knowledge already gained in this important area should help to stimulate further investigation into the pathogenesis of sudden cardiac death and other acute cardiovascular catastrophes. Completely unknown, at present, is the effect on circadian rhythms of more recent interventional strategies, such as thrombolytic therapy, angioplasty, and newer cardioactive medications. The recently reported additive benefit of beta-blockers with thrombolytic therapy in acute myocardial infarction (37) suggests that longer-term studies to clarify the role of beta-blockers and other medical alternatives after invasive interactions will require further study.

REFERENCES

1. Muller JE, Stone PH, Turi ZG, Rutherford JD, Czeisler CA, Parker C, Poole WK, Passamani E, Roberts R, Robertson T, Sobel BE, Willerson JT, Braunwald E, and the MILIS Study Group. Circadian variation in the frequency of onset of acute myocardial infarction. N Engl J Med 1985; 313:1315-22.
2. Muller JE, Ludmer PL, Willich SN, Tofler GH, Aylmer G, Klangos I, Stone PH. Circadian variation in the frequency of sudden cardiac death. Circulation 1987; 75:131-8.
3. Willich SN, Levy D, Rocco MB, Tofler GH, Stone PH, Muller JE. Circadian variation in the incidence of sudden cardiac death in the Framingham heart study population. Am J Cardiol 1987; 60:801-6.
4. Beta-Blocker Heart Attack Trial Research Group. A randomized trial of propranolol in patients with acute myocardial infarction. 1: Mortality results. JAMA 1982; 247:1707-13.
5. Pickering TG. Sleep, circadian rhythms, and cardiovascular disease. Cardiovascular Review and Reports 1980; 1:37-47.
6. Millar-Craig MW, Bishop CN, Raftery EB. Circadian variation of blood-pressure. Lancet 1978; 1:795-7.
7. Burdick JA, Brinton G, Goldstein L, Lazio M. Heart rate variability in sleep and wakefulness. Cardiology 1970; 55:79-83.
8. Mills JN. Human circadian rhythms. Physiol Rev 1966; 46:128-71.
9. Weitzman ED, Fakashima D, Nogeire C, Roffwarg H, Gallagher TF, Hellman L. Twenty-four hour pattern of the episodic secretion of cortisol in normal subjects. J Clin Endocrinol Metab 1971; 33:14-22.
10. Turton MB, Deegan T. Circadian variations of plasma catecholamines, cortisol and immunoreactive insulin concentrations in supine subjects. Clin Chim Acta 1974; 55:389-97.

11. Rosing DR, Brakman P, Redwood DR, Goldstein RE, Beiser GD, Astrap T, Epstein SE. Blood fibrinolytic activity in man. Diurnal variations and the response to varying intensities of exercise. Circ Res 1970; 27:171-84.
12. Petralito A, Mangiafico RA, Gibino S, Cuffari MA, Miano MF, Fiore CE. Daily modifications of plasma fibrinogen, platelet aggregation, Howell's Time, PTT, TT and antithrombin III in normal subjects and in patients with vascular disease. Chronobiologia 1982; 9:195-201.
13. Rocco MB, Nabel EG, Sclwyn AP. Circadian rhythms and coronary artery disease. Am J Cardiol 1987; 59:136-76.
14. Mulcahy D, Cunningham D, Crean P, Wright C, Keegan J, Quyyumi A, Park A, Fox K. Circadian variation of total ischemic burden and its alteration with anti-anginal agents. Lancet 1988; 2:755-9.
15. Marler JR, Price TR, Clark GL, Muller JE, Robertson T, Mohr JP, Hier DB, Wolf PA, Caplan LR, Foulkes MA. Morning increase in onset of ischemic stroke. Stroke 1989; 20:473-6.
16. Peters RW, Muller JE, Goldstein S, Byington R, Friedman LM. Propranolol and the morning increase in the frequency of sudden cardiac death (BHAT Study). Am J Cardiol 1989; 63:1518-20.
17. Davies MJ, Thomas A. Thrombosis and acute coronary-artery lesions in sudden cardiac ischemic death. N Engl J Med 1984; 310:1137-40.
18. Ambrose JA, Tannenbaum MA, Alexopoulos D, Hjemdahl-Monsen CE, Leavy J, Weiss M, Borrico S, Gorlin R, Fuster V. Angiographic progression of coronary artery disease and the development of myocardial infarction. J Am Coll Cardiol 1988; 12:56-62.
19. Muller JE, Tofler GH, Stone PH. Circadian variation and triggers of onset of acute cardiovascular disease. Circulation 1989; 79:1-11.
20. Ambrose JA, Winters SL, Stern A, Eng A, Teichholz LE, Gorlin R, Fuster V. Angiographic morphology and the pathogenesis of stable angina pectoris. J Am Coll Cardiol 1985; 5:609-16.
21. Sherman CT, Lituack F, Grandifest W, Lee M, Hickey A, Chauz A, Kass R, Blanche E, Matloff J, Morganstern L, Ganz W, Swan HJC, Forrester J. Coronary angioscopy in patients with unstable angina pectoris. N Engl J Med 1986; 315:913-19.
22. Constentinides P. Plaque fissures in human coronary thrombosis. J Atheroscler Rev. 1966; 1:1-17.
23. Little WL, Constantinesca M, Applegate RJ, Katcher MA, Burrows MT, Kahl FR, Santamore WP. Can coronary angiography predict site of a subsequent myocardial infarction in patients with mild-to-moderate coronary artery disease? Circulation 1988; 78:1157-66.
24. The Norwegian Multicenter Study Group. Timolol-induced reduction in mortality and reinfarctdion in patients surviving acute myocardial infarction. N Engl J Med 1981; 304:801-7.
25. Hjalmarson A, Elmfeld TD, Herlitz S, Malek I, Nyberg G, Ryden L, Swedberg K, Venin A, Wacgstein F, Waldenstrom A, Waldenstrom J, Wedel H,

Wilhelmsen L. Effect on mortality of metoprolol in acute myocardial infarction: a double blind randomized trial. Lancet 1981; 2:823-7.
26. Yusuf S, Peto R, Lewis J, Collins R, Sleight P. Beta blockade during and after myocardial infarction: an overview of the randomized trials. Prog Cardiovasc Dis 1985; 27:335-71.
27. Lichstein E. Why do beta-receptor blockers decrease mortality after myocardial infarction? J Am Coll Cardiol 1988; 6:972-5.
28. Peters RW. Beta blockers and mortality following myocardial infarction: more questions than answers. Arch Intern Med 1987; 47:33-4.
29. Willich SN, Linderer T, Wegscheider K, Shroder R, and the ISAM STudy Group. Increased risk of myocardial infarction in the mornings. (Abstract) J Am Coll Cardiol 1988; 11:28A.
30. Hjalmarson SN, Gilpin EA, Nicod P, Dittrich H, Henning H, Engler R, Blacky AR, Smith SC Jr, Ricon F, Ross J Jr. Differing circadian patterns of symptom onset in subgroups of patients with acute myocardial infarction. Circulation 1989; 80:267-75.
31. Byington RP. For the Beta-Blocker Heart Attack Trial Research Group. Beta-Blocker Heart Attack Trial: design methods and baseline results. Controlled Clin Trials 1984; 5:382-437.
32. Beta-Blocker Heart Attack Trial Research Group. A randomized trial of propranolol in patients with acute myocardial infarction: II. Morbidity results. JAMA 1983; 250:2814-19.
33. Peters RW, Byington R, Arensberg D, Friedman LM, Romhilt DW, Barker A, Laubach C, Wilner GW, Goldstein S. Mortality in the beta blocker heart attack trial: circumstances surrounding death. J Chron Dis. 1987; 40:75-82.
34. Lichstein E, Morganroth J, Harrist R, Hubble E. Effect of propranolol on ventricular arrhythmia—the Beta Blocker Heart Attack Trial experience. Circulation 1983; 67:1-5.
35. Morganroth J, Lichstein E, Byington R. For the Beta-Blocker Heart Attack Trial Study Group. Beta-Blocker Heart Attack Trial: impact of propranolol therapy on ventricular arrhythmias. Preventive Med 1985; 14:34;6-57.
36. Willich SN, Pohjola-Sintomen S, Bhatia SJS, Shook TL, Tofler GH, Muller JE, Curtis DG, Williams GH, Stone PH. Suppression of silent ischemia by metoprolol without alteration of morning increase of platelet aggregability in patients with stable coronary artery disease. Circulation 1989; 79:557-65.
37. The TIMI Study Group. Comparison of invasive and conservative strategies after treatment with intravenous tissue plasminogen activator in acute myocardial infarction: results of the Thrombolysis in Myocardial Infarction (TIMI): Phase II Trial. N Engl J Med 1989; 320:618-27.

III

Beta-Blockers as Primary Antiarrhythmic Agents in Cardiac Tachyarrhythmias

8

Beta-Adrenergic Blockade and the Treatment of Exercise-Induced Ventricular Arrhythmias

Ruey J. Sung*
San Francisco General Hospital and The Cardiovascular Research Institute, University of California at San Francisco, San Francisco, California

Wei Fan and Motonobu Hayano
Wadsworth Veterans Affairs Medical Center and University of California at Los Angeles School of Medicine, Los Angeles, California

INTRODUCTION

Exercise produces a multitude of metabolic, hemodynamic, and electrophysiological effects, all of which are conducive to the genesis of cardiac arrhythmias (1,2). Clinical studies have noted that exercise stress testing may provoke ventricular arrhythmias not only in patients with arteriosclerotic coronary heart disease and primary or secondary cardiomyopathy, but also in patients without clinical evidence of structural heart disease (3-6). In an attempt to define electrophysiological mechanisms of ventricular arrhythmias, Sung et al. (7) have observed that patients with exercise-provocable sustained ventricular tachycardia generally do not have excessive secretion of catecholamines as plasma epinephrine and norepinephrine levels are within normal limits at rest and those measured during exercise stress testing are comparable to the extent of exercise. Sung et al. (7) suggest that the presence of a low sympathetic threshold and/or an arrhythmia-

*Present affiliation: Director of Electrophysiology and Cardiac Arrhythmia Service, Stanford University Medical Center, and Professor, Division of Cardiovascular Medicine, Department of Medicine, Stanford University School of Medicine, Palo Alto, California

prone anatomic substrate is responsible for the occurrence of exercise-induced ventricular tachycardia. Furthermore, Sung et al. (7-9) have characterized three forms of ventricular tachycardia according to the mode of arrhythmia initiation and termination and the arrhythmia response to various pharmacological agents. Sung et al. (7-9) conclude that the existence of disparate electrophysiological mechanisms explains why exercise-induced ventricular arrhythmias are not uniformly responsive to any specific antiarrhythmic agent (7-13).

Beta-adrenergic blockade also exerts a multitude of metabolic, hemodynamic, and electrophysiological effects and has been shown to be clinically efficacious in the treatment of certain forms of ventricular arrhythmias (14-17). However, the mechanisms by which beta-adrenergic blockade suppresses ventricular arrhythmias remain incompletely understood. Recently, Sung et al. (2) have classified exercise-induced ventricular arrhythmias into subtypes based on clinical presentations as well as electrophysiological characteristics. This classification may be of value in better understanding the role of beta-adrenergic blockade in the treatment of exercise-induced ventricular arrhythmias.

EXERCISE-INDUCED VENTRICULAR ARRHYTHMIAS WITH ONSET CAUSED BY ACUTE MYOCARDIAL ISCHEMIA

Exercise increases sympathetic tone and promotes secretion of catecholamines (1,2). Exercise can thus increase myocardial oxygen demands by accelerating the heart rate, increasing cardiac contractility, and elevating blood pressure, and, as a consequence, exercise may induce acute myo-

Table 1 Exercise-Induced Ventricular Tachyarrhythmias with Onset Caused by Acute Myocardial Ischemia

MECHANISMS:

Exercise

↑ Myocardial O_2 demand

↓ Coronary arterial blood flow

by ↑ Heart rate
↑ Cardiac contractility
↑ Systemic BP

c̄ Coronary arterial spasm

Acute myocardial ischemia

Ventricular tachyarrhythmia

cardial ischemia with or without myocardial infarction (Table 1). Acute myocardial ischemia decreases the ventricular fibrillation threshold and is a potential trigger of an onset of ventricular arrhythmias (18), particularly in patients with arteriosclerotic coronary heart disease. Beta-adrenergic blockade counteracts the effects of catecholamines and can thus decrease myocardial oxygen demands by slowing the heart rate, decreasing cardiac contractility, and lowering blood pressure (19) and may thereby circumvent the development of acute myocardial ischemia and ventricular arrhythmias. However, in addition to beta-adrenergic blockade, an optimal antiischemic regimen should include the use of nitrates and/or calcium channel blocking agents (20), and as clinically indicated, revascularization with the use of percutaneous transluminal coronary angioplasty and/or aorto-coronary bypass grafting should be considered as the ultimate measure of treatment.

Exercise may also cause acute myocardial ischemia by provoking coronary arterial spasm in a small subset group of patients with minimal or no gross arteriosclerotic coronary heart disease (the variant angina syndrome) (see Table 1) (21). Beta-adrenergic blockade alone is contraindicated in this subset group of patients as beta-adrenergic blockade leaves alpha-adrenergic activity unopposed and may thereby facilitate the induction of coronary arterial spasm. The combination therapy with nitrates and calcium channel blocking agents offers protection against development of coronary arterial spasm, but, in selected patients, cardiac sympathetic denervation may be indicated.

Ventricular arrhythmias of an ischemic etiology may manifest as monomorphous or polymorphous ventricular tachycardia (torsade de pointes) (22) and/or ventricular fibrillation (23). Because of the serious nature of these ventricular tachyarrhythmias, repeated exercise stress testing to confirm the arrhythmia reproducibility without treatment is not advisable, and electrophysiological study is of limited value in defining the underlying electrophysiological mechanism. Diagnosis of acute myocardial ischemia as the cause of exercise-induced ventricular arrhythmias depends on careful monitoring and analysis of clinical symptomatology and electrocardiographic ST-T wave changes. It may be necessary to use thallium-201 myocardial senitigraphy to confirm the diagnosis.

EXERCISE-INDUCED VENTRICULAR ARRHYTHMIAS WITH ONSET INDEPENDENT OF ACUTE MYOCARDIAL ISCHEMIA

As a result of the increase in sympathetic tone and secretion of catecholamines (1,2), exercise can enhance diastolic (phase 4) depolarization, improve membrane conductivity, shorten refractory periods of all cardiac tissues (24), and activate the adenylate-cyclase-cyclic AMP system, thereby increasing the transmembrane calcium influx (25). Exercise can thus provoke ventricular arrhythmias of various mechanisms including reentry, automaticity, and triggered rhythmic activity (26).

Exercise-induced ventricular tachycardias not caused by acute myocardial ischemia can be subclassified into verapamil-unresponsive and verapamil-responsive ventricular tachycardias (Table 2) (2,7,8).

Verapamil-Unresponsive Exercise-Induced Ventricular Tachycardia

Based on the mode of arrhythmia initiation and termination during electrophysiology study, this group of patients can be divided into groups IA and IB (Table 2). Group IA patients have ventricular tachycardia that can be provoked and terminated by programmed ventricular stimulation, whereas group IB patients have ventricular tachycardia that cannot be provoked electrically but is provocable with intravenous infusion of isoproterenol.

Group IA patients commonly manifest significant structural heart disease such as arteriosclerotic coronary heart disease with prior myocardial infarction and/or primary or secondary cardiomyopathy (7,8,11). Paroxysms of sustained monomorphous ventricular tachycardia are usually inducible with programmed ventricular stimulation and can usually be

Table 2 Exercise-Induced Ventricular Tachyarrhythmias with Onset Independent of Acute Myocardial Ischemia

Mechanisms:
- ↑ Sympathetic tone and secretion of catecholamines
- ↑ Diastolic (phase 4) depolarization
- ↓ Refractory periods of cardiac tissues
- ↑ Cell membrane conductivity
- ↑ Adenylate cyclase—cyclic AMP system (transmembrane Ca influx)

I. Verapamil-unresponsive
   A. Reentry
   B. Catecholamine-sensitive automaticity

II. Verapamil-responsive
   Triggered rhythmic activity

terminated by overdrive ventricular pacing. The QRS complex of ventricular tachycardia can be of either a right or a left bundle branch block pattern, and the electrophysiological mechanisms of the arrhythmia is believed to be due to reentry involving the border zone of infarcted or fibrotic tissues (26).

The initiation of a reentrant ventricular tachycardia requires induction of unidirectional block in one area and sufficient slow conduction in the other area within the reentrant circuit. In group IA patients, the area of slow conduction is probably composed of tissues of depressed fast sodium channels rather than calcium channel-dependent slow responses as intravenous verapamil (0.15 mg/kg bolus followed by 0.005 mg/kg/min infusion), a calcium channel blocking agent, exerts no effect on the inducibility and sustainability of the arrhythmia (8). In contrast, intravenous procainamide (20 mg/kg followed by 2-4 mg/min), a sodium channel blocking agent, can usually slow the rate of the arrhythmia and may even suppress the inducibility and sustainability of the arrhythmia. Similar to intravenous verapamil, beta-adrenergic blockade with intravenous propranolol (0.2 mg/kg) does not affect the inducibility and sustainability of the arrhythmia (7). At therapeutic doses, beta-adrenergic blocking agents of the oral form do not exhibit significant sodium channel blocking effects (18) and are, therefore, expected to have no effects on reentrant ventricular tachycardia unless the induction and/or sustainability of the arrhythmia depends on intravenous infusion of isoproterenol (catecholamine-sensitive reentry). Clinically the group IA patients often present with chronic recurrent sustained ventricular tachycardia that require amiodarone therapy, surgical ablation of the arrhythmia, and/or implantation of automatic implantable cardioverter/defibrillator.

The group IB patients may manifest no clinical evidence of structural heart disease. Characteristically, ventricular tachycardia cannot be elicited by programmed electrical stimulation but is provocable with intravenous infusion of isoproterenol (1-8 μg/min) (Figs. 1 and 2) and cannot be converted to a sustained sinus rhythm with overdrive ventricular pacing. The QRS complex is more often of a left rather than a right bundle branch block pattern. The electrophysiological mechanism of the arrhythmia is presumed to be due to catecholamine-sensitive automaticity (8).

An automatic rhythm occurs spontaneously and can be enhanced by catecholamines (26). Because of the limitations inherent in the clinical electrophysiology study technique, normal automaticity and abnormal automaticity cannot be differentiated. Of note is the observation that the arrhythmia inducibility can be completely suppressed by beta-adrenergic

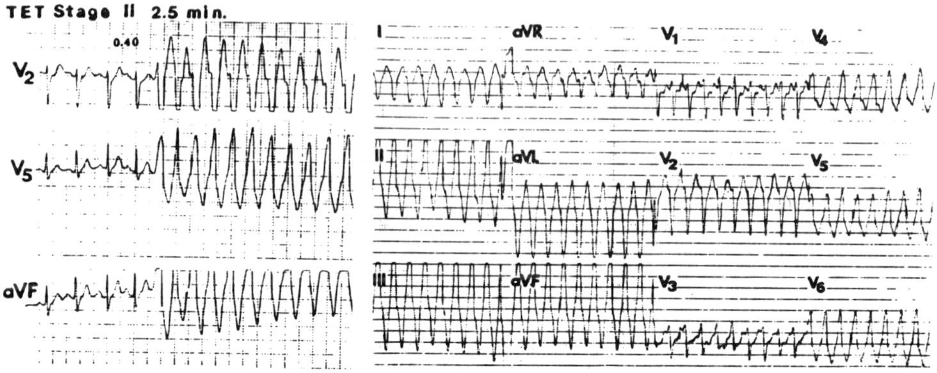

Figure 1 Provocation of ventricular tachycardia (VT) in the verapamil-irresponsive group during treadmill exercise testing. (Left panel) VT emerges during the stage II of treadmill exercise testing (TET) at which time the sinus rate has accelerated to 150 beats/min (cycle length 0.40 sec). Note that attainment of comparable cycle lengths during atrial and ventricular pacing cannot provoke onset of VT as shown in Figure 2A and B. (Right panel) The 12 lead electrocardiogram of the exercise-induced VT corresponding to that demonstrated in the left panel. (With permission from Ref. 7.)

Figure 2 Provocation and suppression of ventricular tachycardia (VT) in the verapamil-irresponsive group (see Table 2) (same patient as in Figure 1). VT cannot be elicited by programmed atrial and programmed ventricular stimulation but is provocable with intravenous infusion of isoproterenol. (A and B) High right atrial (HRA) and right ventricular pacing, respectively, at the cycle length (S-S) of 400 msec (comparable to that which initiates VT during treadmill exercise testing as shown in Fig. 1) cannot elicit the onset of VT. (C) Intravenous infusion of isoproterenol (4 μg/min) accelerates the sinus rate (cycle length shortened to 400 msec) and provokes the onset of VT with a left bundle branch block pattern (frontal axis +120°). The VT has an identical QRS morphology to that provoked by treadmill exercise testing, as shown in Figure 1. The cycle length of VT is 280 msec. (D) After beta-adrenergic blockade with intravenous propranolol (0.2 mg/kg), intravenous infusion of isoproterenol (4 μg/min) can no longer provoke the onset of the arrhythmia. (With permission from Ref. 7.)

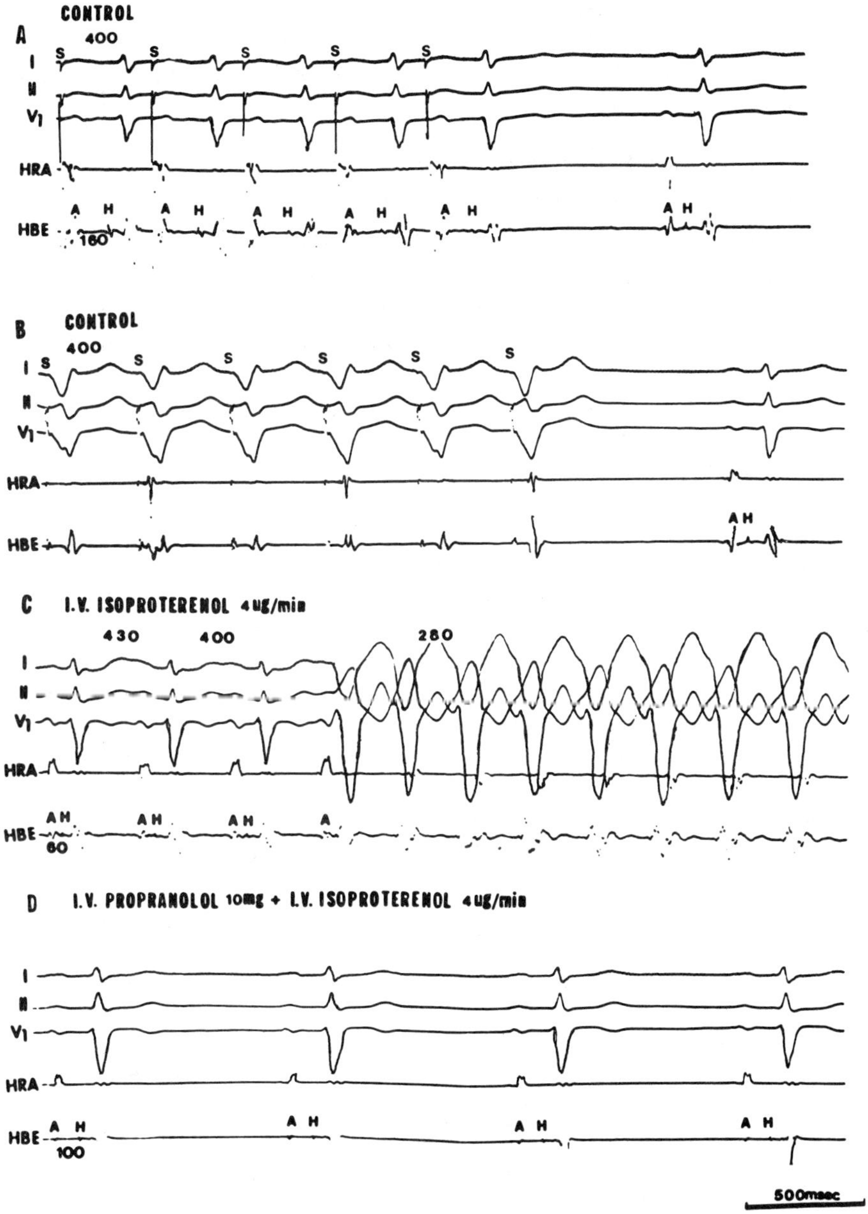
A CONTROL
400
S S S S S
I
II
V1
HRA
HBE
A H A H A H A H A H A H
160
B CONTROL
400
S S S S S S
I
II
V1
HRA
HBE
A H
C I.V. ISOPROTERENOL 4ug/min
430 400 280
I
II
V1
HRA
HBE
A H A H A H A
60
D I.V. PROPRANOLOL 10mg + I.V. ISOPROTERENOL 4ug/min
I
II
V1
HRA
HBE
A H A H A H A H
100
500msec

blockade with intravenous propranolol (see Fig. 2) (7). Intravenous verapamil exerts no effects, but intravenous procainamide may suppress the arrhythmia inducibility presumably by virtue of its depressive action on diastolic (phase 4) depolarization.

Verapamil-Responsive Exercise-Induced Ventricular Tachycardia

Group II patients are usually young and often do not have clinical evidence of structural heart disease. During electrophysiology study, the initiation of arrhythmia requires attainment of a critical range of cycle lengths during sinus, atrial-paced, and/or ventricular-paced rhythm (8). Similar to ventricular tachycardia of the group IA patients, the arrhythmia can be terminated by overdrive ventricular pacing, but unlike ventricular tachycardia of the group IA patients, the arrhythmia can be completely suppressed by intravenous infusion of verapamil (8). The QRS complex can be of either a right or a left bundle branch block pattern with the former being more commonly observed (60% to 40% ratio) (7). The electrophysiological mechanism of the arrhythmia is speculated to be due to triggered rhythmic activity related to delayed afterdepolarizations or due to reentry involving tissues of calcium channel-dependent slow responses within the reentrant circuit (7,8).

The initiation of triggered rhythmic activity related to delayed afterdepolarizations depends on previous depolarizations (27). Within a critical range of cycle lengths, delayed afterdepolarizations can attain the threshold potential and thereby elicit an action potential which, if perpetuated, can lead to a sustained rhythmic activity. The ionic currents responsible for the genesis of delayed afterdepolarizations are believed to be carried by sodium and modulated by calcium. Electrophysiologically, certain aspects of the arrhythmia in the group II patients conform to triggered rhythmic activity related to delayed afterdepolarizations, however, reentry involving tissues of calcium channel-dependent slow responses remains to be a viable mechanism. Notably, intravenous verapamil can totally suppress the inducibility and sustainability of arrhythmia while both intravenous procainamide and beta-adrenergic blockade with intravenous propranolol can only slow the rate of arrhythmia without affecting the arrhythmia inducibility and sustainability (Figs. 3 and 4) (7-9). Beta-adrenergic blockade can suppress arrhythmia inducibility only when the induction of arrhythmia is dependent on intravenous infusion of isoproterenol (catecholamine-sensitive triggered rhythmic activity).

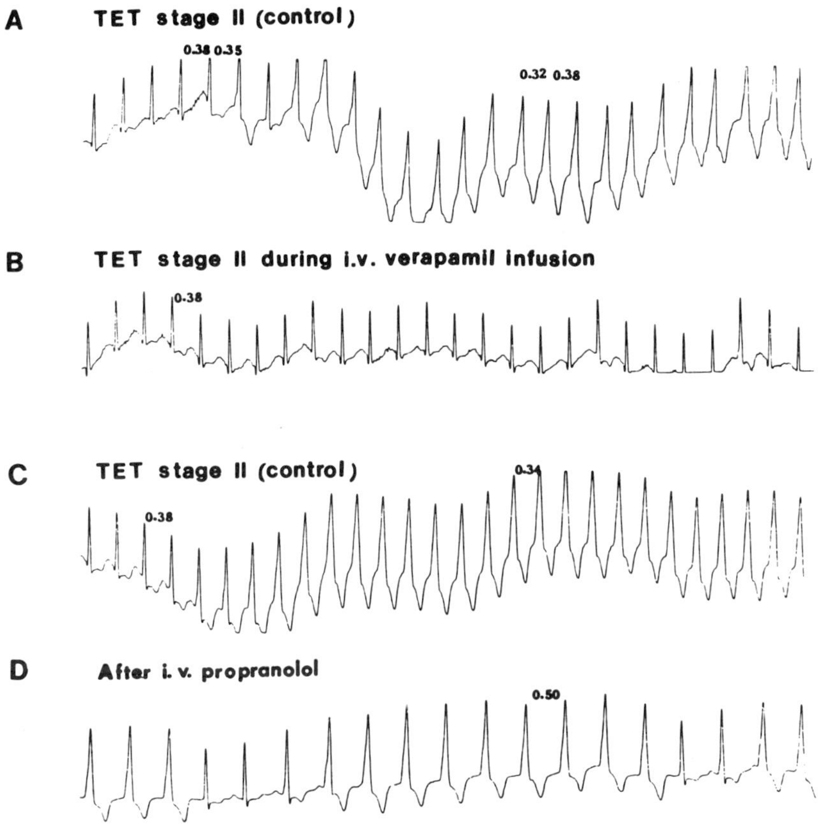

Figure 3 Verapamil-responsive ventricular tachycardia (VT) tested with intravenous verapamil and intravenous propranolol (group II) (see Table 2). (A) At control, treadmill exercise testing (TET) accelerates the sinus rate (cycle length: 0.38 sec) at the stage II and initiates an onset of VT with cycle lengths ranging from 0.32 to 0.38 sec. The QRS complex of VT is of a complete left bundle branch block pattern in lead V_5. (B) Repeated TET during verapamil infusion can no longer initiate the onset of arrhythmia. (C) At control, VT is reproduced by TET at the stage II with sinus rate acceleration (cycle length: 0.38 sec) (TET done on a separate day). The cycle length of VT is 0.34 sec. (D) After beta-adrenergic blockade, the VT slows its rate with a cycle length of 0.50 sec and becomes continuous requiring intravenous verapamil (5 mg) for termination (not shown). (With permission from Ref. 7.)

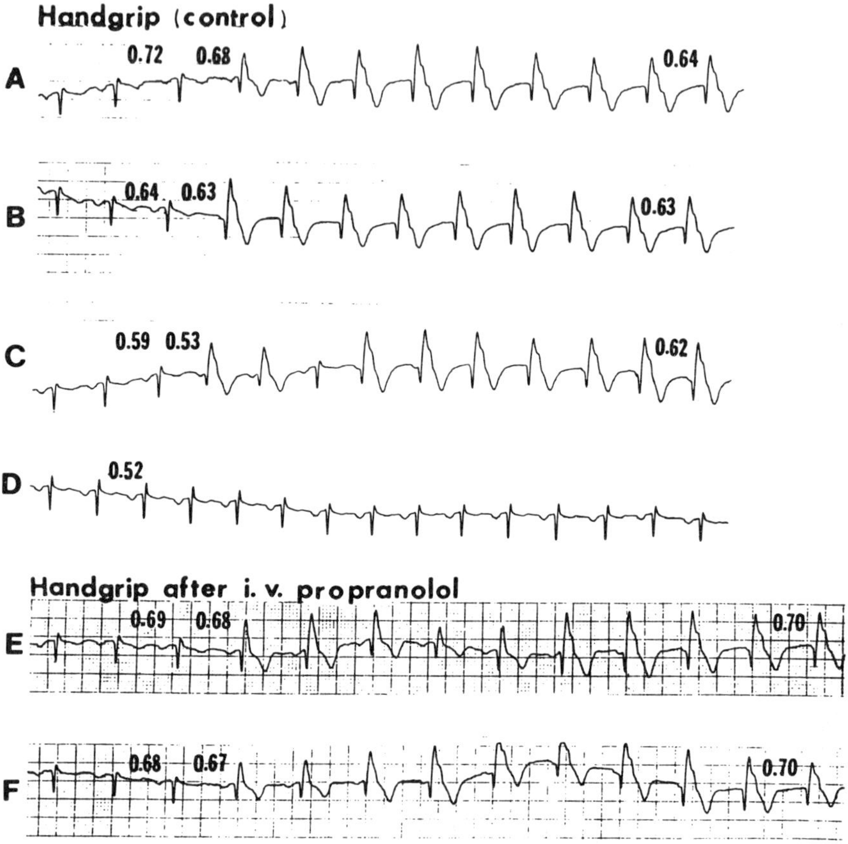

Figure 4 Effects of beta-adrenergic blockade on verapamil-responsive ventricular tachycardia (VT) (group II) (see Table 2). (A-C) At control, repeated handgrips accelerate the sinus rate and trigger an onset of VT. Note that VT starts in late diastole and that there is a progressive shortening of its coupling interval (0.68-0.53 sec) in response to sinus rate acceleration (cycle length 0.72-0.59 sec). Also note that the QRS complex of VT is of a right bundle branch block pattern in lead V_1. (D) Further acceleration of the sinus rate (cycle length 0.52 sec) during handgrip can not initiate the onset of VT. (E and F) After beta-adrenergic blockade with intravenous propranolol (0.2 mg/kg), handgrips continue to trigger the onset of VT at a slower rate (cycle length: 0.70 sec). (With permission from Ref. 7.)

EXERCISE-INDUCED VENTRICULAR ARRHYTHMIAS AS A PROARRHYTHMIC EFFECT OF ANTIARRHYTHMIC THERAPY

Facilitation of the arrhythmia induction during exercise stress testing can be a manifestation of the proarrhythmic effects of antiarrhythmic therapy (28). Antiarrhythmic agents frequently implicated are Class Ic agents such as flecainide and encainide. Postulated mechanisms include drug-induced reentry and/or afterdepolarizations associated with frequency-dependent sodium and/or potassium channel blockade of these antiarrhythmic agents as revealed by acceleration of the sinus rate during exercise stress testing (29,30). Exercise-induced ventricular arrhythmias reflecting a proarrhythmic effect of antiarrhythmic therapy are a distinct clinical entity (28). If the cause of these ventricular arrhythmias is left unrecognized, the occurrence of these arrhythmias may worsen already compromised left ventricular function and may even lead to sudden cardiac death.

CLINICAL APPROACH TO MANAGEMENT OF EXERCISE-INDUCED VENTRICULAR ARRHYTHMIAS: ROLE OF BETA-ADRENERGIC BLOCKADE

Prognostic implications of exercise-induced ventricular arrhythmias remain to be established (31-33). The extent of structural heart disease and the severity of left ventricular dysfunction generally dictate the outcome of these patients. Ventricular premature beats alone may not warrant antiarrhythmic therapy, but nonsustained (lasting shorter than 30 seconds but more than six beats in a row) and, in particular, sustained (lasting longer than 30 seconds or developing circulatory collapse before that time) deserve a complete diagnostic work-up to differentiate between ischemic and nonischemic causes. An aggressive therapeutic approach is justified in certain patients as sudden cardiac death has been reported in those with and those without clinical evidence of structural heart disease (34,35). Myocardial revascularization is not effective in suppressing exercise-induced ventricular arrhythmias not caused by myocardial ischemia even in patients with arteriosclerotic coronary heart disease (11,36). Electrophysiology study with pharmacological testing may be indicated in selected patients (7,8). As has been mentioned, amiodarone therapy, surgical ablation of the arrhythmia, and implantation of automatic implantable cardioverter/defibrillator may be necessary in patients with sustained ventricular tachyarrhythmias refractory to conventional antiarrhythmic treatment. Needless to say, the treatment of exercise-induced ventricular arrhythmias secondary to a proarrhythmic effect of antiarrhythmic therapy is immediate removal of the offending antiarrhythmic agent.

Beta-adrenergic blockade counteracts the effects of catecholamines (19). It is rational and reasonable to use beta-adrenergic blocking agents as the first drugs of choice for treatment of exercise-induced ventricular arrhythmias particularly in patients with arteriosclerotic coronary heart disease (37). It has been shown that beta-adrenergic blockade reduces total mortality during the extended recovery period (1-3 years) after myocardial infarction. The rate of occurrence of reinfarction and sudden death is also reduced by chronic beta-adrenergic blockade in these patients (37). However, beta-adrenergic blockade is not expected to be uniformly effective in suppression of exercise-induced ventricular arrhythmias (8). Beta-adrenergic blockade is specifically useful in the following two clinical settings: (1) exercise-induced ventricular arrhythmias due to acute myocardial ischemia not primarily caused by coronary arterial spasm, and (2) exercise-induced ventricular arrhythmias of catecholamine-sensitive automaticity. In patients with exercise-induced ventricular arrhythmias due to acute myocardial ischemia primarily caused by coronary arterial spasm, beta-adrenergic blockade is contraindicated. Beta-adrenergic blockade generally does not suppress exercise-induced ventricular arrhythmias of reentrant mechanism and those of trigger rhythmic activity related to delayed afterdepolarizations (7,8) unless the induction of these arrhythmias depends on intravenous infusion of isoproterenol (catecholamine-sensitive reentry and catecholamine-sensitive triggered rhythmic activity).

In summary, clinical and electrophysiological mechanisms of exercise-induced ventricular arrhythmias are complex. Developing a rationale for therapy with antiischemic and/or antiarrhythmic agents and tailoring choices to the needs of individual patients should be based on careful analysis of clinical presentations and possible electrophysiological mechanisms.

ACKNOWLEDGMENT

The authors wish to express their appreciation to Mrs. Grace Chen for preparation of this manuscript.

REFERENCES

1. Jelinek MV, Lown B. Exercise stress testing for exposure of cardiac arrhythmia. Prog Cardiovasc Dis 1974; 16:497-522.

2. Sung RJ, Juycke EC, Lai WT, Tseng CD, Chu H, Keung EC. Clinical and electrophysiologic mechanisms of exercise-induced ventricular tachyarrhythmias. PACE 1988; 11:1347-57.
3. Goldschlager N, Cake D, Cohn K. Exercise-induced ventricular arrhythmias in patients with coronary artery disease. Their relation to angiographic findings. Am J Cardiol 1972; 31:434-40.
4. McHenry PL, Fisch C, Jordon JW, Corya BR. Cardiac arrhythmias observed during maximal treadmill exercise testing in clinically normal man. Am J Cardiol 1972; 29:331-6.
5. Mokotoff DM, Quinones MA, Miller RR. Exercise-induced ventricular tachycardia. Clinical features, relation to chronic ventricular ectopy, and prognosis. Chest 1980; 77:10-16.
6. Codini MA, Sommerfeldt L, Eybel CE, Messer JV. Clinical significance and characteristics of exercise-induced ventricular tachycardia. Cather Cardiovasc Diag 1981; 7:227-34.
7. Sung RJ, Keung EC, Nguyen NX, Huycke EC. Effects of beta-adrenergic blockade on verapamil-responsive and verapamil-irresponsive sustained ventricular tachycardia. J Clin Invest 1988; 81:688-99.
8. Sung RJ, Shapiro WA, Shen EN, Morady F, Davis J. Effects of verapamil on ventricular tachycardias possibly caused by reentry, automaticity, and triggered activity. J Clin Invest 1983; 72:350-60.
9. Sung RJ, Huycke EC, Tseng CD, Keung EC. Pharmacologic effects of intravenous procainamide on verapamil-responsive ventricular tachycardia (Abst). Circulation 1988; 78(Suppl II):629.
10. Palileo EV, Ashley WW, Swiryn S, Bauernfeind RA, Strasberg B, Petropoulos AT, Rosen KM. Exercise provocable right ventricular outflow tract tachycardia. Am Heart J 1982; 104:185-93.
11. Sung RJ, Shen EN, Morady F, Scheinmen MM, Hess D, Botvinick EH. Electrophysiologic mechanism of exercise-induced sustained ventricular tachycardia. Am J Cardiol 1983; 51:525-30.
12. Woelfel A, Foster JR, Simpson RJ Jr, Gettes LS. Reproducibility and treatment of exercise-induced ventricular tachycardia. Am J Cardiol 1985; 53: 751-6.
13. Woelfel A, Foster JR, McAllister RG Jr, Simpson RJ Jr, Gettes LS. Efficacy of verapamil in exercise-induced ventricular tachycardia. Am J Cardiol 1985; 56:292-7.
14. Gibson D, Sowton D. The use of beta-adrenergic receptor blocking drugs in dysrhythmias. Prog Cardiovasc Dis 1969; 12:16-39.
15. Taylor RR, Johnston CI, Jose AD. Reversal of digitalis intoxication by beta-adrenergic blockade with pronethalol. N Engl J Med 1964; 271:877-82.
16. Schwartz PJ. The idiopathic long Q-T syndrome. Ann Intern Med 1983; 99:561-2.
17. Ryden L, Ariniego R, Arnman K, Herlitz J, Hjalmarson A,, Holmberg S, Reyes C, Smedgard P, Svedberg K, Vedin A, Waagstein F, Waldenstrom

A, Wilhelmsson C, Wedel H, Yamamoto M. A double-blind trial of metoprolol in acute myocardial infarction: effects on ventricular tachyarrhythmias. N Engl J Med 1983; 308:614-8.

18. Janse MJ, van Capelle FJL, Morsink H, Kleber AG, Schopman FW, Cardinal R, D'Alnoncourt CN, Durrer D. Flow of "injury" current and patterns of excitation during early ventricular arrhythmias in acute regional myocardial ischemia in isolated porcine and canine heart. Evidence for two different arrhythmia genic mechanisms. Circ Res 1980; 47:151-65.
19. Sung RJ, Tai DY, Svinarich JT. Beta-adrenoceptor blockade: electrophysiology and antiarrhythmic mechanisms. Am Heart J 1984; 108:1115-20.
20. Nguyen NX, Yang PT, Huycke EC, Sung RJ. Verapamil and ventricular tachyarrhythmias. PACE 1987; 10:571-8.
21. Kugiyana K, Yasue H, Horio Y, Morikami Y, Fujii H, Koga Y, Kojima A, Takahashi M. Effects of propranolol and nifedipine on exercise-induced attack in patients with variant angina: assessment by exercise thallium-201 myocardial scintigraphy with quantitative rotational tomography. Circulation 1986; 74:374-80.
22. Smith WM, Gallagher JJ. Les torsades de pointes: as unusual ventricular arrhythmia. Ann Intern Med 1980; 93:578-84.
23. Cline RE, Armstrong RG, Stanford W. Successful myocardial revascularization after ventricular fibrillation induced by treadmill exercise. J Thorac Cardiovasc Surg 1973; 65:802-5.
24. Han J, de Jalon PG, Moe GK. Adrenergic effects on ventricular vulnerability. Circ Res 1964; 14:516-24.
25. Brum G, Osterrieder W, Trautwein W. Beta-adrenergic increase in the calcium conductance of calcium myocytes studied with the patch clamp. Pflugers Arch 1984; 401:111-8.
26. Hoffman BF, Rosen MR. Cellular mechanisms of cardiac arrhythmias. Circ Res 1981; 49:1-15.
27. Rosen MR, Reder PF. Does triggered activity have a role in the genesis of cardiac arrhythmias? Ann Intern Med 1981; 94:794-801.
28. Anastasiou-Nana MI, Anderrson JL, Stewart JR, Crevey BJ, Yanowitz FG, Lutz JR, Johnson TA. Occurrence of exercise-induced and spontaneous wide complex tachycardia during therapy with flecainide for complex ventricular arrhythmias: a probable proarrhythmic effect. Am Heart J 1987; 113:1071-7.
29. Ranger S, Talajic M, Lemery R, Roy D, Nattel S. Amplification of flecainide-induced ventricular conduction slowing by exercise: a potentially significant clinical consequence of use-dependent sodium channel blockade. Circulation 1989; 79:1000-6.
30. Rosen MR, Wit AL. Arrhythmogenic actions of antiarrhythmic drugs. Am J Cardiol 1987; 59:10E-17E.
31. Nair CK, Aronow WS, Sketch MH, Pagano T, Lynch JD, Mooss AN, Esterbrooks D, Runco V, Ryschon K. Diagnostic and prognostic significance of

exercise-induced premature ventricular complexes in men and women: a four year follow-up. J Am Coll Cardiol 1983; 1:1201-6.
32. Califf RM, Mckinnins RA, McNeer JF, Harrell FE Jr., Lee KL, Pryor DB, Waugh RA, Harris PJ, Rosati RA, Wagner GS. Prognostic value of ventricular arrhythmias associated with treadmill exercise testing in patients studied with cardiac catherization for suspected ischemic heart disease. J Am Coll Cardiol 1983; 2:1060-7.
33. Sami M, Chaitman B, Fisher L, Holmes D, Fray D, Alderman E. Significance of exercise-induced ventricular rarrhythmia in stable coronary artery disease: a coronary artery surgery study project. Am J Cardiol 1984; 54:1182-8.
34. Wilson FN, Wishart SW, Macleod AG, Barker PS. A clinical type of paroxysmal tachycardia of ventricular origin in which paroxysms are induced by exertion. Am Heart J 1932; 8:155-69.
35. Deal BJ, Miller SM, Scagliotti D, Prechel D, Gallastegui JL, Hariman RJ. Ventricular tachycardia in young population without overt heart disease. Circulation 1986; 73:1111-8.
36. Lehrman KL, Tilkian AG, Hultgren HN, Fowles RE. Effect of coronary arterial bypass surgery on exercise-induced ventricular arrhythmias: long term follow-up of a prospective randomized study. Am J Cardiol 1979; 44: 1056-61.
37. Norwegian Study Group. Timolol-induced reduction in mortality and reinfarction in patients surviving acute myocardial infarction. N Engl J Med 1981; 304:801-7.

9

Clinical Experience with Atenolol in the Treatment of Arrhythmias

Valerie E. Moore and John Malcolm Cruickshank*
ICI Pharmaceuticals, Macclesfield, Cheshire, England

SUPRAVENTRICULAR ARRHYTHMIAS

The types of supraventricular arrhythmias and the response to beta-blockers are illustrated in Table 1.

Sinus Tachycardia

This is not a primary disorder; rather it is secondary to other problems such as fever, infection, hyperthyroidism, phaeochromocytoma, heart failure, pericarditis, pulmonary embolism, anxiety states, or postexercise. Treatment must accordingly be directed to the primary problem. Once this has been diagnosed and treatment instituted, a beta-blocker can be used for controlling heart rate where the rate itself is compromising the patient, e.g., contributing to anginal symptoms in the setting of another disease such as pneumonia.

The slowing of fast heart rates associated with mitral stenosis can prolong diastolic filling time and thus minimize the end diastolic mitral gradient and diminish pulmonary wedge pressures and pulmonary congestion (1). The effect of oral atenolol (100 mg o.d. for 2 weeks) was studied in 13

*Present affiliation: Wythenshawe Hospital, Winslow, Cheshire, and Royal Brompton and National Heart and Chest Hospital, London, England.

Table 1 Expected Response of Supraventricular Cardiac Arrhythmias to Treatment with Beta-Blockers

Supraventricular arrhythmia	Response
Sinus tachycardia	Excellent
Paroxysmal supraventricular tachycardia (including WPW syndrome)	Good—both elective and prophylactic
Chronic ectopic supraventricular tachycardia	Good—sinus rhythm sometimes restored
Atrial fibrillation	Ventricular rate reduced—sinus rhythm rarely restored
Atrial flutter	Ventricular rate reduced—sinus rhythm sometimes restored

Source: Ref. 14.

patients with tight mitral stenosis in a single-blind crossover study. Atenolol resulted in a significant increase in effort tolerance (2).

In a pilot study of the antiarrhythmic action of oral atenolol (50-150 mg/day) or intravenous atenolol (5 mg), all five cases of sinus tachycardia returned to normal sinus rhythm (3), irrespective of etiology (thyrotoxic crisis, alcohol cardiomyopathy, or hyperkinetic heart syndrome).

Reentrant Paroxysmal Supraventricular Tachycardia (PSVT)

This arrhythmia may be divided into two groups: (1) those in which no obvious cause is found and (2) those in which an underlying cause is detected, e.g., Wolff-Parkinson-White syndrome (WPW) and its variants. Both types usually involve reentry involving the AV node.

PSVT (excluding WPW)

Included in this group are AV nodal reentrant and intraatrial reentrant tachycardias. The former use the AV node as an accessory bypass tract. Rare cases are due to reentry at the SA node.

PSVT initiated by programmed stimulation was prevented by intravenous atenolol in four of six (67%) cases (4).

Atenolol (5-10 mg i.v.) was compared with nadolol (0.05-1 mg/kg i.v.) in 46 patients with recurrent SVT. Responders and partial responders to the intravenous beta-blocker continued on oral therapy. Both atenolol and nadolol were effective in the treatment of SVT due to atrioventricular nodal reentry (64%). However, both therapies had limited efficacy in the treatment of SVT due to atrioventricular reentry (5).

Beta-blockers administered orally have also proved useful, particularly where the PSVT is precipitated by emotion or exercise. Patients with chronic PSVT whose programmed stimulated PSVT could be prevented by oral atenolol responded well to chronic prophylactic oral atenolol over a 15- to 20-month period (6). Others have also shown that chronic oral atenolol given over a 6- to 50-month period prevented the recurrence of paroxysmal SVT in seven of 11 patients (7). In 13 patients with paroxysmal SVT, sotalol 120-240 mg/day was superior to atenolol 50-100 mg/day in diminishing the number and duration of episodes of SVT over a 6-week period (8).

Children

Trippel and Gillette (9) have retrospectively evaluated the use of oral atenolol as a single agent in the long-term treatment of children with SVT. Of the 24 patients studied, five had tachycardia due to reentry within the atrioventricular node. Atenolol (0.8-2.0 mg/kg/day) was fully effective in three of these five children, partially effective in one, and ineffective in one.

PSVT Arising from Preexcitation Syndromes (Including WPW Syndrome)

This topic has been reviewed by Gallagher et al. (10). Preexcitation syndromes arise from accessory tracts which bypass the normal pathways linking atria and ventricles, resulting in accelerrated conduction and premature excitation of the ventricles. The classic bypass tract was termed the Bundle of Kent. These events are reflected in the ECG by a short P-R interval and a preexcitation, or delta, wave.

Programmed induction of PSVT in patients with WPW was prevented in three out of five cases with intravenous atenolol (0.07-0.1 mg/kg) (4, 11) but only four out of 14 with propranolol (12).

Children

Trippel and Gillette (9) found that of 14 children with supraventricular tachycardia due to an accessory connection, oral atenolol (0.7-2.0 mg/kg/day) was fully effective in six patients, and partially effective in three. This study demonstrated a lower success rate in children with an accessory connection than those with atrioventricular node reentry.

Atrial Fibrillation (AF)

If the onset of AF is acute or related to high sympathetic drive such as exercise, beta-blockers may convert the AF to sinus rhythm (13,14). Long-standing cases are rarely converted to sinus rhythm (13,15), but a decrease in heart rate can be beneficial (14). Electrophysiologically beta-blockers are not antifibrillatory in the atria.

In eight patients with atrial fibrillation treated with oral atenolol (50-100 mg/day) or intravenous atenolol (5 mg), only two reverted to sinus rhythm, but five patients benefited from a reduction in ventricular rate (3). Similar findings with intravenous atenolol (0.1-0.15 mg/kg) have been reported by other groups (16,17). In a study of the electrophysiological effects of intravenous atenolol (2.5 mg), four of 12 patients showed an increase in episodes of atrial fibrillation (18).

The effects of oral atenolol (50 mg b.i.d.), verapamil (80 mg b.i.d.), and xamoterol (200 mg b.i.d.) have been compared in digitalized patients with chronic atrial fibrillation. All three treatments achieved better control of the ventricular response rate than digoxin (19).

Atrial Flutter

Atrial flutter is rarely restored to sinus rhythm by a beta-blocker. However, the heart is not infrequently usefully slowed with an increase in AV block (14). This effect has been shown for most beta-blockers (14) including atenolol (3). Beta-blockade can be helpful for slowing heart rate in order to identify the type of arrhythmia.

Children

Symptomatic improvement was experienced in five out of five children with atrial flutter treated with oral atenolol (0.8-1.0 mg/kg/day); three children had complete relief of symptoms (9).

Postmyocardial Infarction Supraventricular Arrhythmias

The mode of action of beta-blockers in this condition involves mainly modifications of the ischaemic process and antagonizing catecholamine effects. The topic has been discussed by Singh and Jewitt (14) and Baber (20).

Prophylactic Management

In a retrospective study of 163 patients randomized to either atenolol (initially intravenous 5-10 mg then oral 100 mg o.d. for 10 days) or no beta-blocker early after acute myocardial infarction (i.e., within 12 hours of onset of pain), atrial fibrillation was less common in patients receiving atenolol—one of 85 patients on atenolol developed atrial fibrillation compared with nine of 78 patients receiving no beta blockade (21).

Four hundred and seventy-seven patients suspected of having had acute myocardial infarction within less than 12 hours were randomized to receive intravenous atenolol (5 mg) followed by oral treatment (50-100 mg) for 10 days or to a control group (22). Atenolol-treated patients showed a significant reduction in the incidence of atrial fibrillation and supraventricular tachycardia, and the use of other antiarrhythmic drugs was also significantly reduced.

Others

Trauma and Head Injury

Head injury can be associated with tachyarrhythmias, which may be catecholamine-induced (23). In a double-blind, randomized, between-patient

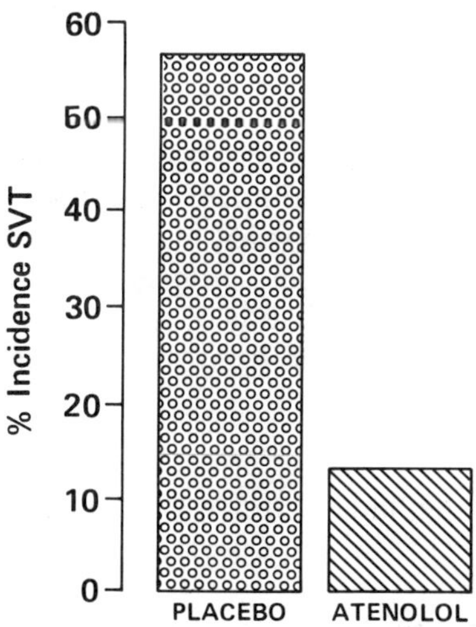

Figure 1 The effect of atenolol on supraventricular tachycardia (SVT) in patients with acute head injury. In a double-blind, randomized study in 114 patients with acute head injury, compared to placebo, atenolol (intravenous 10 mg 6-hourly for 3 days, followed by oral 100 mg daily for 4 days) significantly ($p < 0.0001$) reduced the incidence of SVT in the 95 patients assessed daily by Holter monitoring. (From Refs. 24, 25.)

study in 114 cases of head injury, intravenous atenolol (10 mg 6-hourly for 3 days) followed by oral atenolol (100 mg o.d. for 4 days) was compared to placebo. Sinus tachycardia and supraventricular tachycardia were significantly ($p < 0.001$) less frequent in the beta-blocker-treated group (24,25) (Fig. 1).

VENTRICULAR ARRHYTHMIAS

The presence of ventricular arrhythmias has, generally speaking, a more sinister implication than the presence of supraventricular arrhythmias. VPBs, both simple and complex, and other ventricular arrhythmias must therefore be regarded as potential harbingers of premature death. However, it should be emphasized that to date there is no evidence that suppression of VPBs in any subset of patients leads to prolonged survival. Antiarrhythmic therapy in patients with complex VPBs is based on the expectation that the risk potential might be reduced, but without definitive proof that it is. Thus, the goal of therapy with beta-blockers should be identified—whether it is to reduce symptoms or to enhance survival (or both).

Ventricular Arrhythmias—Idiopathic and Associated with Cardiac Disease

Beta-blockers are generally without effect in ventricular arrhythmias unrelated to sympathetic excess (26). Like all other antiarrhythmic drugs, they can occasionally exacerbate arrhythmias (27). However, in the absence of provocative testing or a therapeutic trial with adequate doses of beta-blocker, it is often impossible to determine the contribution of sympathetic stimulation to the genesis of the arrhythmia. Table 2 shows the expected response of ventricular arrhythmias to beta-blockers.

Ventricular Premature Beats (VPBs)

In 37 patients with chronic ventricular arrhythmias, intravenous atenolol (10 mg) was highly effective in suppressing VPBs, with a peak effect at 1-2 hours and lasting 7 hours (28).

In a placebo-controlled trial the frequency of VPBs was significantly ($p = 0.009$) reduced by oral atenolol (100 mg o.d.) given for 5 days to a group of 45 patients with coronary heart disease (Fig. 2) (29,30).

This was further confirmed by the same clinicians in a randomized comparison of oral atenolol (100 mg o.d.) with prajmalium bitartrate (20 mg t.i.d.) in 37 patients with coronary heart disease (30). Atenolol and

Table 2 Expected Response of Ventricular Arrhythmias to Treatment with Beta-Blockers

Ventricular arrhythmia	Response
Ventricular premature beats (VPBs)	Poor, unless related to digitalis toxicity, exercise or stress, ischemic heart disease, mitral valve prolapse, or the long QT syndrome
Ventricular tachycardia (VT) (sustained)	Fair, but good when due to digitalis toxicity, exercise or stress, or the long QT syndrome
Paroxysmal ventricular tachycardia	Good, particularly in cases unresponsive to other antiarrhythmic therapy
Ventricular fibrillation (VF)	Good if: 1. Due to digitalis toxicity or sympathomimetic amines 2. Refractory to initial defibrillation

Source: Modified from Ref. 14.

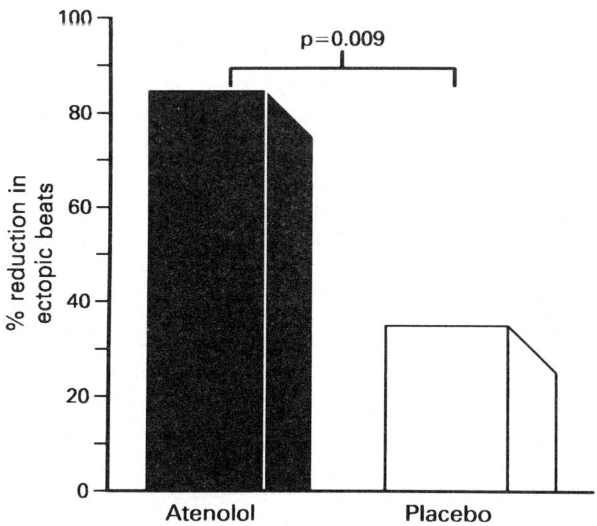

Figure 2 Effect of atenolol on ventricular ectopic beats. (From Refs. 29, 30.)

prajmalium bitartrate reduced VPBs by 91% and 77%, respectively; there was no significant difference between treatments.

Similarly, Heng and Zimmer (31) in a dose-response study have demonstrated that in a group of 25 men with significant ventricular ectopy, oral atenolol (50-200 mg o.d.) given for 2 weeks reduced the frequency of VPBs significantly. These authors suggested that atenolol may be particularly useful in the treatment of chronic ventricular arrhythmias in patients who require a beta-blocker for other associated disorders such as hypertension, angina, or mitral valve prolapse.

In a study involving 54 patients with more than 5000 ventricular extrasystoles per day, oral atenolol (50 mg/day) was compared with propranolol (60 mg/day); both drugs were equally effective in suppressing VPBs (32).

In a comparison of oral atenolol (100 mg o.d. plus diuretic if necessary), tocainide (400 mg t.i.d.), and their combination in 20 patients with hypertension and concomitant ventricular arrhythmias (33), all treatments suppressed VPBs. However only tocainide and the combination did so to a significant extent.

In a randomized trial of treatment of hypertension in 303 elderly patients, oral atenolol (100 mg/day) significantly reduced VPBs in the presence of diuretics and low serum potassium (34). Similar findings were reported in a much smaller study of six elderly hypertensives given oral atenolol (50 mg/day) in combination with chlorthalidone (35).

Ventricular Tachycardia (VT)

Sustained VT is best treated with cardioversion. If drugs are used, intravenous lignocaine is the initial drug of choice, as beta-blockers are often ineffective in this type of arrhythmia and there is also the fear of precipitating heart failure in the presence of severe organic heart disease.

In 37 patients with a mixed background of hypertension, ischemic heart disease, dilated cardiomyopathy, and mitral valve disease, intravenous atenolol (10 mg) was highly effective in suppressing VT in the first 1-2 hours, the effect lasting up to 7 hours (28).

Although beta-blockers have only a limited role in the overall treatment of life-threatening ventricular tachyarrhythmias, some reasonable success has been described with atenolol. For example, good results have been reported with oral atenolol 50-200 mg/day in 25 patients with significant ventricular ectopy treated for 2 weeks (31,36).

In 32 patients with intermittent ventricular tachycardia associated mainly with either coronary artery disease or valvular heart disease, oral atenolol (50-200 mg/day) was effective in suppressing ventricular tachycardia (37).

The frequency of ventricular tachycardia was reduced by at least 75% in eight of 17 patients receiving 50 mg daily, seven of 16 patients receiving 100 mg daily, and eight of 11 receiving 200 mg daily. In this particular study, atenolol was somewhat less effective in reducing ventricular ectopic frequency than in suppressing ventricular tachycardia.

Brodsky et al. (38) have used beta-blockers (metoprolol, atenolol, pindolol) as adjunct therapy in 32 patients with sustained ventricular tachycardia or ventricular fibrillation associated with impaired left ventricular function. Over a mean follow-up of 668 days, patients treated throughout this period with oral beta-blockers had a lower rate of mortality than a control group of patients treated with Class I antiarrhythmic agents alone. The arrhythmia recurrence rate was similar in each group, but the recurrences were less severe and better tolerated in the group receiving beta-blockers. The results of this albeit retrospective analysis suggest that beta-blockers may have been at least partially responsible for an improved prognosis in this group of patients.

The same group (39) have also assessed the efficacy of solitary beta-blocker therapy for ventricular tachyarrhythmia in 30 patients who initially had sustained ventricular tachycardia (70%) or ventricular fibrillation (30%). A variety of beta-blockers were used including atenolol, metoprolol, pindolol, acebutolol, nadolol, and propranolol. Their results suggested that beta-blocker therapy can prevent recurrent VT in patients without coronary artery disease who have normal LV function. However, solitary beta-blocker therapy is unlikely to be an effective long-term antiarrhythmic treatment in patients with significant structural heart disease.

Postinfarction Ventricular Arrhythmias

High catecholamines and tachycardia after acute postmyocardial infarction predispose to ventricular arrhythmias (14,40). Sudden death after myocardial infarction is probably often associated with prior ventricular arrhythmias (41,42) particularly R-on-T VPBs (43,44). Controlled studies on the antiarrhythmic effect of beta-blockers in the postmyocardial infarction period are unfortunately sparse. The topic is reviewed by Baber (20).

Acute Myocardial Infarction

Ventricular Premature Beats (VPBs) The effect of intravenous atenolol on ventricular arrhythmias in acute myocardial infarction was assessed in 182 patients admitted to a coronary care unit within 12 hours of the onset of chest pain. Prophylactic atenolol 5 mg intravenously followed by

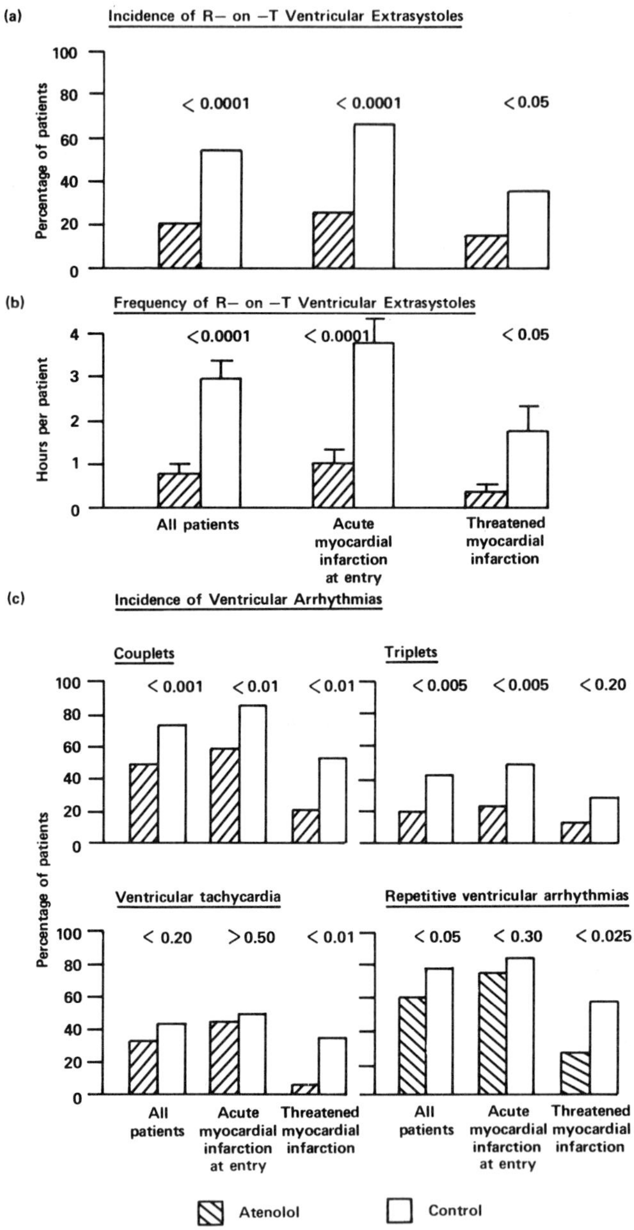

All p values two–tailed (2p)

50 mg orally, then 100 mg/day for 10 days, significantly suppressed VPBs including couplets, triplets, and R-on-T VPBs (Fig. 3) (45). Compared to the control group, deaths were fewer with treatment (22). In a randomized double-blind trial of 388 patients admitted to a coronary care unit within 24 hours of a suspected myocardial infarction, oral propranolol (40 mg t.i.d.) and atenolol (50 mg b.i.d.) did not depress VPBs (46) compared to placebo.

Ventricular Tachycardia (VT) Atenolol 5 mg intravenously followed by 50 mg orally then 100 mg/day for 10 days was effective prophylactically in preventing VT in patients with threatened infarction (45) (see Fig. 3).

Ventricular Fibrillation (VF) VF following induced myocardial infarction in dogs was almost completely prevented by prophylactic atenolol, in contrast to a beta-blocker with high ISA (47).

In the study by Rossi et al. (45) atenolol (5 mg intravenously followed by 50 mg orally then 100 mg/day for 10 days) reduced the occurrence of VF compared to placebo (1 versus 5) but did not achieve statistical significance. Surprisingly, in the large ISIS study (48) involving atenolol, no significant decrease in the incidence of VF or nonfatal cardiac arrest was noted.

Late intervention postmyocardial infarction—prophylactic

Ventricular Premature Beats (VPBs) Hypokalemia has been reported to be associated with an increased incidence of ventricular fibrillation in acute myocardial infarction (49). In a retrospective study, Johansson and Dziamski (50) found an increased incidence of malignant arrhythmias in patients with diuretic-induced hypokalaemia. The incidence of malignant arrhythmias in hypokalemic patients taking nonselective beta-blockers on

---

Figure 3 Effect of atenolol on arrhythmias in acute and threatened myocardial infarction. Comparative effects of atenolol ($n = 95$) (5 mg intravenously plus 50 mg orally immediately and 12 hours later, then 100 mg o.d. orally 2nd to 10th day) and conventional therapy ($n = 87$) in 182 patients with definite (121 patients) or suspected (61 patients) myocardial infarction randomized to treatment within 12 hours of pain onset. The incidence of ventricular arrhythmias was recorded over the first 24 hours: (a) incidence (percentage of patients) of R-on-T ventricular extrasystoles (prematurity index <0.85); (b) frequency (hr/patient) of R-on-T extrasystoles; (c) incidence (percentage of patients developing arrhythmia) of couplets, triplets, ventricular tachycardia, and repetitive ventricular arrhythmias. (From Ref. 45.)

admission was 13.2%, and $beta_1$-selective beta-blockers (including atenolol), 26.1%. However, Nordrehaug (51) could find no relationship between serum potassium concentration estimated on the day of admission to hospital with acute myocardial infarction and the occurrence of malignant ventricular arrhythmias and death over the next 3 months.

In a double-blind crossover study of 103 patients followed up for one year, treatment with oral sotalol 160 mg b.i.d. or atenolol 50 mg b.i.d. was initiated 7-10 days after admission. Although sotalol, a beta-blocker with Class III electrophysiological properties, lengthened QT_c interval and was associated with higher serum potassium levels, both beta-blockers suppressed VPBs to a similar extent (52).

In a randomized double-blind comparison of the efficacy of oral flecainide (100-150 mg b.i.d.) and atenolol (50-100 mg b.i.d.) in 26 patients 1 month after myocardial infarction, a successful response ($\geqslant$70% suppression of ectopic activity or elimination of ventricular tachycardia) was seen in 50% of patients randomized to atenolol compared with 100% of patients receiving flecainide (53).

Ventricular Tachycardia (VT) A positive relationship between infarct size (using enzyme elevation as a rough index of infarct size) and ventricular arrhythmias has been described (54,55). Moreover, atenolol significantly reduces infarct size (22). Postmyocardial infarction patients who develop VT/VF have a longer QT_c interval than those who do not, and patients who die suddenly within one year of discharge have a longer QT_c interval. In a trial of 10 patients with coronary heart disease, atenolol (50-100 mg/day for one week) shortened the QT_c interval in patients with chronic coronary heart disease, but pindolol did not (56).

Other Arrhythmias

Mitral Valve Prolapse

This condition, reviewed by Swartz et al. (57) occurs in young (average age 38 years) patients, 70% of whom are women, and they present with chest discomfort, palpitations, lightheadedness, or syncope.

Oral administration of atenolol (25 mg b.i.d.) in patients with mitral valve prolapse yielded significant reduction in simple and complex ventricular extrasystoles (VES). In fact, 11 out of 12 patients showed a reduction in simple VES and nine out of 12 a reduction in complex VES; the mean reduction was 61 and 47%, respectively (58).

Long QT syndrome (LQTS)

This syndrome comprises a long QT interval on the ECG (even when corrected for heart rate, QT_c) with syncopal attacks as a result of ventricular arrhythmias. The arrhythmias are severe and life-threatening (VF most commonly, with VT and asystole less frequent), and 73% of untreated patients die suddenly (59). Arrhythmias and syncope tend to be triggered by heightened sympathetic activity such as stress, anesthesia, emotion, fright and exercise, or isoprenaline (60). Some patients with mitral valve prolapse have a long QT interval, and this might account for the beneficial effect of beta-blockers in such cases (61).

Children Trippel and Gillette (62) have reviewed the use of oral atenolol as a single agent in children and adolescents with LQTS. The study group included 10 patients aged 1.5-18 years. The maximum dose of atenolol administered ranged from 0.9 to 2.5 mg/kg/day. Therapy was effective in three of 10 patients. Therapy was ineffective in seven of 10 patients.

ANESTHESIA, SURGERY, AND ARRHYTHMIAS

A variety of supraventricular and ventricular arrhythmias may occur during general anesthesia in surgical patients. Factors such as sympathetic hyperactivity, especially during induction of anesthesia, hypoxia, acidosis, hypercapnia, and enhanced sensitivity of the heart to catecholamines because of anesthetic agents or other drugs may all be responsible for arrhythmias during surgery. The role of sympathetic stimulation in the etiology of cardiovascular complications and sudden death during surgery has been emphasized (63).

Postoperative arrhythmias are usually transient and therefore do not require the use of antiarrhythmic drugs. Such arrhythmias include first and second degree heart block and AV dissociation, premature atrial and ventricular beats, and ectopic atrial tachycardias. Arrhythmias that should be treated are:

1. Atrial fibrillation or flutter, junctional tachycardia with rapid ventricular rates
2. Third degree (and sometimes second degree) heart block
3. VT or VF, or complex VPBs such as R-on-T beats

Prophylactic Treatment

Atenolol has been given prophylactically in the immediate postoperative period following coronary artery surgery.

In a randomized, double-blind study (64), 70 patients undergoing aortocoronary bypass grafting received either 5 mg i.v. atenolol ($n = 35$) or placebo ($n = 35$) within 3 hr of surgery. A second i.v. dose was administered 24 hr later, then 50 mg oral atenolol or matching placebo was given for 6 days. Atenolol significantly reduced the number of severe episodes of supraventricular arrhythmia (21 with placebo versus five with atenolol, $p < 0.005$) and the number of moderate episodes (142 with placebo versus 30 with atenolol, $p < 0.005$). Overall, there was a 79% reduction in the number of moderate and severe episodes of supraventricular arrhythmias. There were no significant differences between the two groups with respect to the frequency and severity of ventricular arrhythmias.

In 125 patients undergoing coronary bypass surgery, 50 mg oral atenolol given within 24 hours of surgery and continued for 10 days significantly reduced the incidence of a trial fibrillation/flutter (30.1% in control and 10% with atenolol, $p < 0.01$) (65). When given 2 hours preoperatively to patients undergoing major surgery, oral atenolol or labetalol or oxprenolol decreased the incidence of postoperative ischemia and ventricular premature beats (3% vs. 18% in control) (66).

In a study by Lamb et al. (67), 60 patients who underwent elective coronary artery surgery were randomized to receive 50 mg oral atenolol daily ($n = 30$) or no beta-blocker treatment ($n = 30$). Atenolol was given 72 hr before the operation and for 7 days after operation. In the atenolol group the incidence of supraventricular tachyarrythmias was 3% compared to 37% in the control group ($p < 0.001$). Atrial fibrillation was seen on the first postoperative day in one patient receiving atenolol compared to 10 patients in the control group.

In summary the use of an intravenous followed by an oral beta-blocker such as atenolol markedly diminishes the incidence of postoperative arrhythmias. These (particularly in coronary bypass surgery) may best be avoided by continuing the beta-blocker up to the time of operation (3 hours before surgery) and restarting the beta-blocker approximately 6 hours postsurgery (intravenous followed by oral), thus avoiding a possible withdrawal hypersensitivity state.

COMPARATIVE STUDIES

Comparisons with Other Beta-Blockers

Supraventricular Tachycardias

In a comparison of intravenous atenolol (0.15 mg/kg) and acebutolol (1 mg/kg) in 29 patients, both drugs proved effective (16). Eleven of 12 patients with atrial fibrillation or flutter had their ventricular rate reduced to <100 beats/min, including one cardioversion to sinus rhythm. Sixteen patients had SVT, seven (44%) reverted to sinus rhythm, four (25%) had their rate slowed to <100 beats/min, and five (31%) were unchanged.

Lindsay et al. (5) compared the efficacy and safety of nadolol (0.05-0.1 mg/kg i.v.) and atenolol (5-10 mg i.v.) in 46 patients with recurrent SVT. Responders and partial responders to the intravenous beta-blocker continued on oral therapy. Atenolol or nadolol alone was quite effective in the treatment of SVT due to atrioventricular nodal reentry (64%), while each had limited efficacy in the treatment of SVT due to atrioventricular reentry. On the basis of these results, Lindsay et al. (5) recommended that atenolol or nadolol be considered first-line antiarrhythmic therapy for atrioventricular nodal reentrant tachycardia.

Schofield et al. (8) compared the efficacy of oral atenolol (50-100 mg/day) and sotalol (120-240 mg/day) given for 6 weeks under randomized, crossover conditions in 13 patients with paroxysmal SVT; sotalol was significantly superior in diminishing the number and duration of episodes. This is the first controlled study in patients to demonstrate the Class III supraventricular antiarrhythmic property of sotalol.

Palpitations and tachyarrhythmias associated with thyrotoxicosis are probably best treated with beta-blockers without ISA (14), such as atenolol.

Ventricular Arrhythmias

In 54 patients, oral propranolol (60 mg/day) and atenolol (50 mg/day) were equally effective in suppressing VPBs (32).

Postmyocardial Infarction Ventricular Arrhythmias

In a randomized double-blind study of postmyocardial infarction, 388 patients were randomized to oral placebo, atenolol (50 mg b.i.d.), or propranolol (40 mg t.i.d.) within 24 hours of a suspected myocardial infarction, and the incidence of ventricular arrhythmias was monitored for the first 24 hours after admission; there were no differences from placebo (46). The study was criticized (68) for not giving intravenous beta-blocker and thus quickly achieving optimal blood levels. Subsequently, intravenous atenolol was found to have good antiarrhythmic activity in the acute postmyocardial infarction state (45).

The contribution of intrinsic sympathomimetic activity to the antiarrhythmic effects of 150 mg/day oral atenolol and 160 mg/day oral oxprenolol were compared in 20 patients with myocardial infarction and premature ventricular complexes. Premature ventricular complexes were reduced by 45% with atenolol and by 16% with oxprenolol (69).

In a double-blind, randomized, crossover study in 103 patients followed for one year after discharge following acute myocardial infarction, oral atenolol (50 mg b.i.d.) and sotalol (160 mg b.i.d.) were equally effective in suppressing VPBs, in spite of sotalol lengthening the QT_c interval (52). Despite the clear evidence of a sustained Class III effect of sotalol in this study, there was little evidence of a superior antiarrhythmic effect in comparison with atenolol.

Comparisons with Other Antiarrhythmic Agents

Supraventricular Arrhythmias

In a randomized, crossover study, intravenous atenolol (0.1 mg/kg) was compared with intravenous amiodarone in patients with atrial fibrillation (17); both agents reduced equally the ventricular heart rate.

Lewis et al. (19) have compared the effects of oral atenolol (50 mg b.i.d.), verapamil (80 mg b.i.d.), xamoterol (200 mg b.i.d.), and matching placebo on heart rate and exercise tolerance in digitalized patients with chronic atrial fibrillation. In this four week study, atenolol, verapamil and xamoterol achieved better control of exercise-induced tachycardia than digoxin, but atenolol impaired exercise tolerance whereas verapamil did not. Thus verapamil appeared to be the best adjunct to digoxin in the treatment of atrial fibrillation.

Ventricular Arrhythmias

Oral atenolol (100 mg b.i.d.) and disopyramide (200 mg t.i.d.) have been compared for therapy of established VPBs in 10 patients with mitral valve prolapse (70). Both drugs significantly suppressed VPBs, but the percentage decrease in some patients was judged to be unsatisfactory by the authors.

In 37 patients with ischemic heart disease, oral atenolol was randomly compared with prajmalium bitartrate (a rauwolfia alkaloid derivative) and was at least as effective in suppressing ventricular premature beats (91% vs. 77%, respectively) (30).

The effect of therapy with atenolol (100 mg o.d.; plus 25 mg hydrochlorothiazide and 2.5 mg amiloride if required) and tocainide (400 mg t.i.d.), separately or in combination, was studied in 20 patients with hypertension and concomitant ventricular arrhythmias (33). Tocainide alone significantly reduced the incidence of ventricular arrhythmias without affecting atrial arrhythmias; it also controlled exercise-induced arrhythmias in 54% of patients. Atenolol significantly reduced atrial arrhythmias and had a good effect on exercise-induced ventricular arrhythmias (reduced in 75% of patients), but it did not have a significant effect on non-exercise-induced ventricular arrhythmias. In 13 patients it was necessary to combine atenolol with tocainide in order to reduce ventricular arrhythmias.

Post-myocardial Infarction Ventricular Arrhythmias

The efficacy of oral atenolol (50-100 mg b.i.d.) and flecainide (100-150 mg b.i.d.) in suppressing frequent ventricular ectopic activity and non-sustained ventricular tachycardia was compared in 26 patients one month after myocardial infarction in a randomized, double-blind trial (53). A successful response ($\geq$70% suppression of ectopic activity or elimination of ventricular tachycardia) was seen in 100% of patients randomized to flecainide compared with 50% randomized to atenolol ($p < 0.05$). An arrhythmogenic effect was seen in one patient on atenolol, which resolved on crossover to flecainide.

COMBINATION WITH OTHER ANTIARRHYTHMIC AGENTS

Fifty-six patients with malignant ventricular arrhythmias gained some benefit when exposed to a variety of membrane-stabilizing drugs, i.e., quinidine, procainamide, disopyramide, mexiletine, tocainide, aprinidine, lorcainide, propafenone, and encainide (71). These patients had not benefited from beta-blockers alone, but when these drugs (metoprolol 75-200 mg/day ($n = 27$); propranolol 40-160 mg/day ($n = 20$); atenolol 50-100 mg/day ($n = 6$); pindolol 10-80 mg/day ($n = 2$); and nadolol 40-80 mg/day ($n = 1$)) were added to the membrane-stabilizing agents, further significant suppression of the malignant ventricular arrhythmias occurred both during exercise and on 24-hr ECG monitoring.

In a study of 20 patients with hypertension and concomitant ventricular arrhythmias (33), it was necessary in 13 patients to combine atenolol (100 mg o.d. plus diuretics if necessary) with tocainide (400 mg t.i.d.) in order to reduce ventricular arrhythmias.

Children

Atenolol has been successfully combined with flecainide in the treatment of childhood arrhythmias (72).

REFERENCES

1. D'Annunzio E, Mobilij A. Terapia con betabloccanti nei malati affeti da stenosi mitralica. Minerva Med 1980; 71:3131-7.
2. Klein HO, Sareli P, Schamroth CL, Carim Y, Epstein M, Marcus B. Effects of atenolol on exercise capacity in patients with mitral stenosis with sinus rhythm. Am J Cardiol 1985; 56(10):598-601.
3. Sirbulescu R. Atenolol in the treatment of cardiac dysrhythmia. Acta Ther 1977; 3:109-16.
4. Hombach V, Braun V, Höpp HW, Gil-Sanchez D, Behrenbeck DW, Tauchert M, Hilger HH. Antiarrhythmic effects of acute beta-blockade with atenolol on supraventricular tachycardias at rest and during exercise. Klin Wochenschr 1981; 59:123-33.
5. Lindsay BD, Saksena S, Rothbart ST, Herman S, Barr MJ. Long-term efficacy and safety of beta-adrenergic receptor antagonists for supraventricular tachycardia. Am J Cardiol 1987; 60(6):63D-67D.
6. Miller SM, Hoff JV, Coehlo A, et al. Atenolol vs propranolol in supraventricular tachycardia. Clin Res 1985; 33(4):A813.
7. Pimenta J, Pereira CB. Effects of atenolol in patients with reciprocating supraventricular tachycardia. Clin Cardiol 1986; 9:191-5.
8. Schofield PM, Reid F, Bennett DH. A comparison of atenolol and sotalol in the treatment of patients with paroxysmal supraventricular tachycardia. Br Heart J 1987; 57(1):105.
9. Trippel DL, Gillette PCL. Atenolol in children with supraventricular tachycardia. Am J Cardiol 1989; 64(3):233-6.
10. Gallagher JJ, Pritchett ECL, Sealy WC, Kasell J, Wallace AG. The preexcitation syndromes. Prog Cardiovasc Dis 1978; XX(4):285-327.
11. Hombach V. Höpp H-W, Braun V, et al. Relevance of physical activity to the antiarrhythmic effects of β-blockade on supraventricular tachycardias. Drugs 1983; 25(Suppl 2;):186-92.
12. Denes P, Cummings JM, Simpson R,, Wu D, Amat-Y-Leon F, Dhingra R, Rosen KM. Effects of propranolol on anomalous pathway refractoriness and circus movement tachycardias in patients with preexcitation. Am J Cardiol 1978; 41:1061-7.
13. Gibson DG, Sowton E. The use of beta-adrenergic receptor blocking drugs in dysrhythmias. Prog Cardiovasc Dis 1969; XII(I):16-39.
14. Singh BN, Jewitt DE. Beta-adrenoreceptor blocking drugs in cardiac arrhythmias. Cardiovasc Drugs 1977; 2:119-59.
15. Wit AL, Hoffman BF, Rosen MR. Electrophysiology and pharmacology of cardiac arrhythmias IX. Cardiac electrophysiologic effects of beta-adrenergic receptor stimulation and blockade. Part B. Am Heart J 1975; 90(5):665-75.
16. Winchester MA, Jackson G, Meltzer RS, Bowden RE, Mace JG, Winkle RA, Harrison DC. Intravenous atenolol and acebutolol in the treatment of supraventricular arrhythmias. Circulation 1978; 58(4):182.

17. Bracchetti D, De Garate S, Di Cio G, Carini G, Capucci A, Magnani B. A comparative study with computerised analysis of the effects of amiodarone and of atenolol on R-R intervals in patients with stabilised atrial fibrillation. Boll Soc Ital Cardiol 1978; 23:1591-6.
18. Rasmussen K, Andersen K, Wang H. Atrial fibrillation induced by atenolol. Eur Heart J 1982; 3:276-81.
19. Lewis RV, McMurray J, McDevitt DG. Effects of atenolol, verapamil, and xamoterol on heart rate and exercise tolerance in digitalised patients with chronic atrial fibrillation. J Cardiovasc Pharmacol 1989; 13:1-6.
20. Baber NS. Clinical experience with beta-adrenergic blocking agents in myocardial ischaemia: a dilemma and a challenge. Pharmacol Ther 1981; 13: 285-320.
21. Ramsdale DR, Faragher EB, Bennett DH, Bray CL, Ward C, Cruickshank JM, Yusuf S, Phil D, Sleight P. Ischemic pain relief in patients with acute myocardial infarction by intravenous atenolol. Am Heart J 1982; 103(4) (part 1):459-67.
22. Yusuf S, Sleight P, Rossi P, et al. Reduction in infarct size, arrhythmias and chest pain by early intravenous beta-blockade in suspected acute myocardial infarction. Circulation 1983; 67(Suppl 1):I-32-I-41.
23. McLeod AA, Neil-Dwyer G, Meyer CHA, Richardson PL, Cruickshank J, Bartlett J. Cardiac sequelae of acute head injury. Br Heart J 1982; 47:221-6.
24. Cruickshank JM, Neil-Dwyer G, Degaute JP, et al. Reduction of cardiac morbidity in acute head injuries by early beta-blockade. X World Congress of Cardiology, Washington DC, 14-19 September (abstr), 1986.
25. Cruickshank JM, Degaute JP, Hayes et al. Reduction of stress/catecholamine-induced cardiac necrosis by $beta_1$-selective blockade. Lancet 1987; 2 (8559):585-9.
26. Gettes LS, Chen C-M. Mechanisms and efficacy of beta-blocking agents in the treatment of arrhythmias. In: Schwartz PJ, Brown AM, Malliani A, Zanchetti A, eds. Neural mechanisms in cardiac arrhythmias. New York: Raven Press, 1978:377-99.
27. Velebit V, Podrid P, Lown B, Cohen BH, Graboys TB. Aggravation and provocation of ventricular arrhythmias by antiarrhythmic drugs. Circulation 1982; 65(5):886-94.
28. Morganroth J. Intravenous atenolol for ventricular arrhythmias. Am J Cardiol 1986; 58:499-502.
29. Körst HA, Brandes J-W, Lembcke HJ, Littmann K-P. Atenolol in the treatment of premature ventricular contractions. A double blind study in 68 patients. Z Kardiol 1981; 70:419-24.
30. Körst HA, Brandes JW, Pedersen SU, Littman KP. Atenolol and ventricular ectopic beats. Drugs (Symposium on beta-blockers in the 1980's) 1983; 25(Suppl 2):196-7.
31. Heng MK, Zimmer I. Reduction of ventricular arrhythmias by atenolol. Am Heart J 1985; 109(6):1273-80.

32. Yano K, Hashiba H, Arakawa K, Yanaga N, Hosoda S, Sasaki Y, Ichimaru Y, Ogawa N. Multiclinic evaluation of the antiarrhythmic effect of atenolol on ventricular arrhythmias. Drugs 1983; 25(Suppl 2):195-6.
33. Di Somma S, Savonitto S, Petitto M, Ligouri V, Magnotta C, de Divitiis O. Treatment of hypertensive patients with ventricular arrhythmias: comparison and combination of β-blocker and anti-arrhythmic therapy. J Int Med Res 1989; 17:113-24.
34. Coope JR. Reduction of ventricular ectopic beats in older subjects on atenolol: relation to serum potassium levels. J Hyper 1983; 1(Suppl 2):342-4.
35. Siamopoulos K, Wilkinson R, Campbell R, Boddy K. A combination of chlorthalidone (12.5 mg) and atenolol (50 mg) in the elderly. Drugs (Symposium on beta-blockers in the 1980's) 1983; 25(Suppl 2):88-90.
36. Heng MK, Zimmer I, Udhoji V. Reduction of ventricular arrhythmias by atenolol. J Am Coll Cardiol 1985; 5(2) Pt 2:A439.
37. Fenster PE, Reynolds D, Horwitz LD, et al. Atenolol for ventricular ectopy: a dose-response study. Clin Pharmacol Ther 1987; 41(1):118-23.
38. Brodsky MA, Allen BJ, Bessen M, Luckett CR, Siddiqi R, Henry WI. Beta-blocker therapy in patients with ventricular tachyarrhythmias in the setting of left ventricular dysfunction. Am Heart J 1988; 115:799-808.
39. Brodsky MA, Allen BJ, Luckett CR, Capparelli EV, Wolff LJ, Henry WL. Antiarrhythmic efficacy of solitary beta-adrenergic blockade for patients with sustained ventricular tachyarrhythmias. Am Heart J 1989; 118(2):272-80.
40. Yusuf S, Lopez R, Sleight P. Heart rate and ectopic prematurity in relation to sustained ventricular arrhythmias. Br Heart J 1980; 44:233-9.
41. Cobb LA, Werner JA. Antiarrhythmic therapy, ventricular premature depolarisation and sudden cardiac death: the tip of the iceberg. (Editorial) Circulation 1969; 59:864-5.
42. Lown B, Graboys TB. Sudden death: an ancient problem newly perceived. Cardiovasc Med 1977; 2(3):219-32.
43. Adgey AAJ, Devlin JE, Webb SW, Mulholland HC. Initiation of ventricular fibrillation outside hospital in patients with acute ischaemic heart disease. Br Heart J 1982; 47:55-61.
44. Campbell RWF, Murray A, Julian DG. Ventricular arrhythmias in first 12 hours of acute myocardial infarction. Br Heart J 1981; 46:351-7.
45. Rossi PR, Yusuf S, Ramsdale D, Furze L, Sleight P. Reduction of ventricular arrhythmias by early intravenous atenolol in suspected acute myocardial infarction. Br Med J 1983; 286:506-10.
46. Roland JM, Wilcox RG, Banks DC, Edwards B, Fentem PH, Hampton JR. Effect of beta-blockers on arrhythmias during six weeks after suspected myocardial infarction. Br Med J 1979; 2:518-21.
47. Meesmann W. The possible role of the sympathetic nervous system in the genesis of early post-ischaemia arrhythmias. In: Parratt JR, ed. Early arrhythmias resulting from myocardial ischaemia. Mechanisms and prevention by drugs. New York: MacMillan, 1982:139-51.

48. ISIS-I (First International Study of Infarct Survival) Collaborative Group. Randomized trial of intravenous atenolol among 16,027 cases of suspected acute myocardial infarction: ISIS-I. Lancet 1986; 2:57-66.
49. Nordrehaug JE, Von der Lippe G. Hypokalaemia and ventricular fibrillation in acute myocardial infarction. Br Heart J 1983; 50:525-9.
50. Johansson BW, Dziamski R. Malignant arrhythmias in acute myocardial infarction. Relationship to serum potassium and effect of selective and non-selective beta-blockade. Drugs 1984; 28(Suppl 2):77-85.
51. Nordrehaug JE. Hypokalemia, arrhythmias and early prognosis in acute myocardial infarction. Acta Med Scand 1985; 217:299-306.
52. Cobbe SM, Alexopoulos D, Winner SJ, McCaie CP, Cobbe PC, Johnston J. A comparison of the long-term effects of sotalol and atenolol on QT interval and arrhythmias after myocardial infarction. Eur Heart J 1988; 9(1):24-31.
53. Cripps T, Mannering D, Bennett D. Comparison between flecainide and atenolol in the suppression of complex ventricular ectopic activity after myocardial infarction: results of a double-blind, randomized trial. J Electrophysiol 1988; 2(4):281-8.
54. Morrison GW, Kumar EB, Portal RW, Aber CP. Cardiac arrhythmias 48 hours before, during, and 48 hours after discharge from hospital following acute myocardial infarction. Br Heart J 1981; 45:500-11.
55. Roberts R, Husain A, Ambos HD, Oliver C, Cox JR, Sobel BE. Relation between infarct size and ventricular arrhythmia. Br Heart J 1975; 37:1169-75.
56. Amlie JP, Erikssen J. Exercise-induced changes in QT time and its modification by beta-adrenoreceptor blockade. Eur Heart J 1985; 6(Suppl D):175-84.
57. Swartz MH, Teichholz LE, Donoso E. Mitral valve prolapse. Am J Med 1977; 62:377-89.
58. Kafka W. The incidence, response to therapy and prognostic implication of ventricular arrhythmias in the mitral valve prolapse syndrome. Z Kardiol 1985; 74(4):245-53.
59. Schwartz PJ, Perriti M, Malliani A. The long QT syndrome. Am Heart J 1975; 89(3):378-90.
60. Milne JR, Ward DE, Spurrell RAJ, Camm AJ. The long QT syndrome: effeccts of drugs and left stellate ganglion block. Am Heart J 1982; 104(2): 194-8.
61. Puddu PA, Pasternac A, Tubau JF, Krol R, Farley L, de Champlain J. QT interval prolongation and increased plasma catecholamine levels in patients with mitral valve prolapse. Am Heart J 1983; 105(3):422-8.
62. Trippel DL, Gillette PC. Should atenolol by used in children with long QT syndrome? Circulation 1989; 80(4) (Suppl II):II-388.
63. Lown B, Verrier RL, Rabinowitz SH. Neural and psychologic mechanisms and the problem of sudden cardiac death. Am J Cardiol 1977; 39:890-902.
64. Matangi MF, Strickland J, Garbe GJ, Habib N, Basu AK, Burgess JJ, Maitland A, Busse EFG. Atenolol for the prevention of arrhythmias following coronary artery bypass grafting. Can J Cardiol 1989; 5(4):229-34.

65. Sosa Liprandi A, Iglesias R, Krauss J, Doval HC. Prevention of supraventricular arrhythmias in the immediate post-operative phase of myocardial revascularisation (by-pass surgery). A randomised study with atenolol. Rev Argent Cardiol 1986; 54(1):21-7.
66. Stone JG, Foëx P, Sear J, Johnsonn LL, Khambatta HJ, Triner L. Myocardial ischemia in untreated hypertensive patients: effect of a single dose of an oral beta-blocker. Anesthesiology 1986; 65(3A):A36.
67. Lamb RK, Prabhakar G, Thorpe JAC, Smith S, Norton R, Dyde JA. The use of atenolol in the prevention of supraventricular arrhythmias following coronary artery surgery. Eur Heart J 1988; 9:32-6.
68. Sleight P, Yusuf S. Effects of beta-blockers on arrhythmias. Br Med J 1979; 2:864.
69. Lizarraga JI, Lorenzo AC, Esteve JJ. Intrinsic adrenergic activity and antiarrhythmic efficacy of the beta-blocking agents. 10th World Congress Cardiol, Washington, DC, Sept 14-19, 1986:427.
70. Capucci A, Naccarella F, Catena G, Lamberti C, Marchesini B, Bracchetti D, Magnani B. Confronto disopiramide-atenololo nella terapia della extrasistolia ventricolare stabilizzata in pazienti con prolasso valvolare mitralico. G Ital Cardiol 1981; 11(4):498-505.
71. Hirsowitz G, Podrid PJ, Lampert S, Stein J, Lown B. The role of beta-blocking agents as adjunct therapy to membrane stabilizing drugs in malignant ventricular arrhythmia. Am Heart J 1986; 111:852-60.
72. Rosenthal E, Ladusan EJ, Tynan MJ, Jones O, Curry PVL. Efficacy of flecainide in childhood arrhythmias. Eur Heart J 1987; 8(Abs Suppl 2):193.

10

Antiarrhythmic Effects of Conventional Beta-Blockers in Comparison with Sotalol

Prakash C. Deedwania
University of California at San Francisco School of Medicine, San Francisco, and Veterans Affairs Medical Center, Fresno, California

It is now widely recognized that of the available antiarrhythmic drugs, only treatment with beta-blockers has been effective in reducing the mortality and risk of sudden cardiac death in survivors of acute myocardial infarction. Although it is not established whether this beneficial effect of beta-blocking drugs is related to their antiarrhythmic properties, the results of available studies suggest that beta-blockers are effective in reducing the frequency of spontaneous high-grade ventricular arrhythmias. It has also been shown that there is an increase in the risk of sudden cardiac death in the morning hours. Treatment with beta-blocking agents reduces the circadian rhythmicity of ventricular arrhythmias, and this effect of beta-blockers may indeed be related to their beneficial effect in reducing the risk of sudden cardiac death in the morning hours. The results of Cardiac Arrhythmia Suppression Trial (CAST) showing the deleterious effects of Class IC agents, encainide, and flecainide have promulgated the use of beta-blockers in patients with cardiac arrhythmias. Recent studies have also shown that beta-blockers can be safely used in combination with other antiarrhythmic agents and provide an effective means of controlling ventricular arrhythmias when therapy with a single agent has failed in suppressing the ventricular arrhythmias.

Sotalol is a unique, nonselective beta-blocking agent which has additional Class III electrophysiologic properties. Although it is still an investigational agent in the United States, it has been extensively evaluated in the treatment of patients with spontaneous high-grade ventricular arrhythmias as well as sustained ventricular tachycardia. The results of published reports have shown it to be more effective than conventional beta-blocking agents. Although most of the previous studies compared the effects of sotalol with other beta-blocking agents in a small number of patients, a recent double-blind, placebo-controlled, parallel study compared the antiarrhythmic effects of sotalol and propranolol in 172 patients with frequent (>30/hr) stable ventricular premature contractions (VPCs). The results of this study demonstrated that sotalol was significantly more effective than propranolol in reducing the mean hourly frequency of complex as well as repetitive ventricular premature contractions. Also, a significantly greater percentage of patients receiving sotalol achieved adequate suppression of VPCs when compared with patients randomized to propranolol. The unique Class III antiarrhythmic activity of sotalol combined with its beta-blocking properties might account for its superiority over conventional beta-blocking agents in suppressing ventricular arrhythmias.

INTRODUCTION

Sudden cardiac death continues to be a leading cause of death in the United States. Numerous studies in large numbers of patients have demonstrated that of the currently available antiarrhythmic drugs, only beta-adrenergic blocking agents have been proven effective in reducing the risk of sudden cardiac death after a myocardial infarction (1,2). The beneficial effects of beta-blockers on cardiac mortality are in clear contrast with the deleterious effects of other antiarrhythmic agents which have been shown to be devoid of effect or in some cases associated with an increase in mortality (3). The deleterious effects of Class I antiarrhythmics were best illustrated by the findings of Cardiac Arrhythmia Suppression Trial (CAST) (4). In this large clinical trial conducted by the National Heart, Lung, and Blood Institute (NHLBI), survivors of acute myocardial infarction who had ventricular ectopy were randomized to treatment with placebo, ethmozine, or one of the Class IC agents encainide or flecainide. The data and safety monitoring board of this trial decided to prematurely terminate the treatment with Class IC agents encainide and flecainide because, compared to patients assigned to placebo, those randomized to receive encainide or flecainide had significantly higher risk of death due to any cardiac cause as well as increased incidence of arrhythmic death. These results of CAST as well as the well-demonstrated beneficial effects of beta-blockers on cardiac mortality and certain cardiac deaths have generated considerable recent interest in the use of beta-blocking agents for the treatment of these patients.

Although the precise mechanism by which the beta-blocking drugs reduce the risk of deaths in survivors of acute myocardial infarction is not fully established, it may be due in part to their primary antiarrhythmic action. The antiarrhythmic properties of beta-blockers were first described in 1963 when pronethalol was shown to be effective in controlling ventricular arrhythmias (5). During the last 2 decades a large number of studies with various beta-blocking agents have demonstrated the beneficial effects of these agents in reducing the frequency of spontaneous high-grade ventricular arrhythmias (6-11). The results of recent studies have shown that the use of beta-blockers alone or in combination with other antiarrhythmic agents is also beneficial in preventing the induction of ventricular tachycardia (VT) during electrophysiologic studies (12-14). As discussed in Chapter 8, beta-blockers form the mainstay therapy in patients with exercise-induced ventricular arrhythmias as well as other forms of catecholamine-dependent ventricular arrhythmias. Although currently more than 24 beta-blocking agents are available for clinical or investigational use, sotalol, an investigational compound, has several unique properties that distinguish it, in this class of drugs, for use as an antiarrhythmic agent in the treatment of patients with ventricular arrhythmias (15).

Sotalol is a noncardioselective beta-blocker devoid of membrane-stabilizing or intrinsic sympathomimetic activity and is classified as a Class III antiarrhythmic agent by virtue of its ability to prolong cardiac repolarization. This unique combination of Class II and Class III antiarrhythmic properties has generated considerable interest in investigations of its use in managing patients with ventricular arrhythmias (15,16). Recent reports show that it is an effective antiarrhythmic agent in treating life-threatening and potentially lethal ventricular arrhythmias (17). The suppressant effect of sotalol on ventricular arrhythmias is particularly interesting because it is not known whether this effect is due solely to its beta-blocking action or whether the drug's net suppressant effect in this regard is enhanced by its well-documented propensity to prolong cardiac repolarization.

In this chapter, the available data regarding the suppressant effects of conventional beta-blockers and sotalol on complex and repetitive VPCs will be reviewed. The reasons for superiority of sotalol over conventional beta-blocking drugs in controlling ventricular arrhythmias will be explored and discussed.

PATHOPHYSIOLOGICAL CONSIDERATIONS

Before discussing the effects of beta-blocking drugs on ventricular arrhythmias, it is important to review the roles of catecholamines and adrenergic stimulation and their relation to circadian variations in ventricular arrhythmias and sudden cardiac death.

Catecholamines and Cardiac Arrhythmias

It has been known for many years that the sympathetic nervous system plays a significant role in the genesis and perpetuation of potentially serious ventricular tachyarrhythmias (18). The primary mediators of this neural perpetuation of arrhythmias are adrenergic transmitters. This has been confirmed by experiments demonstrating the prevention of ventricular fibrillation by reserpinization in experimental animals with cardiac glycoside intoxication (18). It has also been shown that regional cardiac sympathectomy and left stellate ganglionectomy can control recalcitrant ventricular arrhythmias in humans (18,19).

The electrophysiologic effects of beta-adrenergic stimulation on Purkinje fibers and ventricular myocardium are well known and complex. These effects depend primarily on the concentrations of the catecholamines released and on the presence or absence of abnormal cardiac tissue. In normal Purkinje fibers, beta-adrenergic stimulation causes no change in the transmembrane potential at rest, the initial portions of the action potential, phase 0 and phase 1, or conduction velocity (20,21). However, when the Purkinje fibers are paced at a rate sufficient to overdrive spontaneous activity, repolarization is altered with pure beta-adrenergic stimulation, resulting in modest shortening of the action potential duration. In contrast, alpha-adrenergic stimulation results in lengthening of the action potential duration (20,21). The most consistent effect of beta-adrenergic stimulation in normal Purkinje fibers is an increased rate of rise of phase 4 depolarization, resulting in increased automaticity.

In normal ventricular fibers, the effects of catecholamines on the action potential are quite similar. There is only a minor effect on the resting transmembrane potential, action potential duration, and conduction velocity, despite a marked increase in contractile force. The diastolic depolarization is not altered, and thus, automaticity is not enhanced. However, in the case of partially depolarized fibers, especially after high concentrations of external potassium, catecholamines may markedly augment the upstroke velocity of the resulting slow-response potentials, increasing their amplitude and significantly prolonging their repolarization phases (21).

Electrophysiologic Effects of Beta Blockade

The electrophysiologic effects of beta blockade have been extensively studied in experimental animals and humans (20,21) and are discussed in detail elsewhere in this book. In concentrations that produce substantial beta blockade, none of the available beta-blocking drugs exerts an effect on the resting transmembrane potential, action potential amplitude, or the maximal rate of rise of the action potential. Thus, these agents do not affect conduction velocity or membrane responsiveness in normal fast sodium-channel-dependent fibers. However, in high concentrations, some of the beta-blockers (e.g., propranolol, oxprenolol, and acebutolol) exert local anesthetic effects on nerves, and they reduce sodium conductance at the cardiac membrane, an effect particularly evident in partially depolarized fibers such as may be found in ischemic myocardium (21). Under these conditions, beta-blockers may depress conduction velocity, shift the membrane responsiveness curve in the hyperpolarizing direction and prolong the effective refractory period (21). The most consistent effect of these drugs is to enhance the rate of rise of spontaneous diastolic depolarization under the influence of catecholamines. The enhanced rate of rise of phase 4 depolarization is depressed by beta-blockers without significant effect on the threshold potential or the amplitude of the action potential. The overall effect is decreased automaticity in these fibers. Although the effects of beta-blockers on triggered automaticity are not well established, propranolol has been demonstrated to decrease the amplitude of delayed afterdepolarizations and stop triggering in atrial muscle or Purkinje fibers exposed to high concentrations of catecholamines or cardiac glycosides (22). This may be one of the main mechanisms by which beta-blocking drugs suppress exercise-induced ventricular arrhythmias (23). Beta-blocking drugs have also been shown to increase ventricular fibrillation threshold under both nonischemic and ischemic conditions (24). In a recent study of five beta-blocking drugs in experimental animals, it was clearly demonstrated that all of the beta-blocking agents studied produced significant increases in ventricular fibrillation threshold, particularly in the ischemic myocardium (Fig. 1) (24). These findings may help explain the beneficial effect of beta-blockers in survivors of acute myocardial infarction by protecting against ventricular fibrillation and sudden cardiac death.

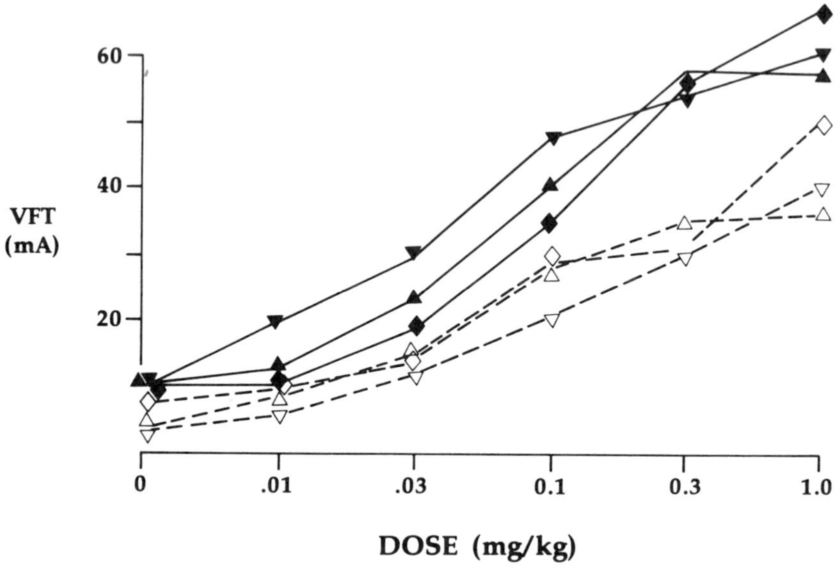

Figure 1 Effect on ventricular fibrillation threshold (VFT) of incremental dosing with labetalol (diamonds), metoprolol (wedges), and propranolol (triangles). The VFT in milliamperes is shown on the ventricular axis and the drug dose on the horizontal axis. Measurements during ischemia are represented by solid symbols and lines. (From Ref. 38 with permission.)

Some other unique features of the electrophysiologic actions of beta-blocking drugs are the differences between the effects of acute and chronic beta blockade on the action potential. It has been shown by Raine and Vaughan Williams (25) that, in animals treated chronically, propranolol and acebutolol produced a modest but significant lengthening of the action potential duration without any effect on the upstroke velocity. It was postulated that these changes during chronic beta blockade represent physiologic adaptation. These data have not been confirmed in clinical studies, since studies in humans show that QTc may be shortened, unchanged, or prolonged during chronic beta-blocker therapy (21). The overall results from available studies indicate that even if chronic beta blockade does prolong the action potential duration, the overall change is minimal with the exception of the changes produced by sotalol. Sotalol is unique in that it causes significant prolongation of the action potential duration in addition to its beta-blocking properties. This property may account for sotalol's superiority in suppressing ventricular arrhythmias (15).

Catecholamines, Beta Blockade, and Circadian Variation in Arrhythmias

Recent studies have demonstrated a circadian rhythmicity for acute myocardial infarction, transient ischemic events, and sudden cardiac death. The increase in sudden cardiac deaths during morning hours may well be due to a significant increase in the frequency of VPCs during the morning hours (26,27). Twenty-four-hour Holter monitorings in patients with ventricular arrhythmias show that the frequency of VPCs increases in the morning hours. It has been postulated that this morning increase in ven-

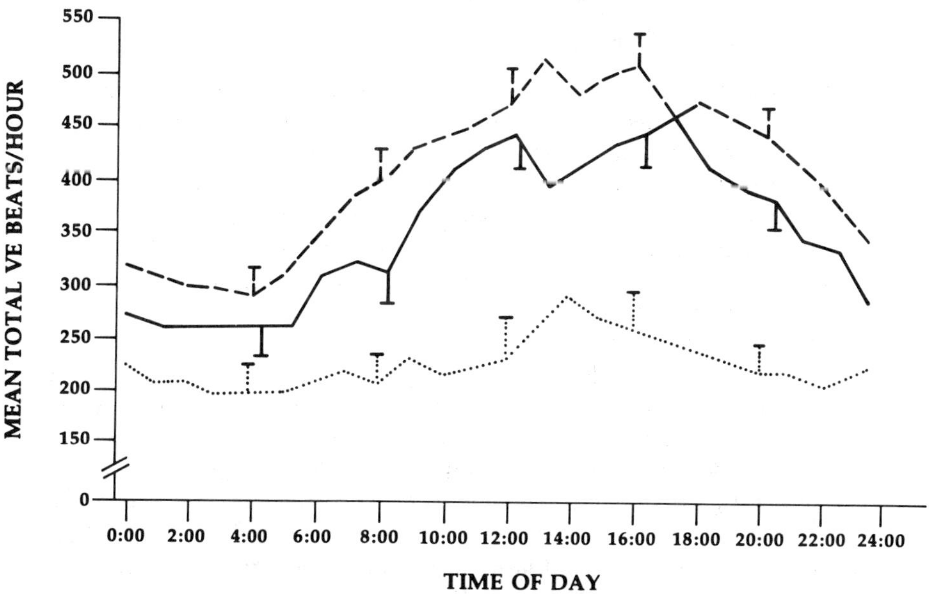

Figure 2 Circadian variation of mean total ventricular premature complexes/hr (mean ± standard error of the mean) at baseline (broken line), during placebo administration (solid line), and with acebutolol (dotted line), Acebutolol markedly attenuated circadian distribution of ventricular premature complexes. VE = ventricular actopic. (From Ref. 38 with permission.)

tricular arrhythmia density, in conjunction with the increases observed in transient myocardial ischemic events and acute myocardial infarctions, may account for the increased risk of sudden cardiac deaths in the morning hours. Although the precise mechanism of circadian rhythmicity of ventricular arrhythmias and ischemic events is not established, it is possible that the morning surge in catecholamines may be responsible for the genesis of these cardiac events and explain the effects of beta-adrenoceptor blockade in the suppressing it. Recent studies demonstrate that beta blockade with acebutolol (Fig. 2) or nadolol attenuates or abolishes the circadian rhythmicity of VPCs (26,27). This decrease in the density of ventricular arrhythmias during morning hours by beta blockade may be responsible for the beneficial effects of these agents in reducing sudden cardiac deaths by removing the trigger for life-threatening ventricular tachycardia or ventricular fibrillation in the setting of coronary artery disease.

ANTIARRHYTHMIC EFFECTS OF CONVENTIONAL BETA-BLOCKERS ON VENTRICULAR PREMATURE COMPLEXES

Recent studies (6-11,26-30) using a variety of conventional beta-blocking agents have evaluated the suppressant effects of these agents on VPCs, including complex and repetitive ventricular ectopy (Table 1). The results from most of these studies demonstrate nearly 50% efficacy of conventional beta-blocking drugs in suppressing VPC frequency, and 40-50% of the patients achieve ≥75% VPC suppression. However, it is difficult to compare the results of these studies because the selection criteria for patients studied, duration of treatment, as well as doses of beta-blocking drugs used varied considerably.

In the study by Woosley et al. (6), 32 patients with stable and frequent ventricular tachyarrhythmias received propranolol given in incremental doses until a defined degree of arrhythmia suppression was achieved, adverse effects developed, or the maximal dose of 960 mg/day was reached. These investigators demonstrated a 70-100% suppression of ventricular arrhythmia with adequate response achieved in 75% of the patients. Eight patients had episodes of VT that responded to lower doses of propranolol than those required to suppress VPCs.

More recently, Nademanee and coworkers (7) reported that, during nadolol treatment with doses titrated up to 640 mg/day, 48% of 36 patients studied achieved ≥75% suppression of ventricular ectopy. Similar to the results of Woosley, these investigators also found that nadolol was

Table 1 Antiarrhythmic Effects of Conventional Beta-Blockers in Benign or Potentially Lethal Ventricular Arrhythmias Relative to Those of Sotalol

Drug used	Maximal VPCs/hr (mg/day)	% Reduction	Patients with efficacy (%)	Ref.
Propranolol	960	70-100	24/32 (75)	6
Acebutolol	1,800	52	—	28
Propranolol	240	47	—	
Metoprolol	200	60	10/20 (50)	29
Acebutolol	1,800	74	14/42 (33)	26
Propranolol	240	60	9/42 (20)	
Nadolol	640	86	17/36 (48)	7
Nadolol	160	85	11/23 (48)	30
Sotalol	160	86	—	32
Sotalol	160	—	5/10 (50)	33
Sotalol	320	58	10/22 (45)	37
Nadolol	160	61	7/22 (32)	
Sotalol	640	83	33/56 (59)	16
Sotalol	640	80	35/63 (56)	38
Propranolol	240	59	22/77 (29)	

VPCs = ventricular premature complexes.

effective in reducing VT events by 75% in all of the 13 patients who had these arrhythmias at baseline. This dramatic effect of nadolol on VT events is unusual and has not been observed in other trials with beta-blockers, and may be due to higher than usual doses of nadolol used. In another study, Morganroth and Duchin (30) evaluated the antiarrhythmic effects of low-dose nadolol in 23 patients with benign or potentially lethal ventricular arrhythmias. Forty-eight percent of patients responded to nadolol with a reduction of >75% in arrhythmia frequency, and several patients responded to a dose of nadolol as low as 10 mg/day.

The antiarrhythmic efficacy of acebutolol and propranolol was evaluated in a double-blind, placebo-controlled, randomized, crossover study by Singh et al. (28). In this study of 31 patients with more than 30 VPCs/hr, both acebutolol and propranolol produced comparable (52 and 47%, respectively) and significant reductions in VPC frequency during both 24-hr Holter monitoring evaluation and exercise testing (51 and 69% VPC suppression, respectively).

Table 2 Summary of Efficacy Results: Acebutolol Versus Propranolol in Ventricular Arrhythmia ($n = 42$)

Parameters	Baseline	Acebutolol Dose titration	Acebutolol Maintenance	Propranolol Dose titration	Propranolol Maintenance	Drug-free
Mean total VPCs/hr	26.5 ± 44.5	63.6 ± 17.2	82.3 ± 22.3	115.3 ± 31.1	140.3 ± 40.3	222.6 ± 41.0
Minimum VPCs/hr	33.8 ± 9.1	8.1 ± 2.5	11.6 ± 3.6	20.1 ± 6.2	27.8 ± 6.2	36.4 ± 10.8
Maximum VPCs/hr	677.5 ± 93.8	299.1 ± 61.9	299.0 ± 65.9	410.3 ± 84.6	375.0 ± 82.0	629.3 ± 80.5
Mean paired VPCs/hr	15.6 ± 4.6	4.3 ± 1.3	5.3 ± 2.7	6.3 ± 2.1	8.8 ± 3.6	8.5 ± 2.6
Mean VT beats/hr	1.0 ± 0.3	0.3 ± 0.2	0.1 ± 0.0	0.3 ± 0.1	0.2 ± 0.1	1.3 ± 0.6
Multiform beats (%)[a]	63.3 ± 6.2	49.4 ± 6.1	56.3 ± 6.0	60.5 ± 6.2	61.4 ± 6.2	66.0 ± 6.2
R-on-T beats (%)	1.7 ± 0.9	1.2 ± 1.2	0.4 ± 0.3	0.1 ± 0.1	0.2 ± 0.1	0.1 ± 0.1
% Below baseline minimal total VPCs[b]	0.0 ± 0.0	73.8 ± 6.9	73.8 ± 6.9	54.8 ± 7.8	59.5 ± 7.8	38.1 ± 7.6
Mean hourly heart rate	73.3 ± 1.4	64.1 ± 1.1	66.7 ± 1.2	63.5 ± 1.2	63.6 ± 1.2	78.6 ± 1.7

[a]Hours noted.
[b]Twenty-five percent of observations are generally expected to be less than the minimum of 3 preceding observations.
Values are mean ± standard error of the mean.
VPC = ventricular premature complexes; VT = ventricular tachycardia.
Source: Ref. 26 with permission.

In a recent report summarizing the results of three large multicenter clinical trials, Chandraratna (26) reported the comparative efficacy of acebutolol, placebo, propranolol, and quinidine in a total of 217 patients with chronic frequent VPCs. As shown in Tables 2 and 3, acebutolol significantly ($p < 0.0002$ to $p < 0.001$) reduced mean total VPCs as well as complex VPCs compared with baseline. The efficacy of acebutolol was superior to placebo and comparable to that of propranolol and quinidine. Also, the number of patients with adequate (≥ 75%) suppression of VPCs was comparable for acebutolol, propranolol, and quinidine.

The results of these studies discussed above indicate that most conventional beta-blocking drugs significantly suppress VPCs in patients with and without organic heart disease. These effects are characterized by the following features: (1) a significant reduction in VPC frequency with adequate (≥75%) suppression in approximately 50% of the patients, (2) a greater response for higher grades (complex VPCs and ventricular couplets) of VPCs, and (3) abolition or marked attenuation of the circadian pattern of VPC distribution (Fig. 2). Another major advantage of beta-blockers in comparison with other antiarrhythmic drugs has been a relatively good safety record with very few adverse effects.

In general, beta-blockers have also not been shown to produce proarrythmic effects. Because of their good safety record and different mechanisms of action, beta-blockers also are frequently used in combination therapy with Class I antiarrhythmic agents. In recent study (31), the effects

Table 3 Summary of Efficacy Results: Acebutolol Versus Quinidine in Ventricular Arrhythmia

	Baseline[a]	Acebutolol[a]	Quinidine[a]	Drug-free
Heart rate (beats/min)				
Resting	83.1 ± 2.7	65.0 ± 1.7	82.4 ± 2.9	81.1 ± 3.1
Peak	110.9 ± 4.0	93.3 ± 2.9	111.6 ± 3.7	111.3 ± 3.7
VPCs (rate/hr)				
At rest (Holter)	223.6 ± 48.4	97.8 ± 37.5	197.5 ± 49.3	145.1 ± 42.7
During exercise[b]	501 ± 73.8	158.4 ± 52.2	262.2 ± 75	305.4 ± 70.2
Higher grade VPCs				
At rest (VPCs/hr)	2.43 ± 0.55	1.14 ± 0.47	0.87 ± 0.21	1.95 ± 0.65

[a]Based on average of two visits.
[b]Computed as rate/hour.
Values are mean ± standard error of the mean.
Source: Ref. 26 with permission.

of beta blockade with nadolol combined with procainamide and quinidine were studied in patients refractory to Class IA agents alone. Although the details of this study are discussed elsewhere in this book, the results demonstrated showed that the combination therapy significantly reduced total VPC frequency during titration as well as during the double-blind phase. A positive response, defined as a decrease of ≥75% in VPCs, was documented in 57% of patients during the titration phase and 63% of patients during double-blind treatment.

ANTIARRHYTHMIC EFFECTS OF SOTALOL

Because of its unique electrophysiologic spectrum of action, sotalol is thought to be superior to conventional beta-blocking agents for the treatment of patients with ventricular arrhythmias. However, as discussed above, most conventional beta-blockers have also been shown to suppress ventricular arrhythmias; thus, to demonstrate the superiority of sotalol, it is essential to compare the relative potency of sotalol to that of conventional beta-blocking agents.

The antiarrhythmic effects of sotalol on VPCs have been known for many years. Most of the earlier studies, however, were performed in small numbers of patients using inadequate dosages of sotalol. In the study by Myburgh et al. (32), optimally titrated doses of sotalol suppressed the frequency of VPCs by 86% in 20 patients with ischemic heart disease. Mary-Rabine et al. (33), reported the long-term effects sotalol in doses of 80-160 mg/day in 10 patients with organic heart disease and symptomatic ventricular ectopy. Serial Holter recordings were obtained before sotalol was started and then at 3- and 6-month intervals during sotalol therapy. Initially, a significant suppression of ventricular ectopy was observed in 9 of 10 patients studied and, during long-term therapy, the efficacy was maintained in 50% of the patients, including suppression of complex and repetitive ectopy.

In a double-blind, placebo-controlled study, Anderson et al. (16) evaluated the suppressant effects of sotalol, given in doses of 320 or 640 mg/day, on complex ventricular ectopy in 56 patients with chronic VPCs. The doses significantly reduced the median arrhythmia frequency by 77 and 83%, respectively ($p < 0.001$), compared with a 6% reduction during placebo administration. Fifty-nine percent of the sotalol group achieved adequate suppression, defined as 75% reduction in ventricular ectopy, compared with an 11% response rate in the placebo group. The effects of sotalol on couplets and runs of nonsustained VT were even more dramatic, showing a 94% ($p < 0.0001$) and 89% ($p < 0.0007$) reduction, respectively.

Another blinded, placebo-controlled study (34) also demonstrated the efficacy of sotalol in suppressing VPCs. Fourteen patients with a history of myocardial infarction and high-density stable VPCs were given 320 mg of sotalol or matching placebo. In 6 of 14 patients, the total number of VPCs decreased by 50% with greater suppression of the higher grades of ventricular ectopy. There were no adverse reactions, and left ventricular ejection fraction was unchanged. In addition, a significant ($p < 0.0005$) correlation was noted between the antiarrhythmic effect and the prolongation of the QTc interval.

Wang et al. (35) examined the significance of the lengthening of cardiac repolarization on heart rate and arrhythmia suppression induced by sotalol. Seventeen patients followed an incremental dose-regimen protocol under serum drug-concentration control. Sotalol at doses of 160, 320, 640, and 960 mg was given once or twice daily. Eleven of the 17 patients achieved antiarrhythmic response with a 70-100% reduction of VPCs at a wide range of plasma concentrations; the responders included eight patients who had poor responses with conventional beta-blocking therapy. The sotalol concentration at which QTc prolongation was noted (2.55 mg/liter) was greater than that required for achieving a 50% reduction in exercise-induced increment in the heart rate (0.80 mg/liter).

The antiarrhythmic effects of sotalol have also been compared with those of Class I antiarrhythmic agents. In a recent study, Lidell et al. (36) compared the efficacy of oral sotalol (160-640 mg/day) and procainamide (1-1.5 g 3 times daily) in 33 patients with chronic, stable VPCs in an open, randomized, crossover study. Sotalol produced <75% reduction of VPCs in 67% of the patients. Procainamide was effective in only 39% of the patients. When VPCs were significantly reduced, both drugs appeared to produce comparable reductions in runs of nonsustained VT. Nine patients responded to both agents, and seven failed to respond to either of the drugs.

The results of these studies indicate that sotalol is an effective antiarrhythmic agent and causes significant reductions in the total VPC frequency as well as complex and repetitive ventricular ectopy. The overall response rates achieved during treatment with sotalol in these studies appear to be better than those reported with conventional beta-blockers in treating patients with chronic ventricular arrhythmias.

COMPARATIVE EFFECTS OF SOTALOL AND CONVENTIONAL BETA-BLOCKERS

Whether sotalol is more effective than conventional beta-blockers can be established only by direct comparison of equiactive beta-blocking doses of sotalol and conventional beta-blocking drugs in a stable population of patients with comparable ventricular arrhythmias. Little data are available for such direct comparison.

In a single-blind, crossover trial, Myburgh et al. (37) compared the suppressant effects of sotalol and nadolol on ventricular ectopy in 22 patients with stable chronic ventricular arrhythmias. All patients had acute myocardial infarction at least 3 months before the study and were required to have ⩾30 VPCs/hr during the 24-hr Holter monitoring at baseline after withdrawal of all antiarrhythmic agents including beta-blocking agents. After a 2-week placebo period, patients began therapy with either 160 mg of sotalol of 80 mg of nadolol once daily in a randomized fashion. After 1 week of active therapy, patients were evaluated, and the dosage of the study drug was doubled in those not achieving a 90% reduction in VPC frequency. Patients were reevaluated after another week of therapy with the effective or highest dosage. This was followed by another 7-day placebo period before crossing over to the other drug, and the sequence of events was repeated exactly as before.

At baseline, the average hourly VPC count was 238 and decreased to 146 (61% reduction) during therapy with 80 mg of nadolol. Seventeen patients were advanced to the higher dose of nadolol (160 mg) because of an inadequate response, and only 2 of the 17 achieved 90% suppression at the higher dose. These data revealed that a higher dose of nadolol was no more effective than the lower dose. In contrast, during sotalol treatment, the baseline average hourly VPC count was 256 and decreased to 199/hr during low-dose administration with a further reduction to 109/hr during high-dose administration of sotalol. The higher dose of sotalol was significantly ($p < 0.02$) more effective than the lower dose. Using ⩾90% suppression as the criterion for adequate suppression, only 7 patients achieved the desired response, but 10 patients (45%) showed ⩾75% VPC suppression during sotalol treatment. Because the highest dose of sotalol used in this study was only 320 mg, one cannot exclude the possibility that even a higher dosage of sotalol than the one used in this study could not have produced greater VPC suppression. This is partially supported by the fact that the average heart rate over 24 hours decreased to only 67 and 65 beats/min (from a baseline heart rate of 85 beats/min) during 160 and 320 mg/day of sotalol compared with 64 and 63 beats/min during 80 and 160 mg/day of nadolol. The QTc interval was not prolonged in these patients during sotalol therapy, further suggesting the possibility of inadequate dosage and the potential for additional benefit from higher doses producing prolongation of the QTc interval.

In a more recent double-blind, placebo-controlled, parallel study, the effects of sotalol and propranolol were compared in 172 patients with chronic stable frequent (average of >30 VPCs/hr) ventricular arrhythmias that would generally warrant treatment in clinical practice (38). Seventy-three percent of the patients were men (mean age 62 years). All antiarrhythmic drugs and beta-blocking agents were discontinued during the initial week and placebo was administered for 7 additional days. Two 24-hour Holter recordings were obtained at the end of the placebo phase, and qualifying

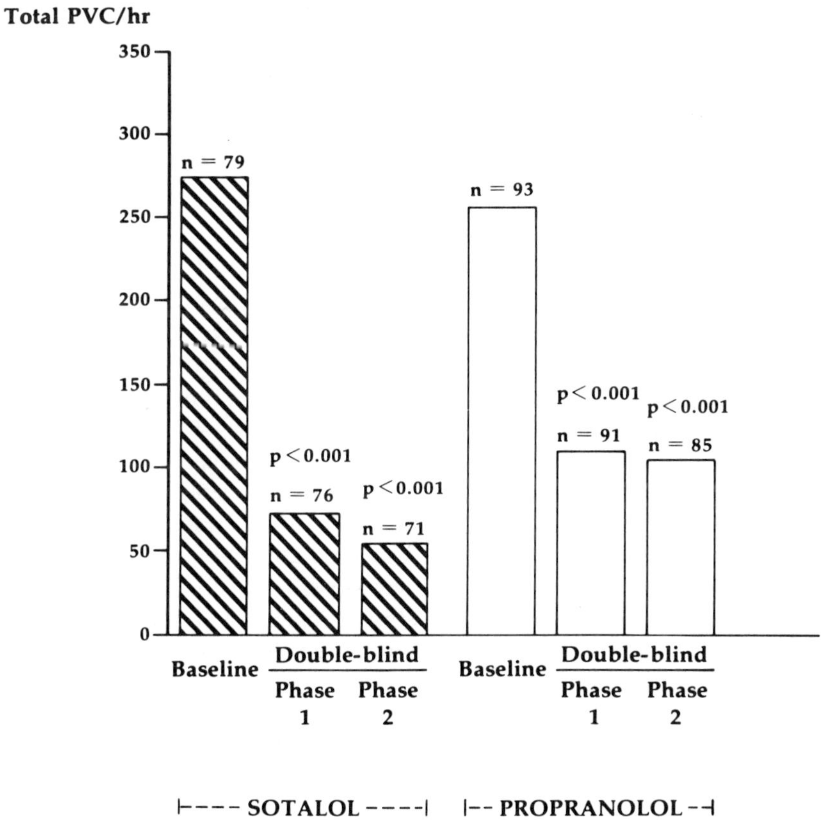

Figure 3 Effects of sotolol and propranolol on mean total hourly ventricular complex (VPC) frequency during initial (phase 1) and final (phase 2) 2 weeks of double-blind treatment. (From Ref. 38 with permission).

patients with an average of ≥30 VPCs/hr were randomized to 160 mg of sotalol twice a day (76 patients) or 40 mg of propranolol 3 times a day (91 patients). Adequate VPC suppression was defined as ≥75% reduction in frequency, and patients not achieving this response during the initial 2-week therapy were advanced to higher doses consisting of 320 mg of sotalol twice daily or 80 mg of propranolol 3 times a day. The treatment was then continued for another 2 weeks, and 24-hour Holter recordings were obtained at the end of this treatment. In the group receiving sotalol, the mean hourly VPC count on two 24-hour Holter recordings was 274 and decreased to 54 (80% reduction) by the end of 4 weeks of therapy (Fig. 3). In contrast, in the propranolol-treated group, the baseline mean hourly VPC count was 255 and decreased to 104 (59% reduction) by the end of 4 weeks of propranolol therapy. Fifty-six percent of patients treated with sotalol achieved adequate suppression (≥75% reduction) of VPCs compared with only 29% of the patients receiving propranolol.

DISCUSSION

The role of beta-blocking agents in improving the survival of patients after an acute myocardial infarction is well established (1-2). The results of several large-scale clinical trials in thousands of survivors of acute myocardial infarction clearly demonstrate that beta-blockers are extremely effective in reducing the overall mortality as well as the risk of sudden cardiac death (1-3). Although none of these studies has established a direct relationship between the antiarrhythmic actions of various beta-blockers used, it is known from the results of other studies that these drugs are effective in reducing the density of spontaneous ventricular arrhythmias. Unlike the recently demonstrated increase in mortality probably due to proarrhythmic effects of the Class IC agents encainide and flecainide in the Cardiac Arrhythmia Suppression Trial (CAST), the administration of conventional beta-blockers is considered safe and is rarely associated with the risk of proarrhythmia. Because of the demonstrated efficacy of beta-blockers in reducing mortality and their relatively safe profile in patients with cardiac arrhythmias, beta-blockers are being used increasingly in the treatment of ventricular arrhythmias particularly in patients with underlying coronary artery disease and prior history of myocardial infarction.

The review of currently available data indicates that sotalol and conventional beta-blocking agents are effective in suppressing VPCs in patients with and without heart disease. Sotalol is unique as an antiarrhythmic agent because in addition to its beta-blocking properties, it also has Class III antiarrhythmic actions and thus it might be superior to the conventional beta-blocker in suppressing ventricular arrhythmias. As discussed above, the results of two comparative studies with sotalol and conventional beta-blocking agents, nadolol and propranolol, indicated that sotalol was more effective than these conventional beta-blockers in suppressing total VPC frequency as well as complex and repetitive ectopy. Although more studies directly comparing sotalol and conventional beta-blockers are needed, the preliminary results from the study of 172 patients with potentially lethal ventricular arrhythmias show significant superiority of sotalol over propranolol in reducing the frequency of chronic stable VPCs. Furthermore, the percentage of patients achieving adequate (≥75%) suppression of VPCs was significantly greater (56%) with sotalol than with propranolol (29%). The results of a recent study demonstrated sotalol's usefulness in patients with symptomatic sustained VT or ventricular fibrillation, even when these arrhythmias were refractory to available conventional antiarrhythmic agents (39). In these patients, sotalol was found to be a powerful suppressant, having selectivity of action, as in the case of most beta-blockers, for the complex and repetitive forms of VPCs.

Although the data appear to be reasonably compelling that sotalol might exert a more powerful suppressant effect on VPCs than conventional beta-blockers, the precise reason for the difference is not clear. Two possibilities should be considered. First, the difference may relate solely to differences in the extent of beta-blocking potencies of the doses of the drugs used chronically. To achieve quantitatively equivalent beta-blocking effects by any two beta-antagonists is notoriously difficult. Sotalol has 100% bioavailability and a rapid onset of action and prolonged duration of activity due to a long elimination half-life. These properties may permit more pronounced and continuous beta blockade than many other beta-blockers, with a consequent effect on arrhythmia suppression. The other possibility that has been suggested (35) is that the associated Class III action of sotalol might contribute to its overall effect in suppressing VPCs. However, Singh (40) indicated that the "isolated" lengthening of the action potential duration (a class III effect) does not necessarily constitute a powerful mechanism for VPC suppression. For example, clofilium, an adrenergic neuron-blocking drug, produces a massive lengthening of cardiac repolarization but is devoid of a suppressant effect on VPCs (40). A synergistic effect between beta blockade and prolonged cardiac repolarization cannot be excluded.

CLINICAL IMPLICATIONS

Whatever mechanism might be established for the apparently greater suppressant effect of sotalol on VPCs relative to conventional beta-blockers, the clinical implications of the observation should be emphasized. There are two consequences of the suppressant effect on VPCs and the pronounced as well as predictable effect on the effective refractory period of cardiac muscle. First, removal of the trigger mechanism by the antiectopic action will reduce the probability of the arrhythmias being initiated. Second, lengthening the refractory period will be associated with an antifibrillatory mechanism resulting from the widening of the tachycardia cycle length. These electrophysiologic mechanisms of sotalol, in conjunection with its known antiischemic actions, are likely to provide the basis for reducing the incidence of sudden death from arrhythmias in patients with coronary artery disease.

REFERENCES

1. Yusuf S, Peto R, Lewis J, Collins R, Sleight P. Beta-blockade during and after myocardial infarction: an overview of the randomized trials. Prog Cardiovasc Dis 1985; 27:335-71.
2. Beta-blocker Heart Attack Trial Group. A randomized trial of propranolol in patients with acute myocardial infarction. JAMA 1982; 247:1707-14.
3. Furberg CD. Effects of antiarrhythmic drugs on mortality after myocardial infarction. Am J Cardiol 1983; 53:32C-36C.
4. The Cardiac Arrhythmia Suppression Trial (CAST) Investigators. Preliminary report: effect of encainide and flecainide on mortality in a randomized trial of arrhythmia suppression after myocardial infarction. N Engl J Med 1989; 321:406-12.
5. Stock JPP, Dale N. Beta-adrenergic receptor blockade in cardiac arrhythmias. Br Med J 1963; 2:1230-3.
6. Woosley RL, Kornhauser D, Smith R, Rede S, Higgins SB, Nros AS, Shand DG, Oates JA. Suppression of chronic ventricular arrhythmias with propranolol. Circulation 1979; 60:819-24.
7. Nademanee K, Schleman MM, Singh BN, Morganroth J, Reid PR, Stritar JA. Beta-adrenergic blockade by nadolol in control of ventricular arrhythmias. Am Heart J 1984; 208:1109-16.
8. Aronow WS, Turbow M, Lurie M, Whittaker K, Van Camp S. Treatment of premature ventricular complexes with acebutolol. Am J Cardiol 1979; 43: 106-10.

9. Gradman AH, Winkle RA, Fitzgerald JW, Meffin PJ, Stoner J, Bell PA, Hanson DC. Suppression of premature ventricular contractions by acebutolol. Circulation 1977; 55:785-9.
10. Podrid PJ, Lown B. Pindolol for ventricular arrhythmias. Am Heart J 1982; 104:491-5.
11. Morganroth J. Short-term evaluation of atenolol in hospitalized patients with chronic ventricular arrhythmias. Drug 1983; 25 (suppl 2):181-6.
12. Mason JW, Winkle RA. Accuracy of the ventricular induction study for predicting long-term efficacy and inefficacy of antiarrhythmic drugs. N Engl J Med 1980; 303:1073-9.
13. Brodskky MA, Allen BJ, Luckett CR, Capparelli EV, Wolff LJ, Henry WL. Antiarrhythmic efficacy of solitary beta-adrenergic blockade for patients with sustained ventricular arrhythmias. Am Heart J 1989; 118:272-80.
14. Friehling TD, Lipshutz H, Marinchak RA, Stohler JL, Kowey PR. Effectiveness of propranolol added to type I antiarrhythmic agents for sustained ventricular tachycardia secondary to coronary artery disease. Am J Cardiol 1990; 65:1328-33.
15. Singh BN, Deedwania P, Nademanee K, Ward A, Sorkin EM. Sotalol: a review of its pharmacodynamic properties, and therapeutic use. Drugs 1987; 34:311-49.
16. Anderson JL, Askings JC, Gilbert EM, Miller RH, Keefe DL. Multicenter trial of sotalol for suppression of frequent, complex ventricular arrhythmias: a double-blind, randomized placebo-controlled evaluation of two doses. JACC 1986; 8:752-62.
17. Nademanee K, Feld G, Hendrickson JA, Singh PN, Singh BN. Electrophysiologic and antiarrhythmic effects of sotalol in patients with life threatening ventricular tachyarrhythmias. Circulation 1985; 72:555-64.
18. Singh BN, Jewitt DE. Adrenoceptor blocking drugs in cardiac arrhythmias. Drugs 1974; 7:426-61.
19. Ebert PA, Allgood RJ, Sabiston DC. The antiarrhythmic effects of cardiac denervation. Ann Surg 1968; 168:728-35.
20. Venditti FJ, Garan H, Ruskin JN. Electrophysiologic effects of beta-blockers in ventricular arrhythmias. Am J Cardiol 1987; 60:3D-9D.
21. Singh BN, Nadamanee K. Antihypertensive compounds as antiarrhythmic agents: focus on beta-blocking drugs in ventricular arrhythmias. Am Heart J 1987; 114:1040-50.
22. Hewett K, Rosen MR. Beta-adrenergic modulation of the digitalis-induced delayed afterdepolarization and triggered activity (abstr). Am J Cardiol 1982; 49:913.
23. Sung RJ, Tai Dy, Svinarich JT. Beta-adrenoceptor blockade: electrophysiology and antiarrhythmic mechanisms. Am Heart J 1984; 108:1115-20.
24. Anderson JL, Rodier HE, Green LS. Comparative effects of beta-adrenergic blocking drugs on experimental ventricular fibrillation threshold. Am J Cardiol 1983; 51:1196-202.

25. Raine AEG, Vaughan Williams EM. Adaptation to prolonged beta-blockade on rabbit atrial, Purkinje and ventricular potentials and papillary muscle contractions. Circ Res 1981; 48:804-12.
26. Chandraratna PAN. Comparison acebutolol with propranolol, quinidine, and placebo: results of three multicenter arrhythmia trials. Am Heart J 1985; 109:1198-204.
27. Mir MA, Tirlapur VG. Circadian rhythm of ventricular arrhythmias and antiarrhythmic efficacy of long-acting beta-adrenergic blocker. In: Hollenberg NK, ed. The hemodynamics of nadolol. Second International Symposium Royal Society of Medicine Series No. 51. New York: Academic Press, and Grune & Stratton, 1982:101-7.
28. Singh SN, DiBianco R, Davidov ME, Gottdiener JS, Johnson WI, Laddu AR, Fletcher RD. Comparison of acebutolol and propranolol for treatment of chronic ventricular arrhythmia: a placebo-controlled, double-blind, randomized crossover study. Circulation 1982; 65:1356-64.
29. Pratt CM, Yepsen SC, Kimbloom MG, Taylor AA, Young JB, Quinones MA. Evaluation of metoprolol in suppressing complex ventricular arrhythmias. Am J Cardiol 1983; 52:73-8.
30. Morganroth J, Duchin KL. Antiarrhythmic effects of beta-adrenergic blocking agents in benign or potentially lethal ventricular arrhythmias. Am J Cardiol 1987; 60:10D-14D.
31. Deedwania P, Olukotun AY, Kuppersmith J, Jenkins P, Golden P. Beta-blockers in combination with class I antiarrhythmic agents. Am J Cardiol 1987; 60:21D-26D.
32. Myburgh DP, Goldman AP, Cartoon J, Schamroth JM. The efficacy of sotalol in suppressing ventricular ectopic beats. Afr Med J 1979; 56:295-8.
33. Mary-Rabine L, Soumagne D, Stiels B. Long-term sotalol therapy in patients with ventricular arrhythmias. Acta Cardiol 1986; 2:89-97.
34. Burchkardt D, Pfisterer M, Hoffman A, Burkart F, Emmenegger H. Effects of the beta-adrenoceptor blocking agent sotalol on ventricular arrhythmias in patients with chronic ischemic heart disease. Cardiology 1983; 70(suppl 1):114-21.
35. Wang T, Bergstrand RH, Thompson KA, Siddoway LA, Duff HJ. Concentration-dependent pharmacologic properties of sotalol. Am J Cardiol 1986; 57:1160-5.
36. Lidell C, Rehnqvist N, Sjogren A, Yli-Uotila RJ, Ronnevik PK. Comparative efficacy of oral sotalol and procainamide in patients with chronic ventricular arrhythmias: a multicenter study. Am Heart J 1985; 109:970-5.
37. Myburgh DP, Smith R, Diamond TH, Faitelson HL, Sommers DK. A comparison of the efficacy of sotalol and nadolol in the suppression of ventricular ectopic beats. S Afr Med J 1983; 63:263-5.
38. Deedwania P. Suppressant effects of conventional beta blockers and sotalol on complex and repetitive ventricular premature complexes. Am J Cardiol 1990; 43A-50A.

39. Nademanee K, Singh BN. Effects of sotalol on ventricular tachycardia and fibrillation produced by programmed electrical stimulation: comparison with other antiarrhythmic agents. Am J Cardiol 1990; 65:53A-57A.
40. Singh BN. Editorial: When is it QT prolongation antiarrhythmic and when is it proarrhythmic? Am J Cardiol 1989; 63:867-9.

11

Beta-Blockers in Combination with Class I Antiarrhythmic Agents: Focus on Nadolol

Prakash C. Deedwania
University of California at San Francisco School of Medicine, San Francisco, and Veterans Affairs Medical Center, Fresno, California

Although a large number of antiarrhythmic drugs are now available for treatment of patients with ventricular arrhythmias, it is becoming increasingly evident that in some patients, treatment with any one of the currently available antiarrhythmic agents may be unsuccessful in effectively controlling the ventricular arrhythmias (1,2). The lack of efficacy of a single agent has led to the development of combination therapy consisting of antiarrhythmic drugs with varying electrophysiologic properties (e.g., combination of a Class IA and IB agent or a Class IA and Class II agent) (3-5). These combinations usually consist of drugs that are ineffective when used individually, and the treatment strategy is based on the hypothesis that these agents given together may produce additive, synergistic, or new effects that exceed those of each drug used alone (3). Most experts agree that combination therapy should not be used as first-line treatment and suggest that lack of adequate response to conventional antiarrhythmic agents given in adequate doses should be demonstrated before such use (2-4). Although combination therapy with antiarrhythmic drugs is

The contents of this chapter have been published in part in Deedwania P, Olukotun A, Kupersmith J, Jenkins P, Golden P. Beta Blockers in combination with class I antiarrhythmic agents. Am J Cardiol 1987; 60:21D-26D and are reproduced with permission from the American Journal of Cardiology.

safe when used appropriately, addition of the second agent may occasionally antagonize the useful electrophysiologic effects of the first drug and may rarely produce additive toxic effects. Thus, careful evaluation and understanding of the mechanisms of arrhythmia to be treated as well as the actions of drugs to be used are essential for the proper selection of effective and safe combinations.

The rationale for use of combination therapy at the mechanistic level is based on several factors. First, an arrhythmia may be caused by one or more of the usual mechanisms, including enhanced automaticity, reentry, reflexion, or triggered automaticity (6). In addition, different classes of antiarrhythmic agents have variable effects on membrane responsiveness, action potential duration, repolarization phase, and other electrophysiologic parameters (7). Accordingly, the most appropriate antiarrhythmic agent or combination of agents will vary depending on the predominant mechanism responsible for the arrhythmia. For example, whereas type I antiarrhythmic agents would probably be chosen initially for the treatment of an ectopic arrhythmia such as ventricular parasystole, treatment with a beta-adrenergic blocking agent would be expected to be more effective for the exercise-induced or catecholamine-dependent arrhythmia. However, a majority of rhythm disturbances may be related to more than one mechanism and thus may respond well to an appropriately selected combination of antiarrhythmic drugs (6). When treatment with a single agent is unsuccessful in effectively controlling the ventricular arrhythmias, combination therapy using drugs with different electrophysiologic properties may be useful (3,6).

Recently, several new antiarrhythmic drugs have been developed and approved for use in patients with ventricular arrhythmia. However, because of the safety concern related to their use, quinidine and procainamide remain the most frequently used antiarrhythmic agents in clinical practice. Although therapy with these agents is frequently considered satisfactory, careful and repeated arrhythmia monitorings will reveal many patients who are inadequately controlled (1-4). Combination therapy with drugs from different classes with varying spectrum of electrophysiologic properties provides an important and often necessary additional approach in the management of refractory patients (2-5,8-12).

Although beta-adrenergic blocking agents have not been used extensively as first-line drugs in the treatment of ventricular arrhythmias, a number of recent and earlier studies have demonstrated their effectiveness in controlling such arrhythmias (13-18). In addition, these agents have been shown to reduce overall mortality and sudden cardiac death in patients after acute myocardial infarction (19-21). Beta-blockers have also been successfully used in combination with quinidine and other Class I agents for treatment of patients with refractory ventricular arrhythmias (8-12). Most of these reports (8-11) however, described results from retrospective review of uncontrolled observations in a small number of patients. In this chapter, the finding of a recently completed double-blind, placebo-controlled trial evaluating the role of combination therapy with beta-blocker nadolol and Class Ia agents quinidine or procainamide will be described in detail (22). The findings of this study will then be compared with the results of other well-controlled trials using beta-blockers in combination with antiarrhythmic agents in the management of patients with ventricular arrhythmias.

STUDY POPULATION

The study group consisted of 18 ambulatory patients (12 men and 6 women). The mean age was 61 years (range 45 to 74). While receiving their usual therapeutic doses of quinidine or procainamide alone, all patients continued to have ventricular premature complexes (VPCs) at a rate of ≥10/hr during 24-hour ambulatory electrocardiographic (Holter) monitoring and had left ventricular ejection fraction >30% by radionuclide ventriculography. Nine patients had coronary artery disease, 4 had hypertensive heart disease, 1 had valvular disease, and 5 had other noncardiovascular diseases. All 18 patients had multiform VPCs, and 5 patients had episodes of nonsustained ventricular tachycardia defined as ≥3 consecutive VPCs terminating spontaneously within 30 seconds. Written informed consent was obtained for each patient before participation in the study. Patients were excluded from the study if they had congestive heart failure, life-threatening ventricular arrhythmias requiring urgent medical treatment, symptomatic bradycardia, symptomatic chronic obstructive lung disease, or type I diabetes mellitus. Patients were discontinued from all other antiarrhythmic agents (except quinidine or procainamide) for at least five drug half-lives before entry into the study. No patient was treated with amiodarone. Abnormalities of serum potassium, calcium, or magnesium were determined and corrected before the qualifying Holter recording.

STUDY DESIGN

The study consisted of three treatment periods: Phase 1, a 2-week placebo lead-in period during which patients received a class I agent alone (quinidine or procainamide); Phase 2, a 2-week open-label nadolol dose-titration period during which increasing doses of nadolol from 40 mg daily up to a maximum of 120 mg daily were gradually added; and Phase 3, a 4-week randomized, placebo-controlled, parallel comparison period during which patients were treated with either a class I agent alone or a combination of a class I agent and nadolol (Fig. 1).

The left ventricular ejection fraction by radionuclide ventriculography and 24-hour Holter recordings were obtained at the end of each treatment period. Holter recordings were analyzed in a blinded fashion by a central laboratory using a Spacelab (ICR 6201) scanner. This semiautomated

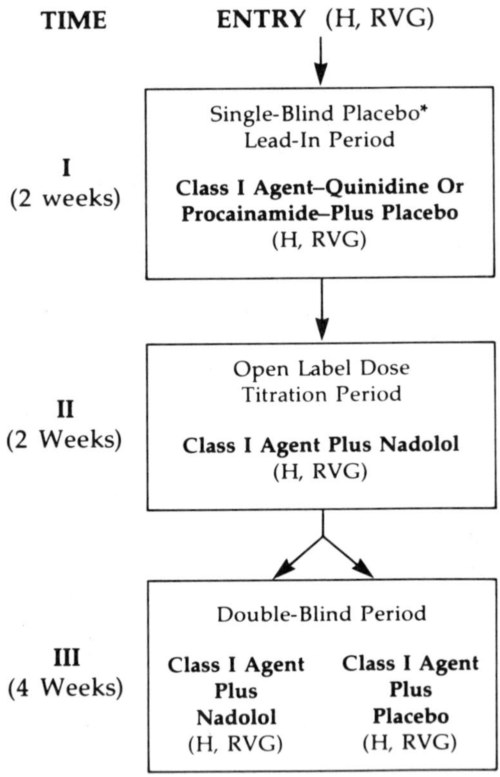

Figure 1 Protocol of beta-blockers in combination with Class 1 antiarrhythmic agents study. H = 24-hour Holter monitoring; * placebo = nadolol matching placebo; RVG = radionuclide ventriculography. (From Ref. 22 with permission from *The American Journal of Cardiology*.)

scanning system had two additional features: an interface with an IBM PC-XT personal computer for the production and storage of reports and an ICR 8003 variprinter that provided full disclosure on compressed write-out of all recorded electrocardiographic data.

The following additional observations and procedures were conducted on entry and at the end of double-blind treatment period: a complete history and physical examination, a standard 12-lead electrocardiogram, complete blood count, urinalysis, T3 and T4 and blood chemistry panel including glucose, creatinine, electrolytes, serum glutamic oxalocetic transaminase, serum glutamic pyruvic transaminase, bilirubin, cholesterol, and triglycerides. Heart rate and blood pressure were measured and adverse drug reactions recorded at the end of each treatment period.

A positive treatment response was defined as a $\geq$75% decrease in VPC frequency. All statistical analyses of change from baseline were performed using Student's paired *t*-tests. A two-way analysis of variance was used to compare mean responses for combination therapy (nadolol plus the Class I agent) versus the Class I agent alone at the end of the double-blind treatment period.

RESULTS

Effects of Combination Therapy on VPCs and Ventricular Couplets

The mean baseline VPC count with a Class I agent alone for the 14 patients with analyzable data during treatment with open-label nadolol in the dose titration phase of the study was 162/hr. With the addition of nadolol, the mean VPC count was decreased by 79% to an average of 34/hr (Fig. 2, top panel). The decrease was statistically significant ($p < 0.01$). A positive response, defined as a decrease of at least 75% in VPCs, was documented in eight (57%) of the patients during combination therapy in the nadolol titration segment. After 4 weeks of double-blind treatment, five of eight patients (62.5%) treated with combination therapy compared with two of seven (28.6%) patients treated with Class I agents alone were positive responders. VPC frequency was decreased on the average by 91.3% for the patients receiving combination therapy ($p < 0.05$) versus 18.9% for the patients receiving Class I agents alone (difference not significant) (Fig. 2, bottom panel).

The baseline frequency of ventricular couplets required for analysis was $\geq$10/day. The mean baseline frequency of ventricular couplets with a Class I agent alone for the eight patients meeting the analysis criteria who

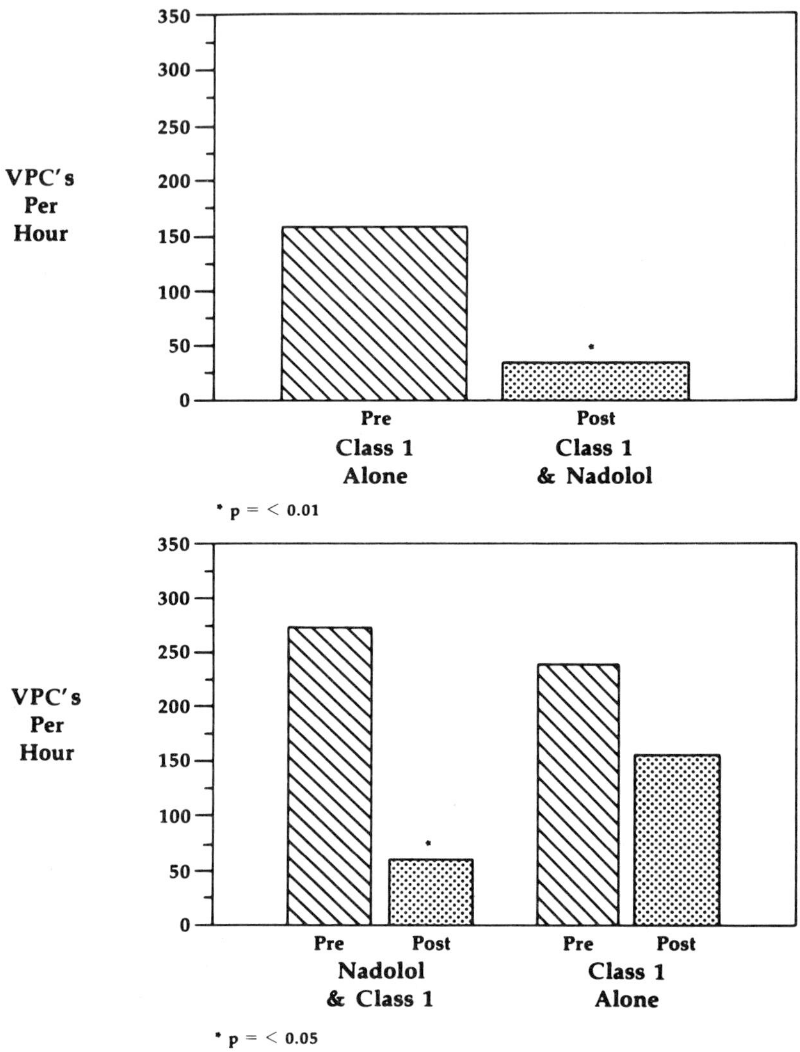

Figure 2 (Top) Mean hourly ventricular premature complex (VPC) frequency at baseline at end of nadolol dose titration. (Bottom) Mean hourly VPC frequency before and after double-blind therapy with nadolol plus a Class I agent or a Class I agent alone. (From Ref. 22 with permission from *The American Journal of Cardiology*.)

were treated with nadolol was 128/day. After nadolol was added, the mean ventricular couplet count decreased by 95% to 6/day, a statistically significant ($p < 0.01$) decrease (Fig. 3, top panel). A decrease of at least 75% in the frequency of ventricular couplets was observed in 7 (88%) of the 8 patients. After 4 weeks of double-blind treatment, 2 (40%) of the 5 patients receiving nadolol plus a Class I agent, but none of the 14 patients who continued to receive a Class I agent alone, experienced a positive response. The mean frequency of ventricular couplets decreased by 91% in patients receiving combination therapy and increased by 156% in patients treated with Class I agents alone (Fig. 3).

Effects on Ventricular Tachycardia

Only five patients had ≥3 runs of nonsustained ventricular tachycardia (VT) per day during baseline Holter recording. Three patients given combination therapy experienced near abolition (>99%) decrease of VT events, while two patients given Class I agents alone had minimal or no decrease in runs of VT. A patient treated with quinidine alone had one run of VT at baseline but developed a marked increase in the number of VT events (32 runs) by the end of the double-blind treatment.

Effects on Heart Rate at Rest and Blood Pressure

Heart rate decreased by approximately 20% ($p < 0.001$) while patients were given combination therapy, but remained at baseline or slightly higher levels while patients were treated with Class I agents alone. Systolic blood pressure decreased by about 10% and diastolic blood pressure by 6% while patients were receiving combination therapy. There was either no change or small increases in systolic and diastolic blood pressure when patients were receiving Class I agents alone.

Adverse Effects

None of the patients developed any evidence of congestive heart failure or left ventricular dysfunction. No patient was discontinued from the study because of serious side effects.

In summary, the results of this study demonstrated that combination therapy with nadolol was effective in suppressing the ventricular arrhythmias refractory to treatment with Class I agents procainamide or quinidine given alone.

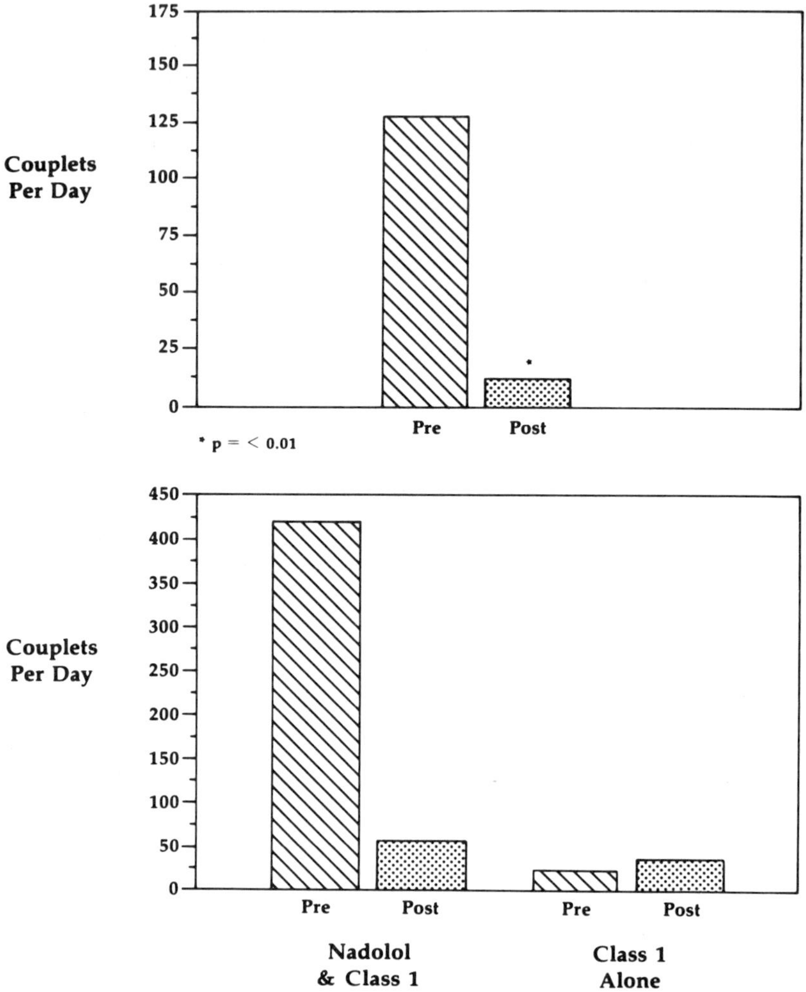

Figure 3 (Top) Mean daily frequency of ventricular couplets at baseline and at end of nadolol dose titration. (Bottom) Mean daily frequency of ventricular couplets before and after double-blind therapy with nadolol plus a Class I agent or a Class I agent alone. (From Ref. 22 with permission from *The American Journal of Cardiology*.)

DISCUSSION

Although the antiarrhythmic effects of the beta-adrenergic blocking agent dichloroisoproterenol were demonstrated more than 25 years ago, beta-blockers have not been as prominent as other antiarrhythmic agents in the treatment of patients with ventricular arrhythmias (13,14). Results from several recent clinical trials (15-18) clearly show that beta-blockers are effective in many patients with ventricular arrhythmias. These drugs are considered to be especially useful in certain subsets of patients, including those with mitral valve prolapse, congenital QT syndrome, exercise-induced ventricular tachycardia, and catecholamine-dependent arrhythmias (14,17,23-25). Beta-blockers have also been shown to reduce mortality in a large number of studies in patients with acute myocardial infarction (19-21). Although it is not clear whether the reduction in mortality in these studies was related to the control of arrhythmia, the treatment with beta-blockers was associated with a more favorable outcome in the subset of patients with demonstrable ventricular arrhythmias (19, 20).

Beta-blockers have also been shown to effectively suppress complex chronic ventricular arrhythmias (15,17,26,27). In a placebo-controlled study of propranolol in 32 patients with chronic high frequency ventricular arrhythmias, Woosley et al. (15) found a 70-100% suppression of ventricular arrhythmias in 75% of the patients. Eight patients in their study had VT at baseline, and treatment with the beta-blocker completely suppressed the VT events. In a recent report, Nademanee and coworkers (26) demonstrated the effectiveness of oral nadolol in controlling ventricular arrhythmias. These investigators evaluated the effectiveness of gradually increased doses (up to 640 mg) of nadolol in 36 patients with ventricular arrhythmias. Nadolol was effective in reducing VPCs in 17 (46%) of the 36 patients studied. Ventricular couplets were decreased by ≥75% in all 13 patients in whom it was present at baseline. Although the dosage of nadolol required for 75% suppression of arrhythmias ranged between 40 and 640 mg daily, the majority of patients responded to doses between 40 and 160 mg daily (26).

More recently, Morganroth and Duchin (27) have demonstrated that nadolol given in doses significantly lower than those used by Nademanee et al. (26) were effective in a majority of their patients. In this study, 23 patients with stable and frequent VPCs (>30/hr) were started on a daily dose of 10 mg oral nadolol, and this dose was doubled at weekly intervals until arrhythmia suppression was achieved, adverse effects appeared, or a maximum dosage of 160 mg daily was reached. In more than half of their patients effective arrhythmia suppression (≥75% reduction in VPCs) was achieved at nadolol dosages of ≤20 mg daily. Based on the results of this study, between 40 and 120 mg daily dosages of nadolol were considered adequate for the combination therapy in the present study.

The main objective of the study described in this chapter was to evaluate the safety and effectiveness of nadolol given in combination with the Class I antiarrhythmic agents procainamide and quinidine. Patients with ventricular arrhythmias refractory to long-term therapy with therapeutic doses of procainamide or quinidine were selected for enrollment. Although the study protocol allowed entry of patients with as few as 10 VPCs/hr while receiving treatment with therapeutic doses of procainamide or quinidine, most patients demonstrated a significantly higher frequency and complexity of VPCs. The average baseline VPC count was 162/hr, and approximately half of the patients had ventricular couplets at baseline. After nadolol was added, highly significant suppression of both VPCs and ventricular couplets was documented. This finding is similar to that reported by Morganroth and Duchin (27). These investigators also showed that ventricular arrhythmias of repetitive type (couplets and nonsustained VT) responded more favorably than the overall frequency of VPCs during treatment with low-dose nadolol (20 mg daily) (27). This type of preferential response to the repetitive forms of ventricular arrhythmia during nadolol therapy may be of considerable clinical importance, because it is now generally believed that suppression of such arrhythmias is more important than mere reduction in the frequency of VPCs.

The response of combination therapy during the double-blind portion of this study is difficult to interpret because the total number of patients completing the 4-week treatment period is small. However, in comparison with those receiving Class I antiarrhythmic agents alone, the patients treated with nadolol in combination with these agents had a substantially better therapeutic response. Another interesting finding is the fact that treatment with nadolol provided adequate control of VPCs during the entire 24-hour period. This is also of practical importance because patient compliance to drugs requiring frequent administration is a major problem in clinical practice. Nadolol is administered once daily, and if such therapy can provide adequate control of arrhythmias for 24 hours, clinicians are likely to achieve greater success in achieving the therapeutic goal for their patients.

Treatment with beta-blockers in combination with quinidine or procainamide can theoretically further depress left ventricular function and result in congestive heart failure. Because of this concern, the effects of combination therapy with nadolol on left ventricular ejection fraction were evaluated as measured by multigated radionuclide ventriculography. Although for safety reasons patients with a left ventricular ejection fraction <30% were excluded from the study, comparisons with placebo treatment as well as with baseline values showed that left ventricular ejection fraction did not change significantly for patients receiving nadolol during the double-blind portion of the study. Also, none of the patients developed any clinical evidence of congestive heart failure during treatment with nadolol.

Other Studies Using Beta-Blockers as Combination Therapy

Combination therapy with beta-blockers and Class I antiarrhythmic agents is not new. Almost 20 years ago, Dreifus et al. (8) described successful treatment of two patients with intermittent VT using a combination of quinidine and propranolol. In a subsequent study, Fors et al. (9) evaluated the effectiveness of propranolol and quinidine in the treatment of patients with quinidine-resistant arrhythmias. Eleven of 14 patients with paroxysmal VT in their series responded to treatment with the combination therapy. In another study, Leahey and coworkers reported success with a combination of mexiletine and propranolol in controlling ventricular tachycardia in patients refractory to long-term mexiletine therapy (10).

Hirsowitz and coworkers evaluated the role of combination therapy with beta-blocking agents in patients with malignant arrhythmias receiving a variety of membrane-stabilizing drugs including quinidine, procainamide, disopyramide, mexiletine, tocainide, aprindine, lorcainide, propafenone, and encainide (12). Although beta-blockers alone did not provide adequate benefit in suppressing the arrhythmia, when one of the beta-blockers was added to the membrane-stabilizing drugs, further significant suppression of malignant ventricular arrhythmias occurred during both the exercise testing and the 24-hour Holter ECG monitorings. Twenty-seven patients were treated with metoprolol (75-200 mg/day), twenty received propranolol (40-160 mg/day), 6 patients were given atenolol (50-100 mg/day), 2 received pindolol (10-80 mg/day), and only 1 patient was given nadolol (40-80 mg/day). The combination of one of these beta-blocking agents and a membrane-stabilizing drug abolished ventricular tachycardia and ventricular couplets in 83 and 86% of exercise tests, respectively, in patients with these arrhythmias present during therapy with membrane-stabilizing drugs alone. During 24-hour Holter monitoring, the addition of a beta-blocker to a membrane-stabilizing drug resulted in abolition of ventricular tachycardia in 43% of the patients. The frequency of VPCs was reduced by more than 50% in 65% of exercise tests and in 52% of Holter monitoring studies. Since beta-blockers given alone failed to reduce the frequency of ventricular arrhythmia, their efficacy during combination therapy with membrane-stabilizing drugs suggests synergistic drug effects of such a combination (12).

Recently, Brodsky and coworkers described the use of beta-blockers (metoprolol, atenolol, and pindolol) as adjunct therapy in 32 patients with sustained ventricular tachycardia or ventricular fibrillation in the presence of left ventricular dysfunction (28). During a mean follow-up of 668 days, patients treated with beta-blocker combinations had a lower mortality compared to a control group of patients treated with Class I antiarrhythmic agents alone. Although the recurrence rate for arrhythmia was not different in the two groups, the patients receiving beta-blockers had less severe arrhythmias and seemed to better tolerate the arrhythmias. Because of the retrospective nature of this study, the precise significance of these findings is limited, but nonetheless these results suggest that adjunctive therapy with beta-blockers has the potential of improving survival in patients with LV dysfunction and life-threatening ventricular arrhythmias. This concept is further supported by the findings of the Beta-Blocker Heart Attack Trial (BHAT) described in Chapter 6 by Lichstein. The results of BHAT clearly showed the maximum survival benefit of treatment with propranolol in those patients who had mechanical complications. In a recent publication, Chaddha and coworkers described the benefits of treatment with beta-blocker therapy in survivors of acute myocardial infarction who had clinical evidence of congestive heart failure (29). Treatment with propranolol was well tolerated and associated with significant reduction in overall mortality as well as risk of sudden cardiac death in patients with CHF and a recent myocardial infarction. Thus, it seems reasonable to consider that despite the known negative inotropic effects of beta-blocking drugs, when used with caution these agents may be utilized and prove beneficial in the treatment of patients with a history of prior MI, CHF, and ventricular arrhythmias.

In the most recent study by Friehling and coworkers the antiarrhythmic effects of propranolol added to a type I antiarrhythmic agent were prospectively evaluated in 38 patients with sustained ventricular tachycardia and coronary artery disease (30). All patients had history of prior myocardial infarction and inducible ventricular tachycardia. In 23 patients who remained inducible in the electrophysiologic laboratory during therapy with Class I antiarrhythmic agents (procainamide, quinidine, propafenon, or disopyramide), intravenous propranolol was administered. The combination therapy with propranolol reduced the rate of ventricular tachycardia by increasing the effective refractory period of the ventricle. Seven of the 23 patients became noninducible after propranolol and 10 had manifested a >100 millisecond increase in the VT cycle lengths. In the remaining 14 patients, propranolol was the initial test drug, and Class I agent was used only if the electrophysiologic testing after propranolol still rendered inducible ventricular tachycardia. Seven of the 14 patients tested were rendered noninducible, 3 with propranolol alone and 4 others with the combination therapy. In 4 additional patients, the cycle length of VT was prolonged >100 milliseconds. Finally, a total of 17 patients were discharged on either propranolol alone (3 patients) or an effective combination (14 patients). During a mean follow-up of 20 months, 1 patient died suddenly, 2 had recurrence of well-tolerated ventricular tachycardia, and 9 patients remained on therapy. Three patients discontinued therapy due to intolerance, and 2 had noncardiac deaths. The results of this study clearly demonstrate the beneficial effects of combination therapy using beta-blockers and a Class I antiarrhythmic agent in patients with sustained inducible ventricular tachycardia. The beneficial effects demonstrated in the electrophysiologic laboratory also predicted a success in reducing the recurrence of sustained VT and sudden cardiac death during the follow-up period. Although these results need to be confirmed in large scale trials, the results of available clinical studies clearly suggest that when used with careful attention to patients' clinical status, combination therapy with beta-blockers and Class I antiarrhythmic agents is safe and effective in the treatment of patients with ventricular arrhythmias.

Clinical Implication

Many patients with ventricular arrhythmias fail to respond to treatment with a single antiarrhythmic agent. When adequate suppression of ventricular arrhythmia is not achieved with a single agent, combination therapy with two or more agents with different antiarrhythmic actions is usually recommended and often successful in achieving the desired response. The results of recent studies clearly suggest that the combination therapy with beta-blockers and Class I antiarrhythmic agents is highly effective in the management of patients with ventricular arrhythmias refractory to treatment with Class I agents given alone.

REFERENCES

1. Lown B, Graboys TB. Management of patients with malignant ventricular arrhythmia. Am J Cardiol 1977; 39:910-18.
2. Bigger JT, Giardina EGV. Rational use of antiarrhythmic drugs alone and in combination. Cardiovasc Clin 1974; 6:103-17.
3. Ross DL, Sze DY, Keefe DL, Swerdlow CD, Echt DS, Griffin JC, Winkle RA, Mason JW. Antiarrhythmic drug combinations in the treatment of ventricular tachycardia. Circulation 1982; 66:1205-10.
4. Dreifus LS, Morganroth J. Antiarrhythmic agents and their use in therapy. Pharmacol Ther 1980; 9:75-106.
5. Winkle RA, Alderman EL, Fitzgerald JW, Harrison DC. Treatment of recurrent symptomatic ventricular tachycardia. Ann Intern Med 1976; 85:1-7.
6. Coumel P. Multiplicity of arrhythmongenic factors. A plea for combined therapies. Int J Cardiol 1983; 4:477-80.
7. Rosen MR, Wit AL. Electropharmacology of antiarrhythmic drugs. Am Heart J 1983; 106:829-39.
8. Dreifus LS, Lim HF, Yatanabe Y, McKnight E, Frank MN. Propranolol and quinidine in the management of ventricular tachycardia. JAMA 1968; 204: 190-1.
9. Fors WJ, Vanderark CR, Reynolds EW Jr. Evaluation of propranolol and quinidine in the treatment of quinidine resistant arrhythmias. Am J Cardiol 1971; 27:190-4.
10. Leahey EB, Heissenbutal RH, Giardina EG, Bigger JT. Combined mexiletine and propranolol for the treatment of refractory ventricular tachycardia. Br Med J 1980; 281:357-8.
11. Stern H, Scheininger M, Theisen K. Antiarrhythmic therapy with flecainide in combination and comparison with propranolol. Drugs 1985; 29(suppl 4): 77-85.
12. Hirsowitz G, Podrid PJ, Lampert S, Stein J, Lown B. The role of beta blocking agents as adjunct therapy to membrane stabilizing drugs in malignant ventricular arrhythmia. Am Heart J 1986; 111:852-60.
13. Lucchesi BR, Hardman HF. The influence of dichloroisoproterenol (DCI) and related compounds upon oubain and acetylstrophanthidine-induced cardiac arrhythmia. J Pharmacol Exp Ther 1961; 132:372-81.
14. Gibson D, Sowton E. The use of beta-adrenergic blocking drugs in dysrhythmias. Prog Cardiovasc Dis 1969; 12:16-39.
15. Woosley RL, Kornhauser D, Smith R, Reele S, Higgins SB, Nies AS, Shand DG, Oates JA. Suppression of chronic ventricular arrhythmia with propranolol. Circulation 1979; 60:819-27.
16. Nixon JV, Pennington W, Retter W, Shapiro W. Efficacy of propranolol in the control of exercise-induced augmented ventricular ectopic activity. Circulation 1978; 57:115-22.

17. Coumel P, Escoubet B, Attuel P. Beta-blocking therapy in atrial and ventricular tachyarrhythmias: experience with nadolol. Am Heart J 1984; 108: 1098-108.
18. Deedwania P, Morganroth J, Lee I, and Sotalol-Propranolol Research Group. Sotalol vs. propranolol in the treatment of potentially lethal ventricular arrhythmia (abstr). Proceedings of the Tenth World Congress of Cardiology. Washington, DC, September 1986:354.
19. Lichstein E, Morganroth J, Harrist R, Hubble E. Effect of propranolol on ventricular arrhythmia-the Beta Blocker Heart Attack Trial experience. Circulation 1983; 67(suppl 1):5-10.
20. Olsson G, Rehnqvist N. Ventricular arrhythmia during the first year after acute myocardial infarction: influence of long term treatment with propranolol. Circulation 1984; 69:1129-34.
21. Frishman W, Furberg CD, Friedwald WT. Beta-adrenergic blockade for survivors of acute myocardial infarction. N Engl J Med 1984; 310:830-7.
22. Deedwania P, Olukotun A, Kupersmith J, Jenkins P, Golden P. Beta Blockers in combination with Class I antiarrhythmic agents. Am J Cardiol 1987; 60: 21D-26D.
23. Schwartz PJ. The long QT syndrome. In: Julbertus HE, Wellens HJJ, eds. Sudden death. The Hague: Martinus Nijhoff, 1980:358-78.
24. Sung R, Shen E, Morady F, Scheinman M, Hess D, Botvinick E. Clinical and electrophysiologic evaluation of patients with exercise-induced sustained ventricular tachycardia. Am J Cardiol 1983; 51:525-30.
25. Winkle RA, Lopes MG, Goldman DJ, Fitzgerald JW, Schroeder JS, Harrison DC. Propranolol for patients with mitral valve prolapse. Am Heart J 1977; 93:422-7.
26. Nademanee K, Schleman MM, Singh BN, Morganroth J, Reid PR, Stritar JA. Beta-adrenergic blockade by nadolol in control of ventricular tachyarrhythmia. Am Heart J 1984; 108:1109-15.
27. Morganroth J, Duchin KL. Effectiveness of low dose nadolol for ventricular arrhythmia. Am J Cardiol 1986; 58:273-8.
28. Brodsky MA, Allen BJ, Luckett CR, Capparelli EV, Wolff LF, Henry WL. Antiarrhythmic efficacy of solitary beta-adrenergic blockade for patients with sustained ventricular arrhythmias. Am Heart J 1989; 118:272-80.
29. Chaddha K, Goldstein S, Byington R, Curb JD. Effects of propranolol after acute myocardial infarction in patients with heart failure. Circulation 1986; 73:503-10.
30. Friehling T, Lipshutz H, Marinchak R, Stohler J, Kowey P. Effectiveness of propranolol added to a type I antiarrhythmic agent for sustained ventricular tachycardia secondary to coronary artery disease. Am J Cardiol 1990; 65: 1328-33.

12

Comparison of Type IA Anti-Arrhythmics and Beta-Blockers in the Treatment of Ventricular Arrhythmias

P. Anthony Chandraratna
University of Southern California School of Medicine, and Los Angeles County & University of Southern California Medical Center, Los Angeles, California

Satish K. Choudhary and Vijay Bhasin
University of Southern California Medical Center, Los Angeles, California

Ventricular arrhythmias continue to be a major cause of morbidity and mortality in the United States. Not all ventricular arrhythmias are responsible for sudden death. Several studies have shown that complex ventricular arrhythmias such as multiform premature ventricular contractions, closely coupled premature ventricular contractions (R on T phenomenon), and nonsustained ventricular tachycardia do not represent an increased risk of sudden death in asymptomatic persons without cardiac disease (1-3). For asymptomatic patients without evidence of heart disease, reassurance and avoidance of alcohol, caffeine, and tobacco is advisable. Sustained ventricular tachycardia is life threatening and can be induced in 85% of patients who have coronary artery disease and in 60% of those who have idiopathic dilated cardiomyopathy.

Chronic ventricular arrhythmias can be classified into three categories: (1) benign, (2) potentially lethal, and (3) lethal, according to the severity of the arrhythmia, left ventricular function, hemodynamic status, and risks of sudden death (4,5) (Table 1).

The decision to initiate long-term treatment of ventricular arrhythmias has always been difficult because of substantial morbidity produced by

Table 1 Classification of Ventricular Arrhythmias

Arrhythmias	Heart disease	Left ventricular function	Hemodynamic status	Risk of sudden death
Benign: PVCs, couplets, nonsustained ventricular tachycardia	Usually absent	Normal	Stable	Minimal
Potentially lethal: frequent PVCs, nonsustained ventricular tachycardia	Usually present	Abnormal	Stable	Moderate
Lethal: sustained ventricular tachycardia, ventricular fibrillation	Present	Abnormal	Unstable	High

antiarrhythmic agents. The Cardiac Arrhythmia Suppression Trial (CAST), a multicenter, randomized, placebo-controlled study, is underway to determine whether or not suppression of arrhythmias will prevent sudden cardiac death (6). Preliminary data revealed that treatment of frequent premature ventricular complexes or short runs of nonsustained ventricular tachycardia with flecainide and encainide may be more dangerous than no treatment (7). Until the final results of CAST are available, the goals of antiarrhythmic therapy are relief of symptoms and reduction of the risk of sudden death. In general, patients with benign and potentially lethal ventricular arrhythmia need not be treated in the absence of symptoms.

Currently available antiarrhythmic drugs act either on different phases of the action potential or on adrenoreceptors (8,9). Antiarrhythmic drugs that act on various phases of the action potential may exert blocking action on sodium channel (Class I antiarrhythmic agents), on potassium channel (Class III antiarrhythmic agents), or on calcium channel (Class IV antiarrhythmic agents). Drugs that act on adrenoreceptors are beta-blockers (Class II antiarrhythmic agents).

Class I agents represent the largest group of antiarrhythmic agents and depending on their effect on phase 0 of the action potential and on repolarization time are subclassified into type IA, IB, and IC agents.

Quinidine and procainamide have been available for many decades, and in the late 1970s, disopyramide was added to the Class IA agents. Quinidine and procainamide are still the most commonly used antiarrhythmic agents in the United States. With type IA agents there is an increase in action potential duration, effective refractory period, and diastolic threshold potential and a decrease in action potential amplitude, membrane responsiveness, and rate of spontaneous phase IV depolarization. As a result there is a decrease in conduction velocity, excitability, and automaticity (Tables 2, 3).

Beta-blocking agents fall into the Class II category of Vaughn Williams's classification of antiarrhythmic agents. Numerous beta-blockers have been used as antiarrhythmic agents, alone or in combination with other drugs. The various beta-blocking drugs are acebutolol, atenolol, esmolol, metaprolol, nadolol, propranolol, and timolol. With beta-blockade, there is a decrease in automaticity and A-V node conduction, and an increase in A-V nodal refractory period and negative inotropic and chronotropic action. In high doses, there is direct membrane depressant action like Class IA agents (Tables 2, 3).

Once it is decided that a patient needs treatment, several factors need consideration:

Table 2 Electrophysiological Comparison of Type 1A Antiarrhythmics and Beta-Blocking Agents

	Action potential amplitude	Action potential duration	Conduction velocity	Effective refractory period	Phase IV automaticity
Type IA agent:					
Quinidine	Decreased	Increased	Decreased	Increased	Decreased
Procainamide	Decreased	Increased	Decreased	Increased	Decreased
Disopyramide	Decreased	Increased	Decreased	Increased	Decreased
Beta-blocking agents					
Propranolol	No effect or decreased	No effect or decreased	No effect	Decreased	Decreased

Table 3 Effects of Type 1A and Beta-Blocking Antiarrhythmic Agents on Electrocardiographic Intervals

	PR interval	QRS interval	QT interval
Type 1A agents			
Quinidine	No effect, increased, or decreased	Increased	Increased
Procainamide	No effect or increased	Increased	Increased
Disopyramide	No effect	No effect or increased	No effect or increased
Beta-blocking agents			
Propranolol	No effect or increased	No effect	No effect or decreased

1. Half-life of the drug: A knowledge of the half-life of the drug or its metabolites is important in calculating the time needed to reach steady state and thereby adjusting the dosage. Approximately 95% of the steady state is achieved after four half-lives.
2. Evaluation of left ventricular function: In patients with ejection fraction >30% and New York Heart Association class one and two, antiarrhythmic drugs rarely produce new onset or worsening of heart failure, whereas in patients with ejection fraction <30% and New York Heart Association class three and four, antiarrhythmic agents can worsen left ventricular function, and certain drugs, especially disopyramide and beta-blockers, should be avoided (10).
3. Side effects of drugs: Proarrhythmia and noncardiac adverse effects are common with Class 1A agents compared to beta-blocking agents (11,12). Manifestations of proarrythmia are: (a) appearance of new ventricular tachycardia or fibrillation which is unrelated to precipitating factors and which is not previously documented, (b) development of Torsade de pointes (the drug should be stopped if corrected QT interval increases by 25%), (c) change in the pattern of ventricular tachycardia (nonsustained to sustained pattern), and (d) marked increase in the frequency of ventricular tachycardia or occurence of premature ventricular complexes.
4. Drugs during pregnancy: The chronic use of propranolol can produce fetal growth retardation. There are no adverse fetal effects

reported with quinidine although it crosses the placenta. Procainamide should be limited in those who do not tolerate or are unresponsive to quinidine because chronic use may produce a lupuslike syndrome. Disopyramide crosses the placenta, however, its safety in pregnancy is unknown.

5. Plasma binding of drugs: Fluctuation of plasma binding of drugs after cardiac surgery should be considered while monitoring the serum level. Therapy with both 1A and beta-blocking agents is often necessary after cardiac surgery. During the first 5 days postoperatively, there is marked fluctuation in the plasma concentration of total protein, albumin, and alpha acid glycoprotein. Thus there are significant changes in plasma binding of drugs (13).

COMPARISON OF BETA-BLOCKERS AND CLASS 1A AGENTS

The comparison of beta-blockers and type 1A agents was done in controlling chronic ventricular arrhythmias in three multicenter arrhythmia trials (14). Acebutolol was compared to placebo, propranolol and quinidine for the suppression of chronic ventricular arrythmia in three double-blind randomized crossover studies. In all three studies, acebutolol significantly reduced mean total and complex premature ventricular contractions. In all measurements, acebutolol was superior to placebo and comparable to propranolol and quinidine. Acebutolol was better tolerated than quinidine.

In this study patients were selected between 21 and 70 years of age who had organic heart disease and/or ventricular arrhythmias, but with adequate cardiac function (New York Heart Association class I and II). Patients were excluded in the presence of type 1 diabetes mellitus, impaired hepatic and renal function, ophthalmic disorders, increased ANA titers, history of spontaneous or drug induced lupus, women of childbearing age, patients requiring antiarrhythmic agents, sedatives, hypnotics and sympathomimetics, history of hypoglycemic attacks, recent myocardial infarction of less than 14 days, and cardiac surgery less than 6 months.

The studies were double-blind during all treatment periods, and patients were randomly assigned to treatment. During the initial 2-week placebo period, three 24-hour Holter recordings, physical examinations, 12 lead electrocardiograms with rhythm strips were obtained. Eligible patients were then randomly assigned to either acebutolol 200 mg three times a day, or placebo for two weeks. Each group was crossed over three times during the study, separated by a one-week weaning period, and received treatment at two different doses of acebutolol (200 mg three times a day and 400 mg three times a day). Patients were evaluated at the conclusion of each treatment interval. At the end of 14 weeks there was an additional 2-week placebo control period in which two 24-hour Holter recordings were made.

In the comparison with propranolol, the initial 2-week baseline period was identical to that of the placebo study. Patients were then randomly assigned to receive either acebutolol 200 mg three times a day or propranolol 30 mg three times a day. Doses of both drugs were increased incrementally at 3-day intervals until the resting heart rate was less than 60 beats per minute or maximum doses of acebutolol 1800 mg per day, or propranolol 240 mg per day were reached. At the end of a one-week dose titration period, patients had physical examination, 12 lead electrocardiogram with rhythm strip, and 24-hour Holter monitoring. If bradycardia (heart rate less than 55 per minute) or hypotension (systolic pressure less than 105 mm of mercury) developed, dose levels were not increased. Patients were maintained for 4-6 weeks at the optimum doses, after which complete physical examination and laboratory studies were done. After the maintenance phase the patients were weaned from the drugs for one week and then entered a single-blind one-week drug-free phase. Patients were then crossed over to the alternate medication and underwent dose titration, maintenance, and weaning phases.

The design of the quinidine comparison was similar to that used in the other studies. Patients received either acebutolol capsules 300 mg three times a day or quinidine 300 mg three times a day, for 4 weeks. At the end of 4 weeks patients were weaned from medication over one week and entered a one-week drug-free period. Patients were then crossed over to the alternate medication for 4 weeks.

In all three studies, medication compliance was determined by counts of returned medication. Efficacy was assessed on the basis of 24-hour Holter recording with quantification of following data: mean total PVCs per hour, mean paired PVCs per hour, mean ventricular tachycardia beats per minute, multiform beats, R on T beats, and mean hourly heart rate.

COMPARISON OF ACEBUTOLOL WITH PLACEBO

Ninety-seven patients were randomly assigned to receive either acebutolol or placebo. Eighty-four patients completed all visits. Among 13 noncompleting patients, 5 patients were withdrawn for administrative reasons during the initial placebo phase, 1 patient died of myocardial infarction while taking placebo, 3 patients on acebutolol and 1 patient on placebo experienced side effects, 1 patient on placebo developed ventricular tachycardia, and 2 patients on acebutolol had worsening of arrhythmias. Of the 84 patients, 6 patients were excluded because of noncompliance, and efficacy was analyzed in 78 patients (Tables 4, 5).

The most common side effects reported by patients were fatigue and nausea. Three patients did not complete the study because of side effects. One patient died of acute myocardial infarction after being weaned from the 600-mg dose of acebutolol.

COMPARISON OF ACEBUTOLOL WITH PROPRANOLOL

Ninety-four patients were randomly assigned to either acetabutolol or propranolol. Seventy-one patients completed all visits. Among 23 noncompleting patients, 5 patients on acebutolol and 6 patients on propranolol were withdrawn because of side effects, 7 acetubolol and 3 propranolol-treated patients were withdrawn for administrative reasons, and 1 acebutolol-treated patient died of myocardial infarction. Of the 71 patients, 29 patients were excluded from analysis (22 for administrative reason and 7 for incomplete Holter monitoring data) (Table 6).

Table 4 Patient Demographics from Three Studies of Acebutolol in Ventricular Arrhythmia

	ABL vs. PLC	ABL vs. PPL	ABL vs. QUI
No. of patients	78	42	20
Sex			
Male	67	35	20
Female	11	7	0
Age (yr)			
Mean	56.2	59.4	55.1
Range	23-77	23-79	44-67
Weight (lb)			
Mean	177.8	167	NA
Range	117-229	124-195	NA

ABL = acebutolol; NA = not available; PLC = placebo; PPL = propranolol; QUI = quinidine.
Source: Ref. 14 with permission.

Table 5 Summary of Efficacy Results: Acebutolol vs. Placebo in Ventricular Arrhythmia

Holter measurement	Baseline (n = 78)	Acebutolol (TDD) 600 mg (n = 73)	Acebutolol (TDD) 1200 mg (n = 75)[a]	Placebo[b] (n = 78)
Mean total PVCs/hr	184.0 ± 24.9	76.6 ± 16.4	36.5 ± 8.8	111.6 ± 23
Mean paired PVCs/hr	28.5 ± 14.1	9.9 ± 7.2	6.6 ± 4.9	25.1 ± 11.6
Mean VT beats/hr	3.2 ± 2.1	1.6 ± 1.5	0.5 ± 0.4	3.0 ± 2.0
Multiform beats (% of hours noted)	61.8 ± 4.3	46.6 ± 4.8	38.1 ± 4.6	54.9 ± 42
R-on T beats (% of hours noted)	2.7 ± 1.3	0.6 ± 0.3	0.3 ± 0.1	2.7 ± 1.1
% Below baseline minimum total PVC[c]	—	63.0 ± 5.7	76.0 ± 5.0	43.0 ± 4.7
Mean hourly heart rate (bpm)	76.7 ± 0.9	67.3 ± 1.0	66.0 ± 0.9	76.8 ± 0.8

TDD = total daily dose.
[a]A complete set of adequate Holter data not available for all patients.
[b]Both placebo periods combined.
[c]Statistical probability of any one of four values to be the lowest is 25%. The actually observed percentages were therefore listed against 25%.
Source: Ref. 14 with permission.

The most common side effects reported for both drugs were fatigue, dizziness, dyspnea, and headache. One died shortly after being weaned from propranolol at the conclusion of the study. Asymptomatic ANA titers of 1:20 to 1:128 developed in 12 patients (8 on acebutolol and 4 on propranolol).

COMPARISON OF ACEBUTOLOL WITH QUINIDINE

Twenty-six patients were randomly assigned to receive either acebutolol or quinidine. Twenty patients completed the study and were analyzed for

Table 6 Summary of Efficacy Results: Acebutolol vs. Propranolol in Ventricular Arrhythmia

Parameters	Baseline	Acebutolol DT	Acebutolol M	Propranolol DT	Propranolol M	Drug-free
Mean total PVCs/hr	236.5 ± 44.5	63.6 ± 17.2	82.3 ± 22.3	115.3 ± 31.1	140.3 ± 40.3	222.6 ±41.0
Minimum PVCs/hr	33.8 ± 9.1	8.1 ± 2.5	11.6 ± 3.6	20.1 ± 6.2	27.8 ± 9.2	36.4 ± 10.8
Maximum PVCs/hr	677.5 ± 93.8	289.1 ± 61.9	299.0 ± 65.9	410.3 ± 84.6	375.0 ± 82.0	629.3 ± 80.5
Mean paired PVC/hr	15.6 ± 4.6	4.3 ± 1.3	5.3 ± 2.7	6.3 ± 2.1	8.8 ± 3.6	8.5 ± 2.6
Mean VT beats/hr	1.0 ± 0.3	0.3 ± 0.2	0.1 ± 0.0	0.3 ± 0.1	0.2 ± 0.1	1.3 ± 0.6
Multiform beats (%)[a]	65.3 ± 6.2	49.4 ± 6.1	56.3 ± 6.0	60.5 ± 6.2	61.4 ± 5.9	66.0 ± 6.2
R-on T beats (%)[a]	1.7 ± 0.9	1.2 ± 1.2	0.4 ± 0.3	0.1 ± 0.1	0.2 ± 0.1	0.1 ± 0.1
% Below baseline minimum total PVCs[b]	0.0 ± 0.0	73.8 ± 6.9	73.8 ± 6.9	54.8 ± 7.8	59.5 ± 7.8	38.1 ± 7.6
Mean hourly heart rate	77.3 ± 1.4	64.1 ± 1.1	66.7 ± 1.3	63.6 ± 1.2	63.6 ± 1.2	78.6 ± 1.7

N = 42; mean ± SEM.
DT = dose titration; M = maintenance.
[a]%Hours noted.
[b]Twenty-five percent of observations are generally expected to be less than the minimum of three preceding observations.
Source: Ref. 14 with permission.

efficacy. Five patients were withdrawn for administrative reason and one patient was not analyzed for efficacy (Table 7).

The side effects were transient and mild. One patient on quinidine was withdrawn because of palpitations. Mild diarrhea developed in three patients on quinidine. Nausea developed in one patient on acebutolol.

On comparison of acebutolol with placebo, mean total PVCs per hour were significantly reduced from baseline for both doses of acebutolol ($p < 0.002$). Mean total PVCs per hour returned to baseline values during the second control period. Compared to both baseline and placebo, acebutolol significantly reduced mean PVCs per hour ($p < 0.001$), paired PVCs per hour ($p < 0.001$), and multiform beats per hour ($p < 0.02$) at both 600 and 1200 mg doses. No statistical differences between the effects of the high and low doses were noted.

On comparison of acetubolol with propranolol, acebutolol significantly reduced mean total PVCs in comparison with baseline PVCs during both dose titration and maintenance (both $p < 0.001$), as did propranolol ($p < 0.01$ and $p < 0.05$, respectively). The reduction in total PVCs induced by acebutolol was significantly ($p < 0.05$) greater than that seen with propranolol during both phases of study.

On comparison of acebutolol with quinidine, both drugs significantly reduced mean hourly PVCs compared to baseline, both at rest (acebutolol, $p < 0.002$, quinidine $p < 0.001$) and during exercise ($p < 0.001$ for both drugs). No significant differences were noted between acebutolol and quinidine.

Table 7 Summary of Efficacy Results: Acebutolol vs. Quinidine in Ventricular Arrhythmias

	Baseline[a]	Acebutolol[a]	Quinidine[a]	Drug-free
Heart rate (bpm)				
Resting	83.1 ± 2.7	65.0 ± 1.7	82.4 ± 2.9	81.1 ± 3.1
Peak	110.9 ± 4.0	93.3 ± 2.9	111.6 ± 3.7	111.3 ± 3.7
PVCs (rate/hr)				
At rest (Holter)	223.6 ± 48.4	97.8 ± 37.5	137.5 ± 49.3	145.1 ± 42.7
During exercise[b]	501 ± 73.8	158 ± 52.2	262.2 ± 75	305.4 ± 70.2
Higher-grade PVCs				
At rest (PVCs/hr)	2.43 ± 0.55	1.14 ± 0.47	0.87 ± 0.21	1.96 ± 0.65

Mean ± SEM.
[a]Based on average of two visits.
[b]Computed as rate per hour.
Source: Ref. 14 with permission.

The data showed that acebutolol was as effective as propranolol and quinidine in suppressing both total and complex PVCs and was superior to placebo. Acebutolol was better tolerated than quinidine. There was a lesser decrease in mean resting heart rate with acebutolol, thus reducing the risk of symptomatic bradycardia. The results clearly showed the efficacy of acebutolol in suppressing ventricular arrhythmia.

REFERENCES

1. Crow R, Prineas R, Blackburn H. The prognostic significance of ventricular ectopic beats among the apparently healthy. Am Heart Journal 1981; 101: 244-8.
2. Elkin KB, Swedlow TA, Myburgh DP. Persistent ventricular ectopic beats: a long term study. S. Afr Med J 1977; 52:564-6.
3. Kennedy HL, Whitlock JA, Sprague MK, et al. Long term follow-up of asymptomatic healthy subjects with frequent and complex ventricular ectopy. N Engl J Med 1985; 312:193-7.
4. Morganroth J. Pre mature ventricular complexes. JAMA 1984; 252:673-6.
5. Bigger JT Jr. Definition of benign versus malignant ventricular arrhythmias: targets for treatment. Am J Cardiol 1983; 52(6):47-54C.
6. The Cardiac Arrhythmia Pilot Study (CAPS) Investigators. The effects of encainide, flecainide, imipramine, and moricizine on ventricular arrhythmias occurring 6 to 60 days after myocardial infarction: results of a randomized, double-blind, multi-center trial. Am J Cardiol 1988; Apr.
7. Cardiac Arrhythmia Suppression Trial. Preliminary Report. Effect of encainide and flecainide on mortality in a randomized trial of arrhythmia suppression after myocardial infarction. N Engl J Med 1989; 321:406-12.
8. Vaughn Williams EM. A classification of antiarrhythmic actions reassessed after a decade of new drugs. J Clin Pharmacol 1984; 24:129.
9. Harrison DC. Antiarrhythmic drug classification: new science and practice application. Am J Cardiol 1985; 56:185.
10. Podrid PJ et al. N Engl J Med 1980; 302:614.
11. Bhandari AK, Rahimtoola SH. Proarrhythmic effects of antiarrhythmic agents. Cl. 6 arrhythmias and conduction disturbances, 1987; 4(9):49-59.
12. Podrid PJ. Am J Card 1987; 59:38E.
13. Davis RF, Dube LM, et al. Perioperative variability of binding of lidocaine, quinidine, and propranolol after cardiac operations. J Thorac Cardiovascular Surg 1988; 96:634-41.
14. Chandraratna PAN. Comparison of acebutolol with propranolol, quinidine, and placebo: results of three multicenter arrhythmia trials. American Heart Journal 1985; 109(5):1198-204.

13

Sotalol: A Unique Beta-Blocker with Class III Antiarrhythmic Properties

Prakash C. Deedwania
University of California at San Francisco School of Medicine, San Francisco, and Veterans Affairs Medical Center, Fresno, California

Bramah N. Singh
Veterans Affairs Medical Center of West Los Angeles, and University of California at Los Angeles School of Medicine, Los Angeles, California

INTRODUCTION

Although sotalol was introduced in 1965 as a specific beta-adrenergic blocking agent (1), it has been somewhat slow in getting recognition as a therapeutic agent in cardiovascular disorders. It is now known that the drug is devoid of membrane-stabilizing or local anesthetic properties, intrinsic sympathomimetic actions, or cardioselectivity (2,3). Although Singh and Vaughan Williams (4) and Singh and Hauswirth (5) drew attention to the drug's unique electrophysiological properties over a decade ago, it is only in the last few years that the broad-spectrum antiarrhythmic properties of the compound have become increasingly recognized (6-9). Sotalol is now regarded as an important Class III antiarrhythmic agent in addition to being a specific beta-adrenoceptor blocking agent with a role in the treatment of hypertension, ischemic myocardial syndromes, and other disorders in which beta-blockade is beneficial. The major focus of this review is the role of the drug in cardiac arrhythmias.

PHARMACODYNAMIC PROPERTIES

Two distinct properties of sotalol are the major determinants of its net pharmacodynamic and therapeutic effects. The first is the well-known property of the agent to competitively antagonize beta-adrenoceptors; the second, its propensity, unlike other beta-antagonists, to selectively lengthen the action potential duration in all cardiac tissues.

BETA-ADRENOCEPTOR BLOCKING PROPERTIES

Sotalol is *d,l*-4-(2-isopropylamino-1-hydroxyethyl) methane sulfonanilide-HCl (Fig. 1). Unlike other *para*-substituted beta-blockers, sotalol is not cardioselective nor does it exhibit intrinsic sympathomimetic activity or local anesthetic actions (10). However, numerous in vitro and in vivo studies have clearly established its beta-blocking propensity (1,10-15).

ELECTROPHYSIOLOGICAL BASIS FOR ANTIARRHYTHMIC ACTIONS

Between 1940 and 1962, the only major antiarrhythmic compounds available were quinidine, lidocaine, procainamide, and disopyramide. These compounds are essentially local anesthetic drugs with variable effects on cardiac repolarization. It was therefore of particular interest when it was found that the beta-blocking drug sotalol (MJ1999) had the additional property of lengthening the cardiac action potential (Fig. 2) and prolonging the QT_c interval of the surface electrocardiogram (4,15,16). The drug also protected experimental animals from ventricular fibrillation due to cardiac glycoside intoxication (4,16). The overall effects of the drug could not be explained on the basis of beta blockade alone nor by the inhibition of the fast-sodium channel since, unlike quinidine or procainamide, sotalol produced no significant changes in depolarization

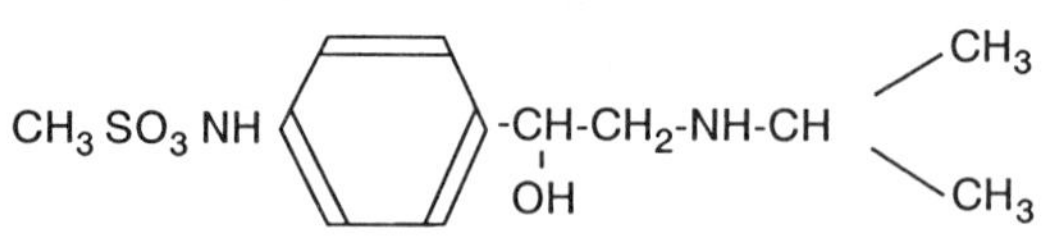

Figure 1 Chemical structure of sotalol.

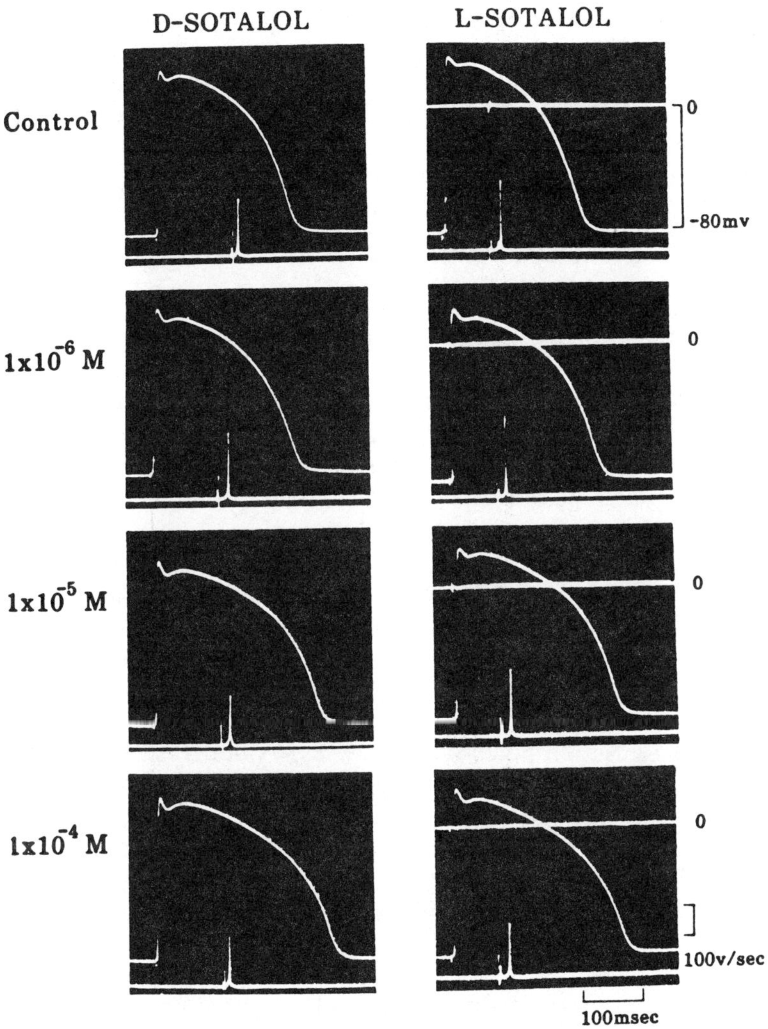

Figure 2 Effects of increasing *d*- (left) and *l*-sotalol (right) concentrations on the action potential in canine ventricular muscle. Note the concentration-related increases in the action potential duration at 50% repolarization time but no reduction in the maximal rate of rise of the action potential with each drug. Voltage and time calibrations are the same for each panel. The time course of the action potentials has been displayed at two sweep velocities. (Reproduced with permission from Ref. 19 and the *American College of Cardiology*.)

(4,16). Thus, it was believed that sotalol exhibited unique electrophysiological properties. It was postulated that the simple lengthening of the action potential duration constituted a significant and discrete mechanism (the so-called Class III action) for the control of cardiac arrhythmias (4, 16). Recent experimental and clinical observations have tended to vindicate the postulated theoretical expectations.

ELECTROPHYSIOLOGICAL EFFECTS IN ISOLATED CARDIAC TISSUES

It is becoming increasingly evident that sotalol is not simply "another beta-blocker." The initial electrophysiological studies, reported by Singh and Vaughan Williams (4) and Strauss et al. (15), indicated that in all cardiac tissues the drug increased the duration of the action potential in a concentration-dependent fashion with a concomitant lengthening of the effective and the absolute refractory period. There was no change in the upstroke velocity of phase 0 of the action potential except when concentrations were 10^{-4}M or greater. The property of lengthening the cardiac action potential exhibited by sotalol cannot be attributed to its actions as a beta-blocker. Although some lengthening of the myocardial action potential duration has been reported in rabbits and in man chronically treated with a number of beta-blockers (17,18), the magnitude of these changes has been trivial compared to those found with sotalol. Therefore, the prolongation of the action potential induced by sotalol is unlikely to be due to beta-blockade. This is now supported by the recent observations that the *d* isomer of the drug (devoid of beta-blocking property) exerts an identical effect (see Fig. 2) on repolarization as does the *l*-sotalol (19).

The fact that the *l* isomer and the *d* isomer (having 1/50 the beta-blocking potency of *l*-sotalol) exerted identical electrophysiologic effects on cardiac muscle clearly established that the observed lengthening of the action potential induced by sotalol was not mediated through an antiadrenergic effect (19,20). For example, at a concentration (10^{-5} M) at which *d*-sotalol had negligible beta-blocking activity, there were no statistically significant differences between the effects of *d*- and *l*-sotalol on the action potential duration at 90% repolarization time either in Purkinje fibers (15% vs. 19%) or in ventricular muscle (14% vs. 20%). Similarly, at this drug concentration, the changes in the effective refractory period in the Purkinje fibers (16% vs. 19%) and in ventricular muscle (14% vs. 21%) did not differ significantly. The effects in the atria were similar. Differences between the actions of propranolol (the reference beta-blocker) and sotalol should be emphasized. For example, Nakaya et al. (3) examined the effects of propranolol (0.3-30 μM) and sotalol (3-300 μM) in canine Purkinje fibers and ventricular muscle fibers using the standard microelectrode techniques. Propranolol shortened the action potential duration in Purkinje fibers but had little or no effect in ventricular muscle; in contrast, sotalol produced a concentration-dependent increase in the action potential duration in both tissues. Furthermore, propranolol decreased the maximal rate of rise of the action potential whereas sotalol had no effect on this parameter except at very high concentrations of the drug emphasizing the relative selectivity of the compound for altering repolarization rather than depolarization in cardiac muscle. The data are concordant with the observations of Shimatori et al. (21), who examined the effects of five different beta-blockers (including sotalol) on sino-atrial conduction time in isolated blood-perfused canine atria.

At concentrations equal to or below 10^{-4}, Carmeliet (20) found that the main electrophysiological effects of sotalol and its isomers were to prolong the action potential duration. At higher concentrations, there was shortening of the action potential duration and a significant reduction in V_{max} due to the inhibition of the tetrodotoxin-sensitive inward sodium current. The voltage clamp studies of Carmeliet (20) have indicated that the lengthening of the action potential duration by sotalol may be due to a substantial reduction in the plateau outward K current in association with a small decrease in the background current. These electro physiological effects raise two theoretical possibilities. First, the lengthening of repolarization will delay the inactivation of the slow-calcium channel, which will tend to augment myocardial contractility. This is consonant with the findings of Kaumann and Olsson (22) and Singh (16), who have reported a positive inotropic effect due to sotalol in the cat papillary muscle in association with markedly lengthened action potential duration. In the case of the dextro-isomer of sotalol, such an effect is likely to be more pronounced since it will not be attenuated by associated beta-receptor blockade. Second, the inhibition of the outward K currents by sotalol and its isomers will lengthen the refractory period. Both isomers of sotalol are thus likely to exert antiarrhythmic actions.

Potential Antiarrhythmic Correlates of the Electrophysiological Effects of *d*- and *l*-Sotalol

Numerous experimental (4,16,23-28) reports have documented a broad range of antiarrhythmic effects in the case of *d,l*-sotalol. Indeed, the spectrum of effects of the compound in arrhythmias is wider than that of conventional beta-blockers (4). For example, unlike conventional beta-blocking drugs, *d,l*-sotalol has been found to be effective in lenghtening the anterograde effective refractory period of the bypass tracts in the WPW syndrome (34,35) and to prevent the reinduction of ventricular tachycardia in experimental animals (28) and in man (6,7). These observations suggest that the additional antiarrhythmic actions of *d,l*-sotalol as compared to those of other beta-blockers may be due to its propensity to lengthen repolarization and refractoriness in cardiac muscle. Although our data have clearly shown that the *d* isomer is equipotent with the *l* isomer and with the racemic compound in prolonging the effective refractory period, the data dealing with the antiarrhythmic actions of *d*-sotalol are limited. However, Lynch et al. (25) recently found that 8 mg/kg intravenous cumulative doses of the l as well as the *d* isomer suppressed the induction of ventricular tachycardia in their conscious-dog ischemic model of sudden death in 50% of the animals. At this dose, only the l-sotalol exerted an antiadrenergic effect such as lengthening of the PR interval of the surface ECG, but both isomers produced equivalent increases of 15-20% in the ventricular effective refractory period. Our in vitro electrophysiological data on the effects of the two isomers on the refractory period of cardiac muscle are in accord with these in vivo experimental findings and with the preliminary clinical experience with intravenously administered *d*-sotalol in man (36).

Clinical Electrophysiological Effects

The clinical effects of sotalol are in accord with those found in isolated tissues and in intact animals. Electrophysiological studies using the intravenous drug have established that sotalol lengthens the monophasic action potential in atria and ventricles in man (18,37,38) and increases the effective refractory period in atria, ventricle, AV node, bypass tracts while lengthening the intranodal but not the infranodal conduction time (6,8, 34,35,39). These properties differ from those of conventional beta-blockers, which have little or no effect on atrial, ventricular, and bypass tract effective refractory period (40). The studies of Nademanee et al. (8) are concordant in this regard. Intravenous sotalol lengthened the ERP in atrial (+24.6%; $p < 0.01$), AV node (+24.9%; $p < 0.01$), and ventricle (+14.9%; $p < 0.01$); it significantly lengthened sinus node recovery time, QT_c, and AH but not the HV interval. Very similar data have been reported by Touboul et al. (39), overall effects being accountable in terms of a summated effects of beta-blockade and those due to the lengthening of the action potential duration without a change in depolarization.

These overall findings thus represent a combination of beta-blocking (Class II) and Class III antiarrhythmic actions, a combination that is likely to confer on the drug a broad spectrum of antiarrhythmic effects and a side effect profile which is essentially predictable on the basis of these two fundamental actions. Although the complete spectrum of the antiarrhythmic actions of sotalol has not been completely delineated (6, 7,29-32,41), the available data allow certain general conclusions regarding the drug's overall clinical utility. These will be delineated later in this chapter.

INOTROPIC AND HEMODYNAMIC EFFECTS

The hemodynamic effects of sotalol and its dose response relationships in patients with varying levels of ventricular functions have not been fully evaluated. The net hemodynamic effects of sotalol are likely to be due to a balance between the depressant actions of the drug due to the blockade of beta receptors and those tending to increase contractility by prolonging the time course of calcium influx due to the prolongation of the action potential duration (42). It appears that lengthening of the action potential duration induced by the drug may augment contractility, a phenomenon that has been demonstrated in isolated cardiac muscle (16,22); such an effect may, in part, offset the depressant effect of beta blockade in a patient with cardiac decompensation. This feature distinguishes sotalol from conventional beta-blocking drugs, and the available clinical data are in agreement with these postulates (43). For example, it has been reported by Brooks et al. (44) that the intravenous drug, unlike other beta-blockers, exerts little or no depressant effect on systemic hemodynamics in patients with heart failure. However, it is known that cardiac failure may be exacerbated in a small number of patients given *d,l*-sotalol. The absence of beta-blocking activity in the *d* isomer would obviate this possibility.

PHARMACOKINETICS OF SOTALOL

The pharmacokinetics of sotalol have been extensively studied in experimental animals and in man. Sotalol concentrations in biological fluids can be measured accurately by high-performance liquid chromatography (45-47). Pharmacokinetically, sotalol conforms to an open linear two-compartment model (48) in which all processes of drug absorption, distribution, and elimination occur by first-order kinetics.

Absorption and Plasma Concentrations

Absorption of sotalol in man is slower than that found for most other beta-blockers (49-51). The time to maximum plasma concentrations following a single dose of 80 mg of sotalol is usually 2-3 hours, whereas values of about 1.5 hours have been found for many other beta-antagonists. After 160-mg single oral doses, peak plasma sotalol concentrations were between 1.4 and 1.7 mg/liter at 2 to 3 hours after administration (52).

The absolute bioavailability of sotalol on oral administration approaches 100%, indicating negligible first-pass effect in the liver. The absorption of sotalol is not significantly affected by antacids (53), but it may be reduced by food (54), especially milk and milk products, which reduce the bioavailability of the drug; it is possible that an interaction with calcium ions may be the major reason for the decreased drug absorption.

Distribution

After single oral doses of sotalol the total apparent volume of distribution was 1.5 times the body weight (52). Protein binding of the drug appears to be negligible (51).

The partition coefficient in octanolol/water determines the lipophilic versus hydrophilic properties of various beta-blockers (55). In anesthetized cats Arendt et al. (56) reported that propranolol had the highest rate of penetration into the cerebrospinal fluid (CSF) with the highest brain:plasma ratio (38.0). In contrast, sotalol, the most hydrophilic drug in the series that was studied, had the slowest CSF entry and the lowest brain:plasma ratio (0.52). Similar findings in human volunteers have shown that after single oral doses of sotalol, the CSF concentrations were only 10% of those in the plasma (51). In a study comparing sotalol and atenolol, the distributions coefficients were similar, but that for atenolol was somewhat lower (57). Ochs et al. (58) studied single-dose kinetics of oral propranolol, metoprolol, atenolol, and sotalol in relation to the lipophilic properties of these beta-antagonists. In vitro lipid solubility of the compounds was highly correlated with their plasma clearance.

Metabolism and Elimination

Plasma clearance of sotalol, unlike that of propranolol, is not dependent on liver enzyme-metabolizing capacity (59), but it may be reduced by drinking alcohol (60). No active metabolites of the drug have been identified (61-63), and urinary excretion occurs by glomerular filtration, with about 75% of the drug being excreted in the urine within 72 hours after single-dose administration (52). After 400-mg single oral dose of sotalol, or following daily doses of 400 mg for 8 days, McDevitt and Shanks (64) found an elimination half-life of 15.5 ± 1.2 and 17.7 ± 2.6 hours, respectively, along with similar plasma concentration curves. Thus, medium-term therapy with the drug did not alter its kinetics.

At present there are no data on the pharmacokinetics of *d*-sotalol in man, although the kinetics of the individual isomers have been studied in dogs (19).

EFFECTS OF AGE AND PREGNANCY ON PHARMACOKINETICS

Ishizaki and Tawara (65) compared the pharmacokinetics and pharmacodynamics of sotalol in young versus elderly subsets of hypertensive patients. In elderly patients the elimination half-life of the drug was prolonged (11 vs. 7 hr, approximately), total plasma clearance was reduced (primarily due to reduced renal clearance; 1.93 vs. 4.10 ml/min/kg), and volume of distribution was decreased. Increased serum concentrations of the drug in elderly patients were attributed both to total reduced plasma clearance and the decreased volume of distribution. There was no evidence of impaired absorption of the drug. There was a significant correlation between the plasma drug concentrations and the reduction in the absolute values of exercise-induced increments in heart rate; however, the pharmacodynamic effects of sotalol outlasted its serum half-life.

Beta-blockers are used widely in the control of hypertension during pregnancy (67). O'Hare et al. (67) have shown that sotalol rapidly crosses the human placenta. The same group later found that the elimination half-life and bioavailability of sotalol were not affected by pregnancy (68). Erkola et al. (69) found sotalol concentrations in the maternal circulation twice that in the umbilical cord. It appears that the more rapid clearance noted during pregnancy may be due to increases in renal plasma flow and glomerular filtration (68).

EFFECTS OF RENAL INSUFFICIENCY ON PHARMACOKINETICS

Since sotalol is not metabolized in the liver, its pharmacokinetics are not affected by impaired hepatic function. However, since it is excreted largely by the renal route, the serum concentrations of the drug for any given dose vary linearly with the creatinine clearance (50,70-74). Berglund et al. (70) studied sotalol kinetics in normal subjects and in those with impaired renal function. In subjects with creatinine clearance ⩾39 ml/min/m^2, mean sotalol plasma clearance was 71 ml/min/m^2, elimination half-life was 8.1 hours, and patients had a renal clearance of sotalol of 46 ml/min/m^2. In patients with creatinine clearance of 8 to 38 ml/min/m^2, the sotalol elimination half-life was 24.2 hours, with a plasma clearance of the drug of 24 ml/min/m^2. In patients requiring dialysis, the elimination half-life was even greater (33.9 hr); however, during dialysis, the elimination half-life was 5.8 hours and was associated with a reduction of 56.7 ± 21% in plasma concentrations.

These data suggest that in patients with moderately reduced renal function, the initial dose of sotalol should be 160 mg/day, and subsequent dose adjustment should be made in light of the clinical response and plasma drug concentrations. In cases with severely diminished renal function, the drug should be avoided or used with a great deal of caution with regular monitoring of serum drug concentrations. In cases of overdosage or excessively high serum drug concentrations, the studies of Blair et al. (71) indicate that hemodialysis may rapidly reverse the effects by reducing the serum drug concentrations.

PHARMACOKINETIC AND PHARMACODYNAMIC CORRELATIONS

Harron et al. (75) determined the effects of varying doses of sotalol on exercise-induced tachycardia as a function of plasma concentration. The maximum effect occurred at 2 or 3 hours and was greater with each increasing dose, although the effect of 50 mg of the drug was negligible. The effects of 400 mg were significantly greater than that of 200 mg. All 4 doses (50, 100, 200, 400 mg) reduced exercise-induced changes in heart rate at 24 hours. The data indicated that the effects of sotalol in blocking beta-receptors occurred as a function of drug dose and plasma concentration, as well as that of the elimiantion half-life.

DOSAGE AND ADMINISTRATION

Sotalol is available as an intravenous as well as oral formulation. In the treatment of supraventricular and ventricular arrhythmias, doses of the drug between 0.2 and 1.5 mg/kg i.v. have been used in patients with normal as well as depressed ejection fraction without problems. As in the case of all intravenous beta-blockers, slow administration is recommended, and for high-risk patients such as those with acute myocardial infarction, careful monitoring of hemodynamic or electrocardiographic changes is recommended.

The lowest minimum clinically effective dosage for orally administered sotalol in arrhythmia treatment is likely to be either 160 mg once daily or 80 mg twice daily, taken before food. Available evidence suggests that 160 mg once daily is probably the appropriate minimum antiarrhythmic dosage, particularly for supraventricular arrhythmias. Although this dosage may be increased every 3 or 4 days to a maximum of 480 mg daily, the efficacy and safety of daily doses higher than this has not been critically evaluated. Furthermore, doses higher than 640 mg daily should be used in conjunction with careful monitoring of the electrocardiographic changes, serum drug concentrations and to the possibility of concomitant hypokalemia (particularly when diuretics are used concomitantly). In the treatment of hypertension and angina pectoris, sotalol should initially be given as either 80 mg twice daily or 160 mg once daily. Should dosage titration be necessary after an adequate trial of the drug (7-10 days), the dose of sotalol may be increased by 40-160 mg; further increments may thereafter be given, if necessary, at intervals of 2 or more weeks.

SOTALOL IN CARDIAC ARRHYTHMIAS

Sotalol is a novel antiarrhythmic agent exhibiting unique electrophysiological properties. The first property is the ability to competitively antagonize beta adrenoceptors and the second is its propensity to selectively lengthen the action potential duration in all cardiac tissue. The effect of sotalol on cardiac action potential and refractoriness are independent of its beta-blocking actions. These unique electrophysiological properties make sotalol a highly suitable antiarrhythmic agent for the treatment of patients with a variety of supraventricular and ventricular tachyarrhythmias.

USE IN SUPRAVENTRICULAR ARRHYTHMIAS

Since sotalol is a beta-blocker, it is likely to be as effective as conventional beta-blockers in suppressing atrial extrasystoles and other ectopic atrial tachycardias, in slowing sinus tachycardia and the ventricular response in atrial flutter and fibrillation, in terminating reentrant supraventricular tachycardia, and in controlling the recurrence of a proportion of such arrhythmias during prophylactic drug administration. It remains to be demonstrated whether the associated property of lengthening action potential duration will make the compound more suitable in this regard compared with conventional beta-blockers. The experience of Teo et al. (76), showing a 100% response demonstrated as conversion of PSVT with intravenous bolus administration of sotalol, indeed suggests that this might be the case. Although the results of this study do not necessarily demonstrate the importance of sotalol's action in lengthening action potential duration, the relationship of such an action can be indirectly estimated by the findings of a study by Brugada and coworkers (77) in which they demonstrated that at a dose of 1.5 mg/kg intravenous sotalol significantly prolonged the right and left atrial refractory periods.

There are situations in which one might expect sotalol to be more effective than conventional beta-blocking agents in patients with SVT. Preliminary observations suggest that, unlike most beta-blockers, intravenously administered sotalol will convert significant numbers of patients with atrial fibrillation and flutter into sinus rhythm, and once restored sotalol will maintain sinus rhythm in these patients restored either by other pharmacological agents or electrical conversion. Orally administered sotalol is also likely to be more effective than conventional beta-blockers in preventing recurrences of paroxysmal supraventricular tachycardias, both with atrioventricular nodal reentry and with accessory pathways. From knowledge of the electrophysiology of the compound discussed earlier, one might also expect sotalol to be of use in the control of atrial flutter and fibrillation in patients with Wolff-Parkinson-White syndrome.

ATRIAL FLUTTER AND FIBRILLATION

Fogelman et al. (30) gave 20 mg of intravenous sotalol to 5 patients with atrial flutter. Although sinus rhythm was not restored in any patient, all had slowing of ventricular (from 167 to 127/min) and atrial (from 334 to 311/min) responses. In 3 of the 5 patients with acute onset of atrial fibrillation who received 20 mg of intravenous sotalol, the arrhythmia converted to sinus rhythm, with a slowing of the ventricular response in the remaining 2. Sinus rhythm was not restored in any of the 9 patients with chronic atrial fibrillation, although the ventricular response was reduced from 127 to 94 beats/min; in 2 patients there was a mild acceleration of the ventricular response. Prakash et al. (29), using widely ranging sotalol doses (9-40 mg intravenously followed by 20-80 mg orally every 6 hours), showed sotalol to produce conversion to sinus rhythm in 1 of 4 patients, with a decrease in the ventricular response in the other 3 patients. In 3 cases of atrial fibrillation in this series, sotalol decreased the ventricular response without producing conversion to sinus rhythm. It should be emphasized that the sotalol doses used by Fogelman et al. (30) or Prakash et al. (29) were low in light of the subsequent experience with sotalol dosage since 1.5 mg/kg of the drug is currently being used in controlling acute arrhythmias. In this regard, in 23 patients treated on 24 separate occasions, only 2 of 6 and 1 of 5 patients with atrial flutter and atrial fibrillation, respectively, reverted to sinus rhythm within 1 hour after intravenous bolus administration (average doses of 0.41 and 0.33 mg/kg, respectively) of sotalol (76). However, 6 of 7 (86%) atrial flutter and 2 of 6 (33%) atrial fibrillation patients reverted to sinus rhythm after a slow intravenous infusion of the drug (average doses of 0.60 and 0.34 mg/kg, respectively). Overall, 62% of the patients with atrial flutter and 27% of those with atrial fibrillation reverted to sinus rhythm, and the greater success rate in atrial flutter was observed with higher doses of the drug. While in this study there was no relationship between therapeutic response and plasma concentrations of the drug, sotalol by infusion appeared to be superior to that by bolus administration in restoring sinus rhythm in the majority of the atrial flutter patients (76).

In a recent study (78) of 74 patients with symptomatic chronic recurrent atrial fibrillation unresponsive to conventional therapy with Class I antiarrhythmic agents (one to five drugs with a median of two drugs), the effects of stepped care treatment with propafenon, sotalol, and amiodarone were evaluated in alleviating the symptoms by controlling ventricular rate and/or conversion to sinus rhythm. The results of this study demonstrated that treatment with sotalol was highly effective (72% success rate) in maintaining sinus rhythm in patients with chronic atrial fibrillation previously refractory to treatment with Class Ia antiarrhythmic agents. Although at 6-month follow-up only 41% of the 74 patients were free from atrial fibrillation while receiving propafenon, a total of 72% of patients receiving sotalol remained free from atrial fibrillation. These data suggest that sotalol may be a suitable drug for maintenance of sinus rhythm in patients refractory to therapy with Class I antiarrhythmic agents.

The effects of oral sotalol in maintaining sinus rhythm after direct current conversion were recently evaluated and compared with quinidine in a large multicenter Swedish clinical trial (79). In this study, 183 patients with chronic atrial fibrillation were randomized to receive sotalol (98 patients) or quinidine (85 patients) 2 hours after conversion to sinus rhythm with direct current conversion. Patients randomized to sotalol initially received 80 mg b.i.d. dosage for 1 week after which, if needed, the dose could be increased to 160 mg twice daily. For patients assigned to quinidine, slow release preparation of quinidine sulfate (Durules, Astra, Sweden) was administered in 600 mg b.i.d. dosage. At the end of the 6-month study period, 49 (52%) of 95 evaluable patients randomized to sotalol were still in sinus rhythm compared to 38 (48%) of 79 patients receiving quinidine. Although some patients were receiving digitalis, the presence or absence of digitalis therapy did not significantly alter the success rate in the two groups of patients. At 1 month, 39 patients were receiving an 80-mg twice daily dose of sotalol and 50 patients received 160 mg twice daily. Sixty-four percent of patients on 80-mg dosage and 50% of the patients at the 160-mg dosage were in sinus rhythm at 6 months. In patients with relapse into atrial fibrillation while on treatment with sotalol and digitalis, the ventricular rate decreased from 80 to 68 beats/min ($p < 0.03$) compared with the baseline recording before DC conversion. In patients treated with digitalis in the quinidine group, the ventricular rate increased from 80 to 109 beats/min ($p < 0.02$) compared to the baseline. Compared to sotalol, a significantly greater number of patients receiving quinidine experienced overall adverse drug reaction as well as the need to withdraw from the study due to intolerable side effects. In the group of patients treated with sotalol, 27 of 97 patients (28%) reported side effects compared with 43 of 86 patients (50%) in the group treated with quinidine ($p < 0.01$). The overall withdrawal rate for intolerable side effects or recurrence of atrial fibrillation was 11% for sotalol patients compared with 27% for patients treated with quinidine ($p < 0.03$). Two patients (one in each treatment group) had proarrhythmic events in early phase of treatment while patients were still in the hospital. A 64-year-old woman who was randomized to 80 mg sotalol twice daily had a polymorphic ventricular tachycardia and circulatory arrest on the second day of therapy. Her heart rate on the previous day was 47 beats/min and the QT_c interval was 595 msec. The serum potassium level was 3.3 mmol/liter after the cardiac arrest. Sotalol was discontinued and no more ventricular arrhythmias occurred. A 47-year-old woman had an episode of ventricular fibrillation 1 day after starting quinidine therapy and recovered after defibrillation.

The results of this large prospective clinical trial are interesting on several accounts. First, the results demonstrated no significant difference between the number of patients maintained in sinus rhythm after 6 months of sotalol or quinidine treatment given after successful DC cadioversion. Second, the patients treated with quinidine had significantly greater incidence of adverse drug experience, and a large percentage (27%) of them were withdrawn due to intolerable side effects of recurrence of atrial fibrillation. Finally, during recurrence of atrial fibrillation, patients treated with sotalol and digitalis maintained a slow ventricular response, whereas those receiving quinidine and digitalis had an increase in their ventricular response during the recurrence. These findings clearly suggest that sotalol is not only equally effective in maintaining sinus rhythm after DC conversion in patients with chronic atrial fibrillation, but it is also better tolerated than quinidine in the chronic treatment of these patients. These results are particularly noteworthy in view of the recent findings (80) that show that in patients with atrial fibrillation, chronic therapy with quinidine is associated with increased mortality. Although not fully established, it is thought that the increased mortality is most likely secondary to the proarrhythmic effects of quinidine. In the study by Juul-Moller et al. (79) the effects of sotalol or quinidine on cardiac mortality could not be evaluated because there was no placebo group. However, chronic maintenance therapy with sotalol appears promising, but further studies are needed to establish the long-term safety and efficacy of sotalol therapy in patients with chronic atrial fibrillation.

PREVENTION OF SUPRAVENTRICULAR TACHYARRHYTHMIAS AFTER CARDIOPULMONARY BYPASS

In a randomized parallel-group study in 40 patients, Campbell et al. (81) compared the effects of disopyramide and digoxin with those of sotalol in the prevention of atrial flutter and fibrillation after cardiopulmonary bypass. Sotalol was given as a 1 mg/kg bolus intravenously followed by 0.2 mg/kg intravenously over 12 hours in one group of 20 patients. The other group received digoxin 0.75 mg intravenously as a bolus and reverters to sinus rhythm continued to receive digoxin 0.25 mg intravenously twice daily. Nonreverters received disopyramide 2 mg/kg as an intravenous bolus with 0.4 mg/kg/hr for 10 hours in addition to 0.75 mg digoxin intravenously. In each group 17 out of 20 patients reverted to sinus or junctional rhythm within 12 hours. However, the time to conversion was significantly shorter in the case of sotalol.

In another preliminary study, the effects of metoprolol and sotalol were evaluated in 151 patients undergoing coronary artery bypass surgery (82): 39 patients were treated with metoprolol, 41 with sotalol, and 50 served as controls. In the metoprolol group 15.3% developed supraventricular tachyarrhythmias compared with only 2.4% of the sotalol group. Eighteen patients (36%) in the control group developed an arrhythmia, 10 of whom received sotalol and 4 metoprolol for arrhythmia conversion. The time to conversion was strikingly shorter in the case of sotalol compared to that after metoprolol. In a recent study (83) of 429 consecutive patients, effects of low (40 mg t.i.d.) and high (80 mg t.i.d.) dosages of sotalol were compared with propranolol in the prevention of supraventricular tachyarrhythmias early after coronary artery bypass operations. Patients with severely depressed LV function and contraindications for beta-blocker therapy were excluded. Seventy-four patients received low-dose sotalol, 66 low-dose propranolol (10 mg Q.i.d.), 133 high-dose sotalol, and 156 high-dose propranolol (20 mg Q.i.d.). The occurrence of any arrhythmias during the entire postoperative period was evaluated and reported every 4 hours, and the nature of arrhythmias was verified by the supervising physician. Supraventricular tachyarrhythmias were observed in 13.9% of patients receiving low-dose sotalol, 18.8% of those receiving low-dose propranolol, 10.9% of patients on high-dose sotalol, and 13.7% of patients on high-dose propranolol. Although no statistically significant difference was demonstrated for the occurrence of supraventricular tachyarrhythmias between patients receiving sotalol versus those on propranolol, the overall findings suggest that supraventricular tachyarrhythmias were less prevalent in patients treated with sotalol.

SOTALOL IN PAROXSYMAL SUPRAVENTRICULAR TACHYCARDIA

The effects of sotalol in a variety of paroxysmal supraventricular tachycardias (reentrant or ectopic) have been evaluated in several studies. Fogelman et al. (30) found that 5 of 6 (83%) patients with supraventricular tachycardia rapidly converted to sinus rhythm following 20 mg intravenous sotalol. In the other patient, tachycardia slowed from 203 to 169 beats/min. Prakash et al. (29) also found 4 of their 6 patients with supraventricular tachycardia converted to sinus rhythm following 10-20 mg intravenous sotalol. It should, however, be emphasized that the dose of sotalol used in these studies was low. Moreover, the precise mechanism of PSVT also could not be determined from the description provided in these studies. Teo et al. (76) reported that 2 of 4 patients given intravenous boluses (average dose 0.69 mg/kg) and 3 of 3 patients given slow intravenous infusions of sotalol (average dose 0.76 mg/kg) reverted to sinus rhythm within 1 hour of drug administration. Furthermore,, Rizos et al. (33) found that intravenous sotalol (1.5 mg/kg) was more effective compared to intravenous metoprolol (0.15 mg/kg) in patients with either atrioventricular reentrant or atrioventricular reciprocating supraventricular tachycardia. sotalol prevented inducible supraventricular tachycardia in 10 of 17 patients (59%) and metoprolol in 4 (28%).

A recent paper (84) summarized the findings of seven open trials using intravenous sotalol (0.4-1.5 mg/kg) in the acute management of patients with PSVT. Of the 106 patients studies in these trials, 47 (46%) patients converted to sinus rhythm (Fig. 3). The conversion rate was significantly less in earlier studies (29,30) and might be accounted for by the low dosage used in these trials. Recent studies (84) have used the current recommended dosage (1.5 mg/kg) which is significantly higher, and the results of these studies reflect a better response rate for the conversion of PSVT. The results of electrophysiological studies in six clinical trials demonstrated that administration of intravenous sotalol (0.6-2.75 mg/kg) prevented reinduction of sustained PSVT in 44 of 74 (59%) patients. In the recent

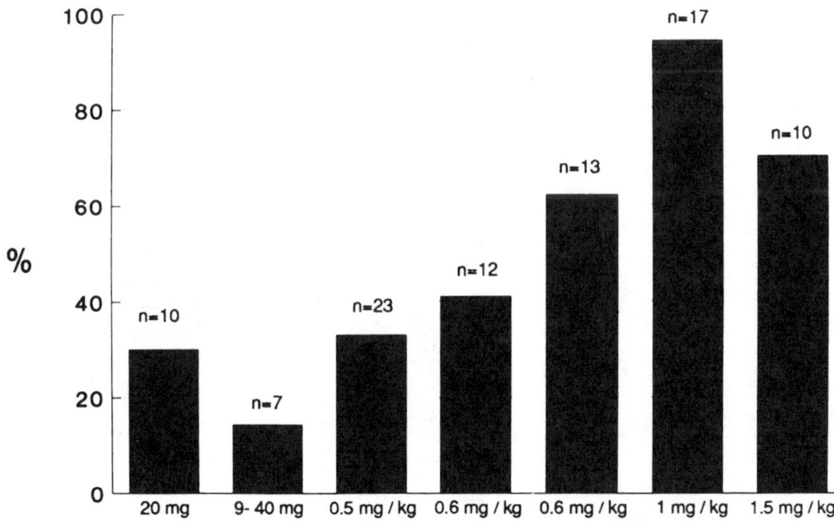

Figure 3 Efficacy of intravenous sotalol in the acute conversion of paroxysmal supraventricular tachycardia. (Reproduced with permission from Ref. 84 and the *American Journal of Cardiology*.)

double-blind, placebo-controlled study, Camm and Paul (84) evaluated the role of oral sotalol in the prophylaxis of PSVT in patients with frequent (>1 attack/month) symptomatic palpitations. Sixty-four patients were enrolled and randomized to receive placebo or sotalol (80 or 160 mg twice daily) during a period of 1-4 weeks depending on the frequency of PSVT during the 3-week baseline period. Of the patients randomized to receive 160 mg of sotalol twice daily, 45% were free from tachycardia recurrence (Fig. 4) during the treatment phase compared to only 5% response rate in the placebo group ($p = 0.0004$). Sotalol (80 mg twice daily) showed a trend toward successful control but did not quite reach statistical significance, with 31% of patients free from relapse of PSVT during the treatment phase. The evaluation of adverse reaction to sotalol was also acceptably low, and only 2 patients were withdrawn. Interestingly, compared to baseline, the QT interval was prolonged in both low- and high-dose sotalol groups, however, the changes were largely rate related, and increases in QT_c were not significant. No proarrhythmic events were observed.

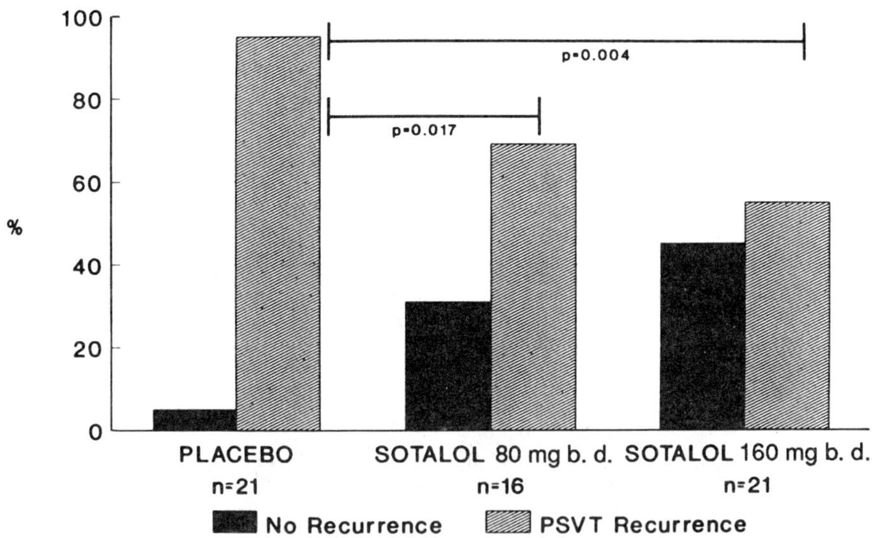

Figure 4 Summary of efficiency of sotalol in intent to treat analysis in the sotalol paroxysmal supraventricular tachycardia (PSVT) study. (Reproduced with permission from Ref. 84 and the *American Journal of Cardiology*.)

WOLFF-PARKINSON-WHITE SYNDROME

Manz et al. (85) studied the effects of intravenous sotalol (80 mg) in 11 patients with the Wolff-Parkinson-White syndrome and in 9 patients with atrioventricular reentrant supraventricular tachycardia. Sotalol lengthened the effective refractory period of the right atrium and ventricle with a depression of conduction in the atrioventricular node and accessory bypass tracts in the anterograde as well as retrograde directions. The rate of reentrant tachycardia was slowed from 182 to 153 beats/min, and the ventricular rate during atrial fibrillation slowed from 148 to 112 beats/min. Sotalol exerted a depressant effect in all parts of the reentrant circuit including the atrium, ventricle, atrioventricular node, and accessory bypass tracts. Although little information is available regarding the long-term effects of sotalol in these patients, uncontrolled observation by Simon and Berman indicates that when given for prophylaxis, sotalol may be of value (9).

In a study of 11 patients with Wolff-Parkinson-White syndrome and 4 with concealed left-sided accessory atrioventricular pathways, intravenous sotalol (1.5 mg/kg over 5 min) prolonged the effective refractory periods of the ventricles and accessory pathways. In addition, the ventricular response to atrial fibrillation was reduced in the patients with the Wolff-Parkinson-White syndrome (86).

Blanc et al. (87) administered 160-320 mg oral sotalol daily in 6 patients with preexcitation for 27-80 days. The mean antegrade effective refractory period of the bypass tract increased from 258 to 318 msec, and was even observed in patients with the shortest periods before treatment. The drug is therefore likely to be effective in preventing the rapid ventricular response to atrial fibrillation in patients with the Wolff-Parkinson-White syndrome as well as in preventing reciprocating tachycardias. It will clearly be of importance to compare the effects of sotalol in this setting with Class I antiarrhythmic agents such as quinidine, disopyramide, and procainamide and with Class III agents such as *N*-acetylprocainamide and amiodarone. In a recent study (88) of 22 patients with Wolff-Parkinson-White syndrome resistant to multiple conventional drugs, the effects of sotalol were evaluated during electrophysiological study as well as long-term prophylactic therapy. Sustained reciprocating tachycardia was rendered noninducible in 13 of 18 patients with inducible tachycardia during electrophysiological evaluation. The anterograde as well as retrograde effective periods of accessory pathways were significantly prolonged by 20% and 28%, respectively. Long-term therapy during a follow-up period ranging from 1 to 47 months revealed a 77% success rate in controlling symptomatic tachycardia. Thus, the results of available studies suggest that sotalol is effective in the prevention and/or slowing the rate or reciprocating tachycardia in patients with Wolff-Parkinson-White syndrome. Further studies are needed to evaluate the long-term efficacy and safety of oral sotalol in the prophylaxis of symptomatic tachyarrhythmias in patients with Wolff-Parkinson-White syndrome.

SOTALOL IN VENTRICULAR TACHYARRHYTHMIAS

Because of its unique electrophysiological properties, consisting of both Class II and Class III antiarrhythmic actions, sotalol has been extensively evaluated in patients with ventricular tachyarrhythmias. Although initially most of these evaluations were made in patients with premature ventricular contractions, a large number of recent studies have reported the safety and efficacy of sotalol therapy in patients with life-threatening ventricular tachyarrhythmias. Although the results of available studies do not help establish the precise mechanism of action of sotalol, it is clear that in patients with ventricular tachyarrhythmias sotalol is far more effective than conventional beta-blockers. Whether the superiority of sotalol's antiarrhythmic activity is primarily due to the drug's Class III effect by virtue of lengthening the myocardial action potential duration is not clear. Perhaps the combined beta-blocking properties and the effect on cardiac repolarization are salutary and both play a significant role in patients with ventricular tachyarrhythmias. Furthermore, it is now well known that sotalol has antifibrillatory properties and increases ventricular fibrillation (VF) threshold in both ischemic and normal myocardium (25,89). In the study by Lynch et al. (25) sotalol significantly reduced the incidence of VF during myocardial ischemic injury in conscious dogs. Marshall et al. (89) described the comparative effects of sotalol and metoprolol given intravenously to anesthetized rats. Although both sotalol and metoprolol significantly increased the VF threshold in the ischemic myocardium after coronary artery occlusion, only sotalol demonstrated an increase in VF threshold in the normal myocardium. These antifibrillatory properties of sotalol along with its well-demonstrated antiarrhythmic actions underscore its potential as an effective antiarrhythmic agent in the management of patients with ventricular tachyarrhythmias.

EFFECTS IN PATIENTS WITH FREQUENT PVCs

The results of several previous and recent studies clearly have shown that sotalol is more effective than other beta-blockers in suppressing premature ventricular contractions. Because this subject has been extensively reviewed and discussed elsewhere in this book, we will primarily focus on the antiarrhythmic effects of sotalol in patients with life-threatening ventricular tachyarrhythmias.

SOTALOL IN LIFE-THREATENING VENTRICULAR TACHYARRHYTHMIAS

Although recently several new antiarrhythmic agents have been approved for the treatment of patients with life-threatening ventricular tachyarrhythmias, none of the currently available antiarrhythmic drugs are usually effective in suppressing these arrhythmias and preventing their recurrence. Sotalol, although still an investigational compound, appears promising in the management of patients with sustained ventricular tachyarrhythmias. Although previous studies (6,7,90-92) were performed in small numbers of patients, several recent studies (93-97) have described the safety and antiarrhythmic efficacy of sotalol in large numbers of patients with life-threatening ventricular tachyarrhythmias.

SOTALOL AND INDUCIBILITY OF VENTRICULAR TACHYCARDIA

Senges et al. (6) performed electrophysiological testing in 18 patients before and after intravenous administration of sotalol (1.5 mg/kg) with double stimuli for the induction of ventricular tachycardia and/or fibrillation (VT/VF). In this study, sotalol prevented reinduction of the tachycardia using two extrastimuli in 12 of 18 (67%) patients. The effect on inducibility was not systematically related to the lengthening of the QT_c interval. Nine of the 12 patients with preventable VT/VF were placed on oral sotalol, and four patients were placed on another regimen. In these 13 patients, successful long-term effects were found in 12 patients and partial response in one patient over a mean follow-up period of 16 (range 8 to 24) months. In three patients, heart failure or sinus node dysfunction developed during the early months of treatment. The authors concluded that the overall antiarrhythmic response exhibited by sotalol was not typical of beta-blockers and related the observed effects of the drug to its property of prolonging the cardiac action potential duration. These data are supported by the study of Nademanee et al. (7) in which the effects of sotalol in preventing inducible ventricular tachycardia as well as recurrent arrhythmia on chronic oral sotalol therapy were evaluated. The study population consisted of 37 patients who had clinically manifest sustained symptomatic recurrent VT/VF. There were 36 men and one woman, mean age was 58 years. Most patients had coronary artery disease and the mean left ventricular ejection fraction was 33.0 ± 14.0%. All patients except one either had inadequate response or did not tolerate one or more (mean number of drugs was 2.8 ± 1) conventional antiarrhythmic drugs. In two patients with recurrent and frequent VT/VF who had not responded to intravenously administered lidocaine, procainamide, and bretylium tosylate, intravenous sotalol was given, but electrophysiological studies were not done either before or after the drug administration because of clinical exigencies. In both patients, sotalol was effective in controlling incessant VT/VT. The remaining 35 patients had electrophysiological (EP) testing; 33 had inducible VT/VF. Sotalol (1.5 mg/kg intravenously) prevented VT/VF reinduction with two extrastimuli in 15 patients (45.5%). Twenty-five of the 33 patients (15 EP positive, 10 EP negative) were given oral sotalol (dosage range, 160-460 mg twice a day).

The clinical outcome of patients with inducible vs. noninducible VT/VF after intravenous administration of sotalol relative to the subsequent oral administration of sotalol was evaluated. In the patients in whom intravenously administered sotalol prevented inducible VT/VT ($n = 15$), the arrhythmia could be controlled in 13 patients (86.7%) by oral sotalol; the drug failed early (within the first month) in 1 patient and appeared to aggravate the condition in another. During chronic therapy (longer than 1 month) arrhythmia recurred in 2 patients (at 8 and 8.4 months), and side effects precluded continued use in an additional 2 patients. Eight patients remained free of arrhythmia and without side effects during a mean follow-up period of 14.5 ± 7.5 (range, 2-23) months.

Steinbeck et al. (90) performed programmed ventricular stimulation and ambulatory ECG monitoring during therapy with sotalol in 39 patients with inducible ventricular tachyarrhythmias (sustained VT in 31, VF in 3, and nonsustained VT in 5 patients). Oral sotalol was started at 80 mg twice daily dose and then gradually increased until a mean daily dose 300 mg (range, 160-480 mg) was reached. In 12 of 34 patients with inducible sustained VT/VF the arrhythmias were suppressed; all 5 patients with nonsustained VT had complete suppression during sotalol therapy. Thus, 17 of 39 patients (44%) had a favorable electrophysiological response during therapy with sotalol. Nonresponders had a higher incidence of previously ineffective drug trials. In 22 patients treated long-term with sotalol, the suppression of arrhythmia inducibility predicted freedom from recurrences (16 of 17 responders), whereas continued inducibility indicated drug failure (5 of 5). The results of serial Holter monitoring did not correlate with the results of electrophysiological testing.

Kienzle et al. (91) evaluated the efficacy of oral sotalol in 9 patients with sustained ventricular tachycardia who had inducible VT while receiving quinidine or procainamide. Eight patients had coronary disease with remote myocardial infarction and 1 had cardiomyopathy. During sotalol therapy (average daily dose 600 ± 103 mg) none of the 8 patients had inducible VT during the repeat electrophysiological study. Five of the 8 chronically treated patients had no recurrence of VT during a mean follow-up of 23 months; sudden cardiac death occurred in 1, and 2 patients had nonfatal VT recurrence. The results indicate that in patients refractory to type I agents procainamide and quinidine, sotalol is effective in suppressing serious ventricular tachyarrhythmias.

In a study by Kopelman et al. (92) the electrophysiological effects of intravenous and oral sotalol were prospectively evaluated in 16 patients with ≥1 episode of clinically documented sustained VT in the absence of acute MI. All patients had ischemic heart disease, the majority (63%) had severe left ventricular dysfunction (LVEF <30%), and most patients had drug-refractory VT. Nine patients received intravenous sotalol, and 11 were given oral sotalol. Both intravenous and oral sotalol caused significant increases in sinus cycle length, AH interval, AV nodal refractoriness, as well as prolonged the atrial and right ventricular effective refractory periods. Although induction of sustained VT was only prevented in 22% of patients receiving intravenous sotalol and 18% of those on oral sotalol, the cycle length of VT significantly increased during both forms of therapy. The slowing of VT rate was accompanied by an increase in the mean arterial blood pressure. These results suggest that even if sotalol is not effective in preventing the induction of sustained VT, it may be of therapeutic benefit by slowing the VT rate and thus preventing the associated hemodynamic consequences. Singh et al. (1988) reported the results of sotalol therapy evaluated by electrophysiological testing and ambulatory ECG recordings in 16 patients with recurrent sustained VT or nonfatal cardiac arrest. The patients were refractory to an average of 4.8 conventional antiarrhythmic agents. At baseline, sustained VT was inducible in 12 of the 14 patients tested. Treatment with oral sotalol (320-960 mg daily) completely suppressed the sustained VT in 7 patients (58%) and modified the VT response in 3 (25%) additional patients. During a mean follow-up of 19 ± 7 months, 12 of the 14 patients receiving long-term sotalol therapy remained clinically free of sustained VT. Only 1 of 14 patients had sudden cardiac death. No significant adverse effects were observed during therapy with sotalol. The results of all of the above-described studies clearly demonstrate that sotalol is highly effective in the management of patients with life-threatening ventricular arrhythmias, and the drug appears to be safe and well tolerated during long-term therapy.

The results of these small-scale trials have been recently confirmed in several large clinical trials conducted in patients with life-threatening ventricular tachyarrhythmias (93-95,98). In the study by Gonzalez et al. (93), 50 patients (43 sustained VT and 7 V.fib) resistant to a mean of 2.8 $\pm$ 1.4 conventional antiarrhythmic drugs were treated with sotalol, and 45 underwent invasive electrophysiological testing before and after sotalol therapy. Twenty-two of the 45 patients had complete or partial response to sotalol therapy; arrhythmia could not be induced in 10 patients and was slower and hemodynamically better tolerated in 12 patients. Twenty-five patients received long-term sotalol therapy during which there was no recurrence of clinical VT in the group with noninducible arrhythmia on the drug. Thirty-seven percent of patients with inducible VT had recurrence of clinical VT or sudden death during the follow-up. Proarrhythmic effects were observed in 2 of the 4 patients with QT interval greater than 600 msec. Based on these findings, the investigators concluded that sotalol is an effective therapy for the subset of patients with sustained VT unresponsive to type 1A drugs. The concordance between the response during electrophysiological testing and lack of recurrence during long-term follow-up suggest that response during EP testing is highly predictive of drug efficacy. The findings of this study are supported by a subsequent report by Ruder et al. (94). In this study, 65 patients with symptomatic, drug refractory, sustained VT or V.fib were treated with oral sotalol (80-480 mg twice daily). Although 11 patients were discontinued in the beginning due to lack of efficacy, the clinical effectiveness of long-term sotalol therapy could be evaluated in the remaining 54 patients followed for 11.5 $\pm$ 6 months. The actuarial incidence of successful sotalol therapy was 54 $\pm$ 13% at 6 months and 47 $\pm$ 13% at 12 months. In 39 patients who had repeat electrophysiological studies while receiving sotalol, the arrhythmia was noninducible in 8 (20%) patients. Exacerbation of ventricular arrhythmia was observed in 6 patients (9%), including one patient in whom there was associated hypokalemia. Their findings and conclusion were almost identical to those previously reported by Gonzalez and coworkers (93) and confirm the effectiveness of sotalol in drug-resistant, sustained ventricular tachyarrhythmias.

In a recent multicenter double-blind, randomized crossover study cited by Nademanee and Singh (98), the effects of intravenous sotalol and procainamide were compared in patients with recurrent VT/VF who had inducible arrhythmia during baseline electrophysiological testing. Forty-nine patients were randomized to treatment with procainamide, and 54 were assigned to receive sotalol. Intravenous administration of proacinamide prevented induction of VT/VF in 11 patients (22%), compared to 33% response rate with intravenous sotalol. In retrospective evaluation of 138 patients with clinically sustained VT or VF or both, Nademanee and Singh (98) compared the effect of various antiarrhythmic drugs in suppressing inducible VT by programmed electrical stimulation. Of all the drugs tested, including amiodarone, treatment with sotalol was the most effective, and it prevented induction of VT in 45% of patients. Interestingly, Class Ic agents flecainide, encainide, recainam, and propafenone had the lowest efficacy rate (range 12-17%). However, the retrospective nature of this study warrants caution from interpretation. Therefore, more controlled studies are needed to compare the antiarrhythmic efficacy of various agents in patients with recurrent ventricular tachyarrhythmias.

In the largest study reported so far, Kehoe et al. (95) examined the effects of oral sotalol in 236 patients with sustained ventricular tachyarrhythmias. In 104 patients the index arrhythmia was a cardiac arrest, and all patients had undergone at least three previous unsuccessful antiarrhythmic drug trials (mean = five drug trials/patient). The effects of sotalol therapy were evaluated by electrophysiological testing in 106 patients. Sotalol completely suppressed induction of sustained VT in 33 (31%) and rendered VT slower (>100 msec prolongation of cycle length) or more difficult to induce in 29 (27%) patients. During 24-hour ambulatory ECG recordings complete- and partial-response rates to sotalol were 51 and 12%, respectively. One hundred and fifty-one patients were discharged on long-term sotalol therapy (mean dose 480 mg/daily). During the mean follow-up of 346 ± 92 days, 27 patients (18%) had recurrence of sustained arrhythmias: 9 had sudden death, 11 had sustained VT, 5 had AICD discharges, and 2 had syncope. Ten patients discontinued sotalol therapy due to significant adverse reactions: 6 due to symptomatic bradyarrhythmias, 2 due to refractory heart failure, 1 due to torsades de pointes, and 1 secondary to bronchospasm. Life table actuarial analyses of sotalol's overall efficacy (prevention of arrhythmias recurrence and absence of serious adverse reactions) at 6, 12, and 18 months was 80, 76, and 72%, respectively (Fig. 5).

During long-term follow-up, sotalol therapy was associated with excellent suppression of recurrent VT/VF as demonstrated by the fact that only 27 patients (18%) had arrhythmia recurrence at a mean follow-up

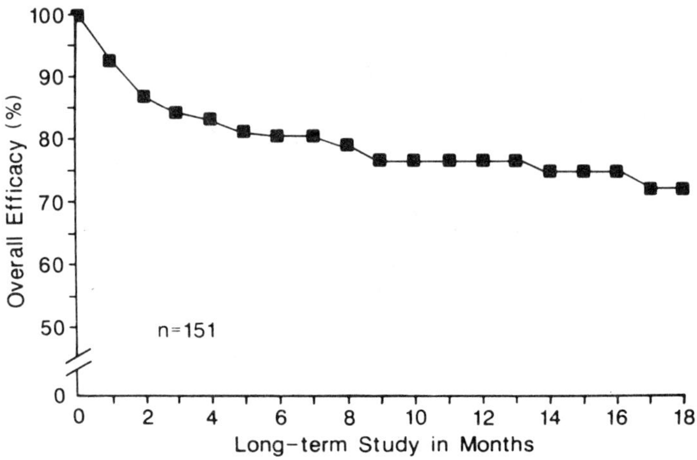

Figure 5 The long-term efficacy of oral sotalol in 151 patients with sustained ventricular tachycardia or ventricular fibrillation in the study by Kehoe et al. (95). Efficacy was defined as suppression of arrhythmic recurrence and absence of serious adverse effects. (Reproduced with permission from Ref. 95 and the *American Journal of Cardiology*.)

of 1 year. After discharge, the arrhythmic mortality in this high-risk population was only 6%, a remarkably low figure considering that 104 of the enrolled patients had prior history of aborted sudden death. Proarrhythmia was observed in 18 patients (7%), 17 during acute phase testing, and only 1 during long-term follow-up. Most (78%) of the proarrhythmic events occurred within 7 days of therapy. Based on the results of this study and those discussed above, it can be concluded that sotalol is an effective and well-tolerated antiarrhythmic agent for suppressing drug refractory, sustained life-threatening ventricular tachyarrhythmias.

ADVERSE EFFECTS

The adverse reactions due to sotalol may be attributed to its beta-blocking actions and to its propensity to lengthen the QT_c interval of the electrocardiogram.

The incidence of side effects due to beta-blockade (tiredness, lassitude, impotence, depression, headache) is similar to that exhibited by other beta-antagonists. Rare cases of retroperitoneal fibrosis as have been documented for other beta-blockers have also been reported (99) with sotalol. As in the case of hydrophilic beta-blockers such as atenolol, the effects of sotalol on the EEG, sleep patterns, and performance in psychological tests have been found to be equivocal and suggest little or no CNS activity of the compound (100,101). Although during long-term oral therapy sotalol has been shown by some investigators to increase serum cholesterol (VLDL plus LDL-cholesterol) and serum triglycerides and decrease HDL-cholesterol (102,103), others have reported no effects on serum lipoproteins or apolipoproteins after treatments as long as 6 months with the drug (104,105).

Blummer and Letzel (106) reported the results of a multicenter field trial of 3 months' treatment with oral sotalol in a total of 6449 (aged 13-95 years) patients. Side effects occurred in 531 (8.2%) patients. In most cases, side effects did not necessitate discontinuation of therapy. Treatment was discontinued prematurely because of adverse side effects in only 188 patients (2.9% of the total number of cases and 35% of 531), and in 123 of these cases adverse effects were noted within the first 6 weeks. For those patients who discontinued therapy, a dosage of 160 mg/day predominated (in 81% of 188). Those cases with side effects in whom treatment was continued without interruption reflected the frequent attempts of the physicians to adjust the dosage and to maintain the dose as well as possible.

In 41% of the 188 patients who discontinued therapy during the study reported by Blummer and Letzel (106), there was very little change in heart rate or diastolic blood pressure. An analysis of heart rate in these patients showed that in addition to the bradycardias, bradycardia with less than 50 beats/min also occurred in a total of 53 patients (0.8% of 6449) at least once during the course of therapy. In 25 of these patients the physician discontinued treatment. Bradycardia was not as frequent a side effect as previously assumed, but in most cases a moderate dosage was used (160 mg/day in 89% of the overall group).

The cardiovascular effects of sotalol include sinus bradycardia, AV block, hypertension, and the exacerbation of heart failure, although the reported incidence of heart failure is lower than that of other beta-blockers. In addition, when sotalol administration involves overdose with concomitant medications such as tricyclic antidepressants, polymorphic ventricular tachycardia, or torsades de pointes may occur.

In recent studies of sotalol in patients with ventricular arrhythmias (6, 7,95,107), the most frequently reported cardiovascular adverse experiences with the drug included bradycardia, dyspnea, congestive heart failure

(1%), and drug-induced proarrhythmias (5%). It should be noted, however, that although side effects are frequently encountered, the drug discontinuation due to adverse experience was rarely (1-4%) necessary except obviously for patients with worsening CHF and drug-induced proarrhythmias. The clinical experience with sotalol and the related key safety parameters in 1288 patients with cardiac arrhythmias were recently described by Soyka et al. (107). The most serious adverse event noted was proarrhythmia, occurring in 56 patients (4.3%). Of these, 27 had hemodynamic compromise due to malignant ventricular arrhythmias. Most patients who encountered proarrhythmia had prior history of sustained VT, myocardial infarction, CHF, dilated cardiomyopathy, or a combination of these. The remaining 29 patients had less severe proarrhythmic events, and 38% of these continued taking sotalol. Proarrhythmia was manifested by torsades de pointes in 24 of the 56 patients. Because of its uniqueness and practical significance, the clinical features and predisposing factors in patients with torsades de pointes will be discussed later in a separate section.

AGGRAVATION OF CONGESTIVE HEART FAILURE

In general, because of their negative inotropic properties, all beta-blockers have the potential of worsening heart failure in patients with preexisting left ventricular dysfunction. The results of several clinical studies, however, suggest that sotalol does not cause significant myocardial depression. In a study by Milei et al. (108), the safety of sotalol treatment was evaluated in 38 high-risk patients with heart failure and angina pectoris. During the 3-month treatment period no adverse effect in terms of worsening heart failure was noted. The investigators did not, however, provide any objective data, such as angiographic findings, regarding the left ventricular function. In a crossover blinded study of 15 patients with stable angina, Lessem (109) evaluated and compared the effects of sotalol, propranolol, and metoprolol on left ventricular ejection fraction by gated radionuclide ventriculography and two-dimensional echocardiography. After 4-6 weeks of therapy, mean LVEF did not change significantly from the baseline value with either drug. More recently, Mahmarian et al. (43) evaluated the hemodynamic effects of oral sotalol in 27 patients with chronic stable ventricular premature depolarizations. The hemodynamic evaluations were performed at baseline and after 4 weeks of drug therapy using gated radionuclide angiogram at rest and during supine bicycle exercise. Sotalol was given initially at a daily oral dose of 320 mg for 2 weeks, then increased to 640 mg/day if the ventricular ectopy was not reduced by 75% of the baseline value. The mean baseline LVEF was 43 ± 15% with 11 patients having LVEF < 40%. None of these patients, however, had clinical evidence of CHF. Sotalol significantly increased the mean LVEF (mean increase 4%) at rest and had a favorable trend towards increase during exercise. Only 1 patient from the group with baseline LVEF < 40% had a decrease in EF at rest during sotalol therapy. Some of the patients were treated with sotalol for 3 months (12 patients) and others for 1 year (6 patients); the hemodynamic evaluation of these patients revealed no significant change in their resting mean LVEF during long-term therapy. There were 2 patients in whom overt congestive heart failure developed while taking sotalol. Both of these patients had markedly dilated LV chamber size and low LVEF (18 and 23%).

In a report by Soyka et al. (107) of the 1288 patients with cardiac arrhythmias treated with sotalol, drug-related CHF requiring discontinuation of therapy was noted in only 19 patients (1% incidence). The predisposing conditions included low baseline LVEF, history of prior CMF, cardiomegaly, cardiomyopathy or both, male gender, and old age (>65 years). Heart failure usually occurred within 7-30 days of initiating therapy. Kehoe et al. (95) reported that only 2 out of 151 patients receiving long-term therapy with sotalol for life-threatening ventricular arrhythmias had refractory heart failure requiring discontinuation of therapy.

The results of available clinical studies appear to suggest that clinically significant aggravation of heart failure occurs far less frequently with sotalol than with other beta-adrenergic blockers. Although not fully established, this may be partially explained by the in vitro positive inotropic effects of sotalol recently described by Antonaccio and Gomoll (42). The positive inotropic effect of sotalol appears to be related to sotalol's ability to prolong the action potential duration and is primarily noted in the isolated ventricular, but not a trial preparation. This positive inotropic effect of sotalol is not blocked by beta or alpha blockade or reserpine pretreatment and appears to be related to sotalol's effect on calcium ion currents and is inversely proportional to the heart rate. Further work is needed to evaluate the safety and clinical efficacy of sotalol therapy in patients with CHF and cardiac arrhythmias. This is of particular clinical importance since it is now well known that sudden cardiac death is the leading cause of death in these patients (110). Furthermore, the results of subanalysis in the Beta Blocker Heart Attack Trial (BHAT) patients with CHF by Chaddha et al. (111) clearly demonstrated the largest benefit of beta-blocker therapy in reducing the risk of sudden cardiac death in survivors of acute myocardial infarction who had congestive heart failure. At present, clinical data are lacking regarding the efficacy and hemodynamic effects of sotalol in patients with acute MI. In a small placebo-controlled study of 30 patients with acute myocardial infarction, the safety and efficacy of intravenous sotalol given at a mean of 6 hours after onset of chest pain have been reported by Lloyd et al. (112). Sotalol was given in the undiluted form starting with 40 mg intravenously over 10 minutes, and if no untoward effects were noted, two further doses of 40 mg were similarly given to a maximum total dose of 120 mg. Thereafter, the patients received the maximum tolerated dose every 6 hours for 72 hours. The heart rate, blood pressure, and pulmonary capillary wedge pressure (PCWP) were monitored continuously during initial dosage, and subsequent evaluations were made on frequent intervals. During the monitoring period, treatment with sotalol was associated with significant decreases in heart rate, blood pressure, and the incidence of ventricular tachycardia without elevating pulmonary capillary wedge pressure or increasing enzymatic infarct size. The left ventricular volumes measured by radionuclide technique also did not reveal any increase in the LV volume during sotalol therapy. These results are extremely encouraging, particularly in light of the recent findings of the Cardiac Arrhythmia Suppression Trial (113) indicating an increase in the number of arrhythmic deaths secondary to treatment with Class Ic agents encainide and flecainide in survivors of acute myocardial infarction with ventricular ectopy. These findings, along with well-demmonstrated cardioprotective effects of beta-blockers in patients with acute MI, as described in Chapters 5 and 6, clearly suggest that the beta-blocking drugs are safe and effective in reducing the cardiac mortality and risk of sudden cardiac death in survivors of acute myocardial infarction. More work is needed to evaluate the safety and clinical benefits of sotalol therapy in these patients.

SOTALOL-INDUCED QT_c PROLONGATION: TORSADES DE POINTES

Although sotalol has significant antiarrhythmic effects (4,6,7,39), it has also been reported to be associated with life-threatening ventricular arrhythmia, particularly in patients with renal failure, hypokalemia, and bradycardia at high concentrations of the drug and also in situations when there is preexisting lengthening of the QT_c interval (114-124). All drugs that prolong the QT_c interval may cause proarrhythmias, particularly the torsades de pointes or polymorphous ventricular tachycardia (Krikler and Curry 1976). In this regard, Neuvonen and coworkers (123) have reported a correlation between the serum sotalol concentration and prolongation of the QT_c interval.

Severe ventricular arrhythmias, including ventricular tachycardia and fibrillation, were initially reported in 5 of 6 cases of sotalol poisoning and correlated with the prolongation of QT_c interval and serum sotalol concentration (123). Most other cases of torsades de pointes following sotalol therapy have also been observed with overdosage (116,119-121, 125,126), although a case was reported in the context of so-called therapeutic serum concentration; this patient was, however, using an additional inappropriate concomitant medication (118). McKibbin et al. (122) reported a series of 13 patients who developed syncope and prolonged QT interval while taking therapeutic doses of sotalol. Polymorphous ventricular tachycardia was observed in 12 patients and criteria typical of torsades de pointes were present in 10 patients. Interestingly, 12 of 13 patients in this series had been treated with a combination of sotalol and hydrochlorothiazide without adequate potassium supplementation, which resulted in reduced serum potassium concentrations. Four patients were also taking other drugs (three on disopyramide and two on tricyclic antidepressants) known to cause prolongation of QT interval. The QT interval returned to normal in all patients after withdrawal of the drugs and the correction of the hypokalemia. Sotalol can induce life-threatening ventricular arrhythmias, particularly when given in combination with hydrochlorothiazide without potassium supplementation. However, when the dose of the drug is kept low and the patient's electrolyte (especially potassium) status is monitored carefully, the incidence of torsades de pointes is low (6,7). The use of sotalol in the setting of renal failure or with concomitant therapy with drugs known to prolong the QT interval (e.g., quinidine, disopyramide, phenothiazines, or tri- and tetracyclic depressants) is not advisable due to greater risk of proarrhythmia, and when absolutely necessary it should only be done under close medical supervision.

The risk of torsades de pointes in patients with ventricular arrhythmia has been described in several recent studies (95,107). In a study by Kehoe et al. (95) 236 patients with sustained ventricular tachyarrhythmias were treated acutely with sotalol, and 151 received long-term oral sotalol therapy. Proarrhythmia was documented in 18 patients (7%), 17 during the acute phase and 1 during long-term follow-up. Eleven patients had torsades de points, and most proarrhythmic events occurred within 7 days of therapy. Summarizing the data derived from 181 clinical studies of 5856 patients treated with sotalol, Soyka et al. (107) described the incidence of sotalol-induced proarrhythmic events in 1288 patients with ventricular arrhythmias. The overall incidence of proarrhythmic events in these patients was 4.3% (56 patients), and 24 of the 56 patients had torsades de pointes. Although no universal relationship was found with previously described factors such as bradycardia, hypokalemia, and long QT interval, the patients with proarrhythmic events had longer mean QT_c interval at baseline as well as at 1 week during therapy with sotalol. The results of available studies also indicate that overall, the risk of proarrhythmic events including torsades de pointes is greater in patients with sustained ventricular tachyarrhythmias, left ventricular dysfunction, marked bradycardia, and prolonged QT interval. Because most of the proarrhythmic events occur within the first 7 days and in general respond to reduction in dosage or discontinuation of sotalol, it is advisable that the high-risk patients be hospitalized and given sotalol therapy under close supervision and continuous ECG monitoring.

SUMMARY

The role of sotalol as an antiarrhythmic agent should be considered, in light of its property, as a nonselective beta-antagonist with less of a depressant effect on myocardial performance than most other beta-blockers and the fact that the compound selectively prolongs myocardial refractoriness by lengthening the action potential duration in all cardiac tissues.

By reason of its combined beta-blocking activity (Class II antiarrhythmic action) and its property of prolonging the action potential duration in myocardial tissues (Class III antiarrhythmic action), sotalol demonstrates a wide spectrum of action in ventricular and supraventricular tachyarrhythmias—a spectrum of activity that differs from that of other beta-blocking drugs. The difference is particularly marked in the case of life-threatening ventricular arrhythmias. The available data, particularly in recent studies of large numbers of patients, indicate that sotalol is an effective antiarrhythmic compound for a significant number of patients with life-threatening ventricular tachycardia/ventricular fibrillation who are refractory to conventional antiarrhythmic drugs. Sotalol appears to have a low arrhythmogenic potential, and since it has a rapid onset of action with a predictable long-term outcome on the basis of intracardiac electrophysiological testing, it appears to be quite suitable in the acute and long-term management of patients with ventricular tachyarrhythmias. By virtue of its beta-blocking properties, sotalol also has antihypertensive and anti-ischemic effects, and thus it may be a preferable antiarrhythmic agent in patients with coronary artery disease and ventricular arrhythmias. In light of the recent data from the CAST (113), which clearly demonstrated proarrhythmic effects of Class Ic drugs encainide and flecainide in patients with acute myocardial infarction, there is a need for evaluation of drugs like sotalol in the treatment of survivors of acute myocardial infarction who have significant ventricular arrhythmias. Clearly more work is needed in this area, but the available data indicate that sotalol is an effective antiarrhythmic agent in patients with life-threatening ventricular tachyarrhythmias.

REFERENCES

1. Lish PM, Weikel JH, Dungan KW. Pharmacological and toxicological properties of two new beta-adrenergic receptor antagonists. J Pharmacol Exp Ther 1965; 149:161-8.
2. Singh BN, Collett JT, Chew CYC. New perspectives in the pharmacologic therapy of cardiac arrhythmias. Prog Cardiovasc Dis 1980; 20:242-301.
3. Nakaya H, Kumura S, Nakao Y, Kanno M. Effects of nipradilol(K-351) on the electrophysiologic properties of canine cardiac tissues: comparison with propranolol and sotalol. Eur J Pharmacol 1984; 104:335-44.
4. Singh BN, Vaughan Williams EM. A third class of antiarrhythmic action. Effects on atrial and ventricular intracellular potentials and other pharmacological actions on cardiac muscle, of MJ 1999 and AH 3474. Br J Pharmacol 1970; 39: 675-87.
5. Singh BN, Hauswirth O. Comparative mechanisms of action of antiarrhythmic drugs. Am Heart J 1974; 87:367-82.
6. Senges J, Lengfelder W, Jauernig R, Czyfan E, Brachmann J, Rizos I, Cobbe S, Kubler W. Electrophysiologic testing of therapy with sotalol for sustained ventricular tachycardia. Circulation 1984; 69:577-83.
7. Nademanee K, Feld G, Hendrickson JA, Singh PN, Singh BN. Electrophysiologic and antiarrhythmic effects of sotalol in patients with life-threatening ventricular tachyarrhythmias. Circulation 1985; 72:555-64.
8. Nademanee K, Feld G, Noll E, Hendrickson JA, Singh BN. Effects of sotalol, Class III antiarrhythmic agent on conduction and refractoriness of the His Purkinje system in man. J Coll Cardiol 1985; 4:38.
9. Singh BN, Nademanee K. Control of cardiac arrhythmias by selective lengthening of repolarization: theoretic considerations and clinical observations. Am Heart J 1985; 109:421-30.
10. Aberg G, Dzedin T, Lundholm L, Olsoon L, Svedmyr N. Comparative study of some cardiovascular effects of sotalol (MJ1999) and propranolol. Life Science 1969; 8:353-65.
11. Blinks JR. Evaluation of the cardiac effects of several beta-adrenergic blocking agents. Ann NY Acad Sci 1967; 139:673-90.

12. Parmley WW, Rabinowitz B, Chuck L, Bonorris G, Katz JP. Comparative effects of sotalol and propranolol on contractility of papillary muscles and adenyl cyclose activity of myocardial extracts of cat. J Clin Pharmacol 1972;12:127.
13. Gomoll AW, Braunwald E. Comparative effects of sotalol and propranolol on myocardial contractility. Arch Int Pharmacodyn 1973; 205:338-54.
14. Goldstein RE, Hall CA, Epstein SE. Comparison of relative inotropic and chronotropic effects of propranolol, practolol and sotalol. Chest 1973; 64: 619-27.
15. Strauss HC, Bigger JT, Hoffman BF. Electrophysiological and beta-receptor blocking effects of MJ 1999 on dog and rabbit cardiac tissue. Circ Res 1970; 26:661-70.
16. Singh BN. A study of the pharmacological actions of certain drugs and hormones with a particular reference to cardiac muscle. Ph.D. thesis, University of Oxford, England, 1971.
17. Raine AEG, Vaughan Williams EM. Adaptational responses to prolonged B-adrenoceptor blockade in adult rabbits. Br J Pharmacol 1980; 70:205-15.
18. Edvardsson N, Olsson B. Effects of acute and chronic beta-receptor blockade on ventricular repolarization in man. Br Heart J 1981; 45:628-36.
19. Kato R, Yabek S, Ikeda N, Singh BN. Electrophysiologic effects of dextro- and levo-isomers of sotalol in isolated cardiac muscle. J Am Coll Cardiol 1986; 7:116-24.
20. Carmeliet E. Electrophysiologic and voltage clamp analysis of effects of sotalol in isolated cardiac muscle and Purkinje fibers. Circulation 1983; 68: 111-297.
21. Shimatori M, Kobayashi M, Chiba S. Comparative study of five beta-adrenoceptor blocking agents on sino-atrial conduction time in isolated blood-perfused canine atria. Arch Int Pharmacodyn 1985; 274:240-52.
22. Kaumann AJ, Olsson CB. Temporal relationship between longlasting aftercontractions and action potentials in cat papillary muscles. Science 1968; 163:293.
23. Schmid JR, Hanna C. A comparison of the antiarrhythmic actions of two new synthetic compounds, iproveratril and MJ1999, with quinidine and pronethalol. J Pharmacol Exp Ther 1967; 156:331-38.
24. Kaumann A, Aramendia P. Prevention of ventricular fibrillation induced by coronary ligation. J Pharmacol Exp Ther 1968; 164:326-32.
25. Lynch JJ, Wilber DJ, Montgonery DG, Hsieh TM, Patterson E, Lucchesi BR. Antiarrhythmic and antifibrillation actions of the levo- and dextro rotatory isomers of sotalol. J Cardiovasc Pharmacol 1984; 6:1132-41.
26. Patterson E, Lucchesi BR. Antifibrillatory properties of the beta-adrenergic receptor antagonists, nadolol, sotalol, atenolol and propranolol in the anesthetized dog and rabbit cardiac tissue. Pharmacol 1984; 28:121-9.
27. Patterson E, Lynch JJ, Lucchesi BR. The antiarrhythmic and antifibrillatory actions of the beta-adrenergic receptor antagonist, d,l-sotalol. J Pharmacol Exper Therap 1984; 230:519-26.

28. Cobbe SM, Hoffman E, Ritzenhoff A, Brachmann J, Kubler W, Senges J. Action of sotalol on potential re-entrant pathways and ventricular tachyarrhythmias in conscious dogs in the late post myocardial infarction phase. Circulation 1983; 68:865-71.
29. Prakash R, Parmley WW, Allen HN, Matloff JM. Effect of sotalol on clinical arrhythmias. Am J Cardiol 1972; 29:397.
30. Fogelman F, Lightman SL, Sillett RW, McNicol MW. The treatment of cardiac arrhythmias with sotalol. Eur J Clin Pharmacol 1972; 5:72.
31. Simon A, Berman E. Long-term sotalol therapy in patients with arrhythmias. J Clin Pharmacol 1979; 19:547.
32. Myburgh DP, Goldman AP, Cartoon J, Schamroth JM. The efficacy of sotalol in suppressing ventricular ectopic beats. Afr Med J 1979; 56:295.
33. Rizos I, Senges J, Jauernig R, Lengfelder W, Czygan E, Brachmannn J, Kubler W. Differential effects of sotalol and metoprolol on induction of paroxysmal supraventricular tachycardia. Am J Cardiol 1984; 53:1022.
34. Ward DE, Camm AJ, Spurrel RAJ. The acute cardiac electrophysiological effects of intravenous sotalol hydrochloride. Clin Cardiol 1979; 2:185-90.
35. Nathan W, Hellestrand KJ, Bextan RS, Ward DE, Spurrell RAJ, Camm AJ. Electrophysiological effects of sotalol-just another B-blocker? Br Heart J 1982; 47:575-20.
36. Rowland E, Perrins J, Donaldson RM, Rickards AF. The clinical electrophysiologic effects of d-sotalol—a new Class III antiarrhythmic drug. JACC 1984; 5:498 (abstract).
37. Edvardsson N, Hirsch L, Emmanuelsson H, Ponten J, Olsson SB. Sotalol-induced delayed ventricular repolarization in man. Eur Heart J 1980; 1:335-40.
38. Echt DS, Berte LE, Clusin WT, Samuelsson RG, Harrison DC, Mason JW. Prolongation of the human cardiac monophasic action potential by sotalol. Am J Cardiol 1982; 50:1082-6.
39. Touboul P, Atallah G, Kirkorian G, Lamaud M, Moleur P. Clinical electrophysiology of intravenous sotalol, a beta blocking drug with class III antiarrhythmic properties. Am Heart J 1984; 107:888-95.
40. Horowitz LN, Josephson ME, Kastor JA. Intracardiac electrophysiologic studies as a method for the optimization of drug therapy in chronic ventricular arrhythmias. Prog Cardiovasc Dis 1980; 23:81-98.
41. Lidell C, Rehnquist N, Sjogren A, Yli-Uotila RJ, Rounnevik PK. Comparative efficacy of oral sotalol and procainamide a patients with chronic ventricular arrhythmias: a multicenter study. Am Heart J 1985; 109:970-5.
42. Antonaccio MJ, Gomoll A. Pharmacology, pharmacodynamics, and pharmacokinetics of sotalol. Am J Cardiol 1990; 65:12A-21A.
43. Mahmarian J, Verani M, Pratt C. Hemodynamic effects of Management Committee. The Australian therapeutic trial in mild hypertension. Lancet 1980; 1:1261-9.
44. Brooks H, Banas J, Meister S, Szucs M, Dalen J, et al. Sotalol-induced betablockade in cardiac patients. Circulation 1970; 42:99-110.

45. Karkkainen S. High performance liquid chromatographic determination of sotalol in biological fluids. J Chromatog 1984; 336:313-19.
46. Lefebvre MA, Girault J, Saux MC, Fourtillan JB. Fluorometric high performance liquid chromatographic determination of sotalol in biologic fluids. J Pharma Sci 1980; 68:1216-19.
47. Poirier JM, Jaillon P, Cheymol G. Quantitative liquid chromatographic determination of sotalol in human plasma. Ther Drug Monitor 1986; 8:474-7.
48. Ritschel WA. Compilation of pharmacokinetic parameters of beta-adrenergic blocking agents. Drug Intell Clin Pharmacy 1980; 14:746-56.
49. Anttila M, Arstila M, Pfeffer M, Tikkanen R, Vallinkoski V, et al. Human pharmacokinetics of sotalol. Acta Pharmacologica et Toxicologica 1976; 39: 118-28.
50. Meier J. Pharmacokinetic comparison of pindolol with other beta-adrenoceptor-blocking agents. Am Heart J 1982; 104:364-73.
51. Sundquist H. Basic review and comparison of beta-blocker pharmacokinetics. Curr Ther Res 1980; 28:338-448.
52. Sundquist H, Attila MS, Simon A, Reich JW. Comparative bioavailability and pharmacokinetics of sotalol alone and in combination with hydrochlorothiazide. J Clin Pharmacol 1979; 19:557-64.
53. Kahela P, Anttila M, Sundquist H. Antacids and sotalol absorption. Acta Pharmacol Toxicol 1981; 49:181-3.
54. Kahela P, Anttila M, Tikkanen R,, Sundquist HK. Effect of food and food constituents and fluid volume on the bioavailability of sotalol. Acta Pharmacol Toxicol 1979; 44:7-12.
55. Cruickshank JM. The clinical importance of cardioselectivity and lipophilicity in beta-blockers. Am Heart J 1980; 100:160-78.
56. Arendt RM, Greenblatt DJ, deJong RH, Bonin JD, Abernethy DR. Pharmacokinetics, central nervous system uptake, and lipid solubility of propranolol system uptake, and lipid solubility of propranolol acebutolol and sotalol. Cardiology 1984; 71:307-14.
57. Taylor PJ, Cruickshank JM. Distribution coefficients of atenolol and sotalol. J Pharmacy Pharmacol 1984; 36:118-19.
58. Ochs HR, Greenblatt DJ, Arendt RM, Schafer-Kortin M, Mutschler E. Single-dose kinetics of oral propranolol, metoprolol, atenolol and sotalol: relation to lipophilicity. Arzneim-Forsch 1985; 35:1580-2.
59. Sotaniemi EA, Anttila M, Pelkonen O, Jarvenivu P, Sundquest H. Plasma clearance of propranolol and sotalol and hepatic drug-metabolizing enzyme activity. Clin Pharmacol Ther 1979; 26:153-61.
60. Sotaniemi EZ, Anttila M, Rautio A, Stengard J, Saukko P, et al. Propranolol and sotalol metabolism after a drinking party. Clin Pharmacol 1981; 29: 705-10.
61. Brown HC, Carruthers SG, Kelly JG, McDevitt DG, Shanks RG. Observations on the efficacy and pharmacokinetics of sotalol after oral administration. Eur J Clin Pharmacol 1976; 9:367-72.

62. Lish PM, Shelanski MV, Labudde JA, Williams WR. Inhibition of cardiac chronotropic action of isoproterenol by sotalol of cardiac chronotropic action of isoproterenol by sotalol (MJ1999) in rat, dog and man. Curr Ther Res 1967; 9:311-42.
63. Schnelle K, Klein G, Schinz A. Studies on the pharmacokinetics and pharmacodynamics of the beta-adrenergic blocking agent sotalol in normal man. J Clin Pharmacol 1979; 19:516-22.
64. McDevitt DG, Shanks RG. Evaluation of once daily sotalol administration in man. Br J Clin Pharmacol 1977; 4:153-6.
65. Ishizaki T, Tawara K. Relationship between pharmacokinetics and pharmacodynamics of beta-adrenergic blocking drug, sotalol, in dogs. J Pharmacol Exper Therap 1979; 211:331-6.
66. Lewis PJ, DeSwiet M, Chamberlain GVP, Bulpitt CJ. The management of hypertension in the pregnant woman. In: Lewis, ed. Therapeutic problems in pregnancy. Lancaster: MTP Press, 1977:530-62.
67. O'Hare MF, Murnaghan GA, Russell CJ, Leahey WJ, Varma MPS, et al. Sotalol as a hypotensive agent in pregnancy. Br J Obstet Gynaecol 1980; 87:814-20.
68. O'Hare MF, Leahey W, Murnaghan GA, McDevitt DG. Pharmacokinetics of sotalol during pregnancy. Eur J Clin Pharmacol 1983; 24:521-4.
69. Erkkola R, Lammintausta R, Liukko P, Anttila M. Transfer of propranolol and sotalol across the human placenta. Acta Obstet Gynecol Scand 1982; 61:31-4.
70. Berglund G, Descamps R, Thomis JA. Pharmacokinetics of sotalol after chronic administration to patients with renal insufficiency. Eur J Pharmacol 1980; 18:321-6.
71. Blair AD, Burgess ED, Maxwell BM, Cutler RE. Sotalol kinetics in renal insufficiency. Clin Pharmacol Ther 1981; 29:457-63.
72. Sundquist H, Anttila M, Arstila M. Antihypertensive effects of practolol and sotalol. Clin Pharmacol Ther 1974; 16:465-71.
73. Sundquist HK, Anttila M, Forrstrom J, Kasenan A. Serum levels and half-life of sotalol in chronic renal failure. Ann Clin Res 1975; 7:442-6.
74. Tjandramaga TB, Thomas J, Verbeeck R, Berbesselt R, Verberckmoes R, et al. The effect of end-stage renal failure and hemodialysis on the elimination kinetics of sotalol. Br J Clin Pharmacol 1976; 3:259-65.
75. Harron DWG, Balnave K, Kinney CD, Wilson R, Russell CJ, et al. Effects of exercise tachycardia during forty-eight hours of a series of doses of atenolol, sotalol and metoprolol. Clin Pharmacol Ther 1981; 29:295-302.
76. Teo KK, Harte M, Horgan JH. Sotalol infusion in the treatment of supraventricular tachyarrhythmias. Chest 1985; 87:113-18.
77. Brugada P, Smeets JLRM, Brugada J, Farre J. Mechanism of action of sotalol in supraventricular arrhythmias. Cardiovasc Drugs Ther 1990; 4:619-24.
78. Antman EM, Beamer AD, Cantillon C, McGowan N, Friedman PL. "Stepped care": antiarrhythmic therapy for refractory symptomatic atrial fibrillation. Circulation 1988; 78:II-62 (Abstract).

79. Juul-Moller S, Edvardsson N, Ahlberg NR. Sotalol versus quinidine for the maintenance of sinus rhythm after direct current conversion of atrial fibrillation. Circulation 1990; 82:1932-9.
80. Coplen SE, Antman EM, Berlin JA, Hewitt P, Chalmers TC. Efficacy and safety of quinidine therapy for maintenance of sinus rhythm after cardioversion: a meta-analysis of randomized control trials. Circulation 1990; 82: 1108-16.
81. Campbell TJ, Garaghan TP, Morgan JJ. Intravenous sotalol for the treatment of atrial fibrillation and flutter after cardiopulmonary bypass: comparison with disopyramides and digoxin in a randomized trial. Br Heart J 1985; 54:86-90.
82. Janssen JH. Prevention and treatment of supraventricular tachycardia early following coronary artery bypass surgery. Angiology 1983; 36:573-6.
83. Suttorp MJ, Kingma JH, Gin RMTJ, van Hemel NM, Koomen EM, Defauw JAM, Adan AJM, Ernst SMPG. Efficacy and safety of low- and high-dose sotalol versus propranolol in the prevention of supraventricular tachyarrhythmias early after coronary artery bypass operations. J Thorac Cardiovasc Surg 1990; 100:921-6.
84. Camm AJ, Paul V. Sotalol for paroxysmal supraventricular tachycardias. Am J Cardiol 1990; 65:67A-73A.
85. Manz M, Kuhl AJ, Luderitz B. Sotalol bei supraventricularer Tachycardie elektrophysiologische Messungen bein Wolff-Parkinson-White Syndrom und AV-Knoten-reentrytachykardie. Kardiologie 1985; 74:500-5.
86. Bennett D. Acute prolongation of myocardial refractoriness by sotalol. Br Heart J 1982; 47:521-6.
87. Blanc JJ, Boschat J, Ollivier JP, Penther PH. Effets du sotalol per os sur la conduction des voies accessoires auriculo-ventriculaires. Archives des Maladies du Coeur et des Vaisseaux 1985; 78:1097-102.
88. Scott Millar RN. Efficacy of sotalol in controlling reentrant supraventricular tachycardias. Cardiovasc Drugs Ther 1990; 4:625-30.
89. Marshall RJ, Muir AW, Winslow E. Effects of antiarrhythmic drugs on ventricular fibrillation thresholds of normal and ischemic myocardium in the anesthetized rat. Br J Pharmacol 1983; 78:165-71.
90. Steinbeck G, Bach P, Haberi R. Electrophysiologic and antiarrhythmic efficacy of oral sotalol for sustained ventricular tachyarrhythmias: evaluation by programmed stimulation and ambulatory electrocardiogram. J Am Coll Cardiol 1986; 8:949-58.
91. Kienzle MG, Martin JB, Wendt DJ, Constantin L, Hopson R, McCue ML. Enhanced efficacy of oral sotalol for sustained ventricular tachycardia refractory to type I antiarrhythmic drugs. Am J Cardiol 1988; 61:1012-17.
92. Kopelman HA, Woosley RL, Lee JT, Roden DM, Echt DS. Electrophysiologic effects of intravenous and oral sotalol for sustained ventricular tachycardia secondary to coronary artery disease. Am J Cardiol 1988; 61:1008-11.

93. Gonzalez R, Scheinman MM, Herre JM, Griffin JC, Sauve MJ, Sharkey H. Usefulness of sotalol for drug-refractory malignant ventricular arrhythmias. J Am Coll Cardiol 1988; 12:1588-72.
94. Ruder MA, Ellis T, Lebsack C, Mead RH, Smith NA, Winkle RA. Clinical experience with sotalol in patients with drug-refractory ventricular arrhythmias. J Am Coll Cardiol 1989; 13:145-52.
95. Kehoe R, Zheutlin T, Dunnington C, Mattioni T, Yu G, Spangenberg R. Safety and efficacy of sotalol in patients with drug-refractory sustained ventricular tachyarrhythmias. Am J Cardiol 1990; 65:58A-64A.
96. Trappe HJ, Klein H, Lichtlen P. Sotalol in patients with life-threatening ventricular tachyarrhythmias. Cardiovasc Drugs Ther 1990; 4:1425-32.
97. Obel IWP, Jardine R, Haitus B, Scott Millar RN. Efficacy of oral sotalol in reentrant ventricular tachycardia. Cardiovasc Drugs Ther 1990; 4:613-18.
98. Nademanee K, Singh BN. Effects of sotalol on ventricular tachycardia and fibrillation produced by programmed electrical stimulation: comparison with other antiarrhythmic agents. Am J Cardiol 1990; 65:53A-57A.
99. Laakso M, Arvala I. Tervonen S, Sotarauta M. Retroperitoneal fibrosis associated with sotalol. Br Med J 1982; 285:1085-6.
100. Bender W, Greil W, Ruther E, Schnelle K. Effects of the beta-adrenoceptor blocking agent sotalol on CNS: sleep, EEG, and psychophysiologic parameters. J Clin Pharmac 1979; 19:505-12.
101. Johnston GD, Finch MB, NcNeill JA, Shanks RG. A comparison of the cardiovascular effects of (+)-sotalol and (±)-sotalol following intravenous administration in normal volunteers. Br J Clin Pharmacol 1985; 20: 507-10.
102. Lehtonen A, Viikari J. Long term effect on plasma lipids. Clin Sci 1979; 57:4055-75.
103. Lehtonen A, Hietanen E, Marniemi J, Peltonen P, Nikkila EA. Effect of sotalol withdrawal on serum lipids and lipoprotein lipase activity. Int J Clin Pharmacol, Ther Toxicol 1983; 21:73-6.
104. Frisk Holmberg M, Juhlin Dannfelt A, Kaiser P, Rossner S, Eliason K, et al. Therapeutic and metabolic effects of sotalol. Clin Pharmacol Ther 1984; 36:174-82.
105. Northcote RJ, Packard CJ, Ballantyne D. The effect of sotalol on plasma lipoproteins and apoliproteins. Clin Chim Acta 1986; 158:187-92.
106. Blummer E, Letzel H. Arterielle Hypertonie: Vertraglichkeit der Betablockertherapie. Ergebnisse einer dreimonatigen Multi-center-Studie mit dem Betablocker Sotalol an 6449 Patienten. Therapiewoche 1982; 32:6477-80.
107. Soyka L, Wirtz C, Spangenberg R. Clinical safety profile of sotalol in patients with arrhythmias. Am J Cardiol 1990; 65:74A-81A.
108. Milei J, Zelasco JF, Fortunato MR. Action of a new beta-blocking agent, sotalol, on high risk anginal patients. Proceedings of advances in beta-adrenergic blocking therapy. Experpta Medica 1974; 2:43-6.

109. Lessem J. Beta-blocker therapy evaluated by radionuclide angiography: A study in chronic stable angina. Clin Cardiol 1982; 5:366-70.
110. Deedwania PC. Significance of arrhythmias in congestive heart failure. Postgrad Med 1988; 83:223-30.
111. Chaddha K, Goldstein S, Byington R, Curb JD. Effect of propranolol after acute myocardial infarction in patients with heart failure. Circulation 1986; 73:503-10.
112. Lloyd EA, Charles RG, Gordon GD, Adam CM, Mabin TA, Commerford PJ, Opie LH. Beta-blockade by sotalol in early myocardial infarction decreases ventricular arrhythmias without increasing left ventricular volume. S Afr Med J 1988; 74:5-10.
113. Echt DS, Liebson PR, Mitchell LB, et al. Mortality and morbidity in patients receiving encainide, flecainide, or placebo. The Cardiac Arrhythmia Suppression Trial. N Engl J Med 1988; 21:1568-72.
114. Bennett JM, Gourassas J, Konstabtibides S. Torsades de pointes induced by sotalol and hypokalemia. S Afr Med J 1985; 68:591-2.
115. Blanc P, Bontemps T, Chabanier A, Richard A, Virot P, et al. Trouble du rythme ventriculaire grave apres prise de sotalol: a propos de 3 observations. Therapie 1986; 41:219-22.
116. Elonen E, Neuvonen PJ, Tarssanen L, Kala R. Sotalol intoxication with prolonged QT interval and severe tachyarrhythmias. Br J Med 1979; 1: 1184.
117. Kontopoulos A, Filindris A, Manoudis F, Metaxias P. Sotalol induced torasade de pointes. Postgrad Med 1981; 57:321-3.
118. Krapf R, Gertsch M. Torsades de pointes induced by sotalol despite therapeutic concentrations. Br Med J 1985; 290:1784-5.
119. Laakso M, Pentikainen PH, Lampainen E. Sotalol, prolonged Q-T interval, and ventricular tachyarrhythmias. Ann Clin Res 1981; 13:439.
120. Laakso M, Pentikainen PH, Pyorola K, Neuvonen PJ. Prolongation of the Q-T interval caused by sotalol-possible association with ventricular tachyarrhythmias. Eur Heart J 1981; 2:355.
121. Laakso M, Pentikainen PJ, Pyorala K. Sotalol and QTc interval. Lancet 1981; 2:1168.
122. McKibbin JK, Pocock WA, Barlow JB, Scottmillar RN, Obel IWP. Sotalol hypokalemia, syncope and torsade de pointes. Br Heart J 1984; 51:157-62.
123. Neuvonen PH, Elonen E, Vuorenmaa T, Laasko M. Prolonged QT interval and severe tachyarrhythmia, common features of sotalol intoxication. Eur J Clin Pharmacol 1981; 20:85-89.
124. Neuvonen PH, Eonen E, Tanskanen A, Tuomilehto J. Sotalol prolongation of the QTc interval in hypertensive patients. Clin Pharmacol Ther 1982; 7:25-32.
125. Belton P, Sheriden J, Mulcahy R. A case of sotalol poisoning. Irish J Med Sci 1982; 151:126-7.
126. Montagna M, Groppi A. Fatal sotalol poisoning. Arch Toxicol 1980; 43:221-6.

Index

About the Editor

PRAKASH C. DEEDWANIA is Clinical Professor of Medicine at the University of California School of Medicine at San Francisco, and Chief of the Cardiology Section, Veterans Affairs Medical Center, Fresno, California. The author or coauthor of more than 150 articles, book chapters, and abstracts in leading journals, Dr. Deedwania is involved in research on antiarrhythmic drugs, silent myocardial ischemia, and newer treatment regimen in congestive heart failure. He is a Fellow of the American College of Cardiology; the American College of Physicians; the American College of Chest Physicians; and the Clinical Council of Cardiology, the Cardiopulmonary Council, and the Lannec Society of the American Heart Association. He is a member of the American Thoracic Society, the American Federation of Clinical Research, the New York Academy of Sciences, and the American Association for the Advancement of Science, among others. Dr. Deedwania received the M.B.B.S. degree (1969) from the University of Rajasthan, Jaipur, India, and is a Diplomate of the American Board of Internal Medicine with certifications in internal medicine, pulmonary disease, and cardiovascular disorders.